Everything
You Need to
Know about
Medical
Treatments

Everything
You Need to
Know about
Medical
Treatments

Springhouse Corporation
Springhouse, PA

STAFF

Senior Publisher
Matthew Cahill

Clinical Manager
Cindy Tryniszewski, RN, MSN

Art Director
John Hubbard

Senior Editor
Stephen Daly

Drug Information Editor
George J. Blake, RPh, MS

Editors
Kathleen Agone, Kathleen Beans, Kathy
Goldberg, Crystal Norris

Copy Editors
Cynthia C. Breuninger (manager), Priscilla
DeWitt, Mary T. Durkin, Lynette High, Nancy
Papsin, Christina P. Ponczek, Doris Weinstock

Designers
Stephanie Peters (senior associate art director),
Lesley Weissman-Cook (book designer), Elaine
Ezrow, Donald G. Knauss, Mary Ludwicki,
Kaaren Mitchel

Manufacturing
Deborah Meiris (director), Pat Dorshaw, T.A.
Landis

Production Coordinator
Margaret A. Rastiello

Editorial Assistants
Mary Madden, Beverly Lane

EYNKT-010595

℞ A member of the Reed Elsevier plc group

Library of Congress Cataloging-in-Publication Data
Everything you need to know about medical treatments.
   p. cm.
   Includes index.
   1. Medicine, Popular.   I. Springhouse Corporation.
RC81.E9156 1996
616 — dc20   95-10231
ISBN 0-87434-821-8   CIP

CONTENTS

ADVISORY BOARD

John J. O'Shea, MD
Chief, Lymphocyte Cell Biology Section
Arthritis and Rheumatism Branch
National Institute of Arthritis and
Musculoskeletal and Skin Diseases
National Institutes of Health
Bethesda, Md.

Ara G. Paul, PhD
Dean and Professor, College of Pharmacy
University of Michigan
Ann Arbor

Kristine A. Bludau Scordo, RN, PhD
Clinical Director
Clinical Nurse Specialist
The Cardiology Center of Cincinnati

Barbara Brandon Shell, PT, BS
Physical Therapist and Consultant
Chair, Texas Board of Physical Therapy Examiners
Former Director, Rehabilitation Medicine Services
M.D. Anderson Cancer Center
Houston

CONTRIBUTORS & CONSULTANTS

Sherri Izes Becker, RN, MBA, CCRN, Clinical Consultant, Blue Bell, Pa.

Barbara Gross Braverman, RN, MSN, CS, Psychiatric Clinical Nurse Specialist, Medical College of Pennsylvania, Philadelphia; Geropsychiatric Clinical Nurse Specialist, Abington (Pa.) Memorial Hospital

Lillian S. Brunner, MSN, ScD, Litt D, FAAN, Nurse and Author, Brunner Associates, Inc., Berwyn, Pa.

Vicki L. Buchda, RN, MS, Director, Special Care Unit, Maryvale Samaritan Medical Center, Phoenix, Ariz.

Janice M. Buelow, RN, MS, Clinical Nurse Specialist, Surgical Epilepsy Program, Rush-Presbyterian-St. Luke's Medical Center, Chicago

Mary Ann Cali-Ascani, RN, MSN, OCN, Nurse Manager, Oncology Unit, Easton (Pa.) Hospital

Jeanette K. Chambers, RN, PhD, CS, Renal Medicine Clinical Nurse Specialist, Riverside Methodist Hospitals; Adjunct Instructor, College of Nursing, Ohio State University, Columbus

David Chaussard, BSN, MBA, CURN, Director of Nursing, Memorial Hospital, Manhattan, Kan.

Luther P. Christman, RN, PhD, FAAN, Former Vice-President, Nursing Affairs, Rush-Presbyterian-St. Luke's Medical Center, Chicago; Former Dean, College of Nursing, Rush University, Chicago

Carla M. Clark, RN, MS, Nurse Research Clinician, Good Samaritan Regional Medical Center, Phoenix, Ariz.

T. Forcht Dagi, MD, MPH, FACS, Staff Neurologist, Walter Reed Army Medical Center, Washington, D.C.; Assistant Professor of Surgery, Uniformed Services University of the Health Sciences, Washington, D.C.

Brian B. Doyle, MD, Acting Director, Psychiatry Residency Program, Georgetown University School of Medicine, Washington, D.C.

Stephen C. Duck, MD, Associate Professor, Pediatrics, Northwestern University Medical School, Evanston, Ill.

Stanley J. Dudrick, MD, FACS, Program Director and Associate Chairman, Department of Surgery, St. Mary's Hospital, Waterbury, Conn.

Sandra D. Durkin, RD, MS, Consulting Dietitian, Nutrition Consult Services, Inc., Washington Crossing, Pa.

Susan Ezzone, RN, MS, OCN, Clinical Nurse Specialist, Bone Marrow Transplant, The Arthur G. James Cancer Hospital and Research Institute, Columbus, Ohio

Nancy M. Flynn, RN,C, MSN, Clinical Educator, Bryn Mawr (Pa.) Hospital

Gunter R. Haase, MD, Neurologist, Pennsylvania Hospital, Philadelphia

Marcia Jo Hill, RN, MSN, Manager, Department of Dermatology, Baylor College of Medicine Methodist Hospital, Houston

Frank Hyland, PT, MS, Director of Physical Therapy, Good Shepherd Rehabilitation Hospital, Allentown, Pa.

Kristina Algiere Kasprisin, RN, MS, Quality Attainment Coordinator (Nursing), Saint Francis Hospital, Tulsa, Okla.; Assistant Clinical Professor (Nursing), University of Oklahoma, Oklahoma City

Joyce LeFever Kee, RN, MSN, Associate Professor, College of Nursing, University of Delaware, Newark

Selma Kendrick, RN, MS, ONC, Director, Oncology and Hematology, Good Samaritan Regional Medical Center, Phoenix, Ariz.

Paul M. Kirschenfeld, MD, FACP, FCCP, Medical Director, Intensive Care Units; Program Director, Internal Medicine Residency Program, Atlantic City (N.J.) Medical Center

Kathleen A. Kucer, MD, Dermatologist, Grand View Hospital, Sellersville, Pa.

Lixing Lao, MD, PhD, RAc, Research Assistant Professor, University of Maryland Pain Center, Baltimore

Gizell Maria Rossetti Larson, MD, Staff Neurologist, Nicolet Clinic, Neenah, Wis.

Dennis E. Leavelle, MD, Associate Professor, Mayo Medical Laboratories, Mayo Clinic, Rochester, Minn.

Anne Doyle McClure, RN, BA, MSN, Biomedical Writer, Lansdale, Pa.

Daniel Edward McGunegle, MD, Associate Professor and Director of Ob/Gyn Services, Truman Medical Center East, Kansas City, Mo.

Deirdre P. Mountjoy, RN, MSN, Family Practice, CIGNA Health Plan of Arizona, Inc., Phoenix

Teresa E. Omert, RN, MS, Clinical Nurse Specialist for Neuroscience, Chicago Neurosurgical Center at Columbus Hospital

Ara G. Paul, PhD, Dean, College of Pharmacy; Professor of Pharmacology, University of Michigan, Ann Arbor

Jody Pelusi, RN, RT, MSN, OCN, Clinical Nurse Specialist, Oncology, Maryvale Samaritan Medical Center, Phoenix

Norman E. Peterson, MD, Professor, Department of Surgery, University of Colorado Health Sciences Center; Associate Director of Surgery, Urology Division Chief, Denver General Hospital

Rose Pinneo, RN, MS, Professor Emeritus, University of Rochester (N.Y.) School of Nursing

Frances W. Quinless, RN, PhD, CCRN, Chairperson, Department of Nursing Education and Services, University of Medicine and Dentistry of New Jersey, School of Health Related Professions, Newark

Grace M. Redheffer, RN, MSN, CEN, Emergency Nursing Consultant, Norristown, Pa.

Pamela Sue Reed, RN, MS, Clinical Nurse Specialist, Medical-Surgical, St. Joseph Mercy Hospital, Pontiac, Mich.

Frank N. Ritter, MD, Clinical Professor of Otolaryngology, University of Michigan Medical Center, Ann Arbor

Mary Faut Rodis, RN, MS, ONC, Assistant Professor, College of Nursing, Rush University, Chicago

Thomas E. Rubbert, BSL, LLB, JD, Attorney-at-Law, Pasadena, Calif.

Harrison J. Shull, Jr., MD, FACP, Assistant Professor of Medicine, Vanderbilt University, Nashville, Tenn.

Gwendolyn A. Smith, RN, MBA, MSM, Clinical Coordinator, Nathan Speare Regional Burn Treatment Center, Crozer-Chester Medical Center, Chester, Pa.

Marilyn Sawyer Sommers, RN, PhD, CCRN, Assistant Professor, College of Nursing and Health, University of Cincinnati

Audrey Stephan, RN, MSN, PhD, Assistant Professor of Nursing, Bergen Community College, Paramus, N.J.

Julie N. Tackenberg, RN, MA, CNRN, Department of Neurology, University Medical Center, Tucson, Ariz.

William M. Valenti, MD, Associate Professor of Medicine—Infectious Diseases, University of Rochester (N.Y.) School of Medicine and Dentistry

Naomi Walpert, RN, MS, CDE, Clinical Nurse Specialist, Endocrinology, Sinai Hospital, Baltimore

FOREWORD

Transplants, laser treatments, and new weapons in the fight against AIDS seem to make the headlines month after month. But these high-profile procedures are just some of the literally hundreds of treatments performed every day.

Drug treatments, for instance, are used by millions of people suffering from high blood pressure, asthma, diabetes, and dozens of different infections. Special diets help us cut down on cholesterol, get more fiber, and avoid food allergies. Surgery is commonplace for repairing hernias, replacing defective heart valves, and restoring vision and hearing. Increasingly, alternatives to surgery have become available to remove gallbladders, clear out clogged coronary arteries, and shatter kidney stones. These alternative procedures often cause less trauma to a person and allow a quicker recovery.

Beyond these treatments, there are therapies for psychological problems, sexual difficulties, pain, and many other conditions. In all, well over 300 treatments are discussed in this book, and they're covered in a clear, accurate, and easy-to-understand way.

In effect, *Everything You Need to Know about Medical Treatments* helps you become informed and prepared for virtually any treatment that you, a family member, or a loved one may undergo. Prepared with the help of more than 60 doctors and medical authorities, this comprehensive reference offers information and advice that can't be found in any other reference for concerned consumers.

For each treatment in the book, you'll find clear answers, usually in a page or two, to essential questions like these:

- Why is this treatment done?
- When shouldn't this treatment be done?
- What happens before the treatment?
- What happens during the treatment? After the treatment?
- What are the side effects or complications of the treatment?

Besides this core information, you'll find special features, each of them marked by a small picture. For instance, you'll find:

- *Self-Help:* what you can do to feel better and care for yourself after surgery and other treatments
- *Advice for Caregivers:* what you can do if you're caring for someone who has undergone a treatment
- *Insight into Treatment:* how a treatment achieves its therapeutic goal — all clearly spelled out in words and illustrations.

With all of these features, *Everything You Need to Know about Medical Treatments* will prove informative and invaluable every time you use it. There's no other book for the general public that rivals its thoroughness, reliability, and ease of use. It's a book no home should be without.

Carol Warfield, MD
Beth Israel Hospital
Harvard Medical School
Boston

1

TREATING HEART & CIRCULATION DISORDERS

DRUG THERAPIES

ACE INHIBITORS

The newest class of drugs used to treat high blood pressure, ACE inhibitors (angiotensin-converting enzyme inhibitors) are widely used to treat high blood pressure and heart failure. Doctors frequently prescribe them because most people do not experience side effects when taking them.

What are ACE inhibitors used for?

ACE inhibitors have become one of the most popular treatments for high blood pressure. They prevent the body from forming angiotensin, a protein that constricts blood vessels. Angiotensin also acts indirectly on the kidneys to cause the body to retain fluid. Both of these effects serve to raise blood pressure. By preventing the activation of angiotensin, ACE inhibitors can:

- promote vasodilation (relaxing of the blood vessels)
- reduce fluid retention
- decrease the workload of the heart.

Researchers have recently discovered that ACE inhibitors are also a highly effective treatment for heart failure. Because these drugs decrease the force against which the heart must pump, people with heart failure dramatically improve after ACE inhibitor therapy.

What are some commonly used ACE inhibitors?

- benazepril, known by the brand name Lotensin
- captopril, known by the brand name Capoten
- enalapril maleate, known by the brand name Vasotec
- fosinopril, known by the brand name Monopril
- lisinopril, known by the brand names Prinivil and Zestril
- quinapril, known by the brand name Accupril
- ramipril, known by the brand name Altace

What are the possible side effects?

The most common side effects of ACE inhibitors include:

- headache
- rapid heart rate

> *ACE inhibitors have become one of the most popular treatments for high blood pressure.*

- altered taste sensation
- dizziness (especially when you rise from a sitting or lying position).

Most of these side effects disappear after a few days or weeks of therapy.

Other side effects include:

- allergic reactions
- swelling of the neck
- elevated blood potassium levels
- kidney problems
- persistent, nonproductive cough.

What are the guidelines for taking ACE inhibitors?

- Most doctors will study the results of blood tests before prescribing an ACE inhibitor. These tests may be repeated periodically to monitor for early signs of side effects.
- Make sure your doctor and pharmacist know all of the other drugs you're taking, to prevent unwanted interactions. Other blood pressure–lowering medicines, nitroglycerin, diuretics (water pills), and certain drugs used to treat gout may increase the actions of ACE inhibitors, which may lower your blood pressure too much.
- Some nonprescription medicines may block the blood pressure–lowering effects of the drug. Examples of these drugs include cold and allergy remedies, anti-inflammatory drugs, and common pain killers.
- Certain salt substitutes, potassium supplements, and some potassium-sparing diuretics may cause your blood potassium levels to rise to dangerous levels. Never use these products without first checking with your doctor.
- Don't stop using this drug without first checking with your doctor. If side effects become intolerable, the doctor may prescribe another drug.
- Take a missed dose as soon as possible, but never double the dose.
- Because food interferes with absorption, take the drug on an empty stomach. Or take it 1 hour before or 2 hours after meals.
- Watch for and immediately report any signs of infection (such as fever and sore throat) or swollen hands or feet.
- Report excessive sweating, vomiting, or diarrhea. These conditions can predispose you to dizziness or low blood pressure.
- Minimize the risk of dizziness or fainting by rising slowly from a sitting or lying position. This is especially important during the first few days of therapy.

VASODILATORS

These drugs are often used after other antihypertensive medications haven't been effective in lowering blood pressure. Because they have some annoying side effects, many doctors won't use them as first-line treatment of high blood pressure.

Vasodilators act directly on the blood vessels, causing them to relax. As the vessels open, blood pressure drops because there is less resistance to blood flow.

What are vasodilators used for?
These drugs are used to treat moderate to severe high blood pressure.

What are some commonly used vasodilators?
- hydralazine, known by the brand names Apresoline and (in Canada) Novo-Hylazin
- minoxidil, known by the brand names Loniten and Minodyl

What are the possible side effects?
- Heart problems, including chest pain, palpitations, and a rapid or irregular heartbeat
- Gastrointestinal disturbances, including diarrhea, nausea, vomiting, and dry mouth
- Skin problems, including flushing and sweating
- Behavioral changes, such as anxiety and depression
- Headache
- Water retention, swelling of the hands or feet, weight gain
- Lupus-like syndrome (weakness, joint pain, itching, blisters, rash, sore throat, and fever)
- Numbness and tingling in the extremities

Additionally, up to 80% of patients receiving minoxidil develop elongation, thickening, and darkening of hair on the temples, eyebrows, forehead, and sideburn areas. This extra hair typically appears within the first 6 weeks of therapy but disappears 1 to 6 months after discontinuation of the drug. You may remove unwanted hair by shaving or using depilatory creams.

Vasodilators act directly on the blood vessels, causing them to relax. As the vessels open, blood pressure drops because there is less resistance to blood flow.

What are the guidelines for taking vasodilators?

- Make sure your doctor and pharmacist know what other drugs you're taking, including nonprescription drugs. Some nonprescription medicines may block the blood pressure–lowering effects of these drugs. These drugs may include cold and allergy remedies, anti-inflammatory drugs, and common pain killers.
- Don't discontinue this drug without first checking with your doctor. If side effects become intolerable, the doctor may prescribe another drug.
- Take a missed dose as soon as possible, but never take two doses at the same time.
- Because food interferes with absorption, take the drug on an empty stomach. Or take it 1 hour before or 2 hours after meals.
- Watch for and immediately report any signs of infection (such as fever and sore throat) or swollen hands or feet.
- Report excessive sweating, vomiting, or diarrhea. These conditions can predispose you to dizziness or low blood pressure.
- Minimize the risk of dizziness or fainting by rising slowly from a sitting or lying position. This is especially important during the first few days of therapy.
- Take your pulse for 1 minute every morning before getting out of bed. Call the doctor promptly if your pulse rate is greater than 100 beats per minute or less than 60 beats per minute, or if the rhythm is abnormal.
- Call the doctor immediately if you have difficulty breathing, chest pain, dizziness, fainting, swollen feet or hands, easy bruising, joint pain, or a rash.
- Weigh yourself weekly at the same time of day, on the same scale, and wearing the same amount of clothing. Promptly report a weight gain of 3 pounds (1.4 kilograms) or more.
- Take the drug with food to increase absorption.
- If you're taking hydralazine, be sure to report for all follow-up doctor's appointments. Blood tests are needed to monitor for early signs of side effects.
- If you're taking minoxidil, know that fluid retention is common. If the doctor also prescribes a diuretic (water pill), be sure to take it as directed. Follow the low-salt diet that has been prescribed for you.
- Hydralazine is sometimes given intravenously to hospitalized patients because it works very rapidly.
- Minoxidil is also used as a topical solution to treat certain types of baldness.

BETA BLOCKERS

Beta blockers (also called *beta-adrenergic blockers)* act directly on the heart to decrease the force and speed of contractions and reduce the heart rate. They also have direct actions on the kidneys, blood vessels, respiratory tract, and other important organs. Because of their potent effects on the heart and blood vessels, beta blockers are used to treat a variety of conditions.

What are beta blockers used for?
- To relieve high blood pressure
- To relieve the pain of angina
- To control an irregular or rapid heart rate

What are some commonly used beta blockers?
- acebutolol, known by the brand names Sectral and (in Canada) Monitan
- atenolol, known by the brand name Tenormin
- betaxolol, known by the brand name Kerlone
- bisoprolol, known by the brand name Zebeta
- carteolol, known by the brand name Cartrol
- metoprolol, known by the brand names Lopressor, Toprol XL, and (in Canada) Apo-Metoprolol, Betaloc Durules, Lopresor SR, and Novometoprol
- nadolol, known by the brand names Corgard and (in Canada) Syn-Nadolol
- penbutolol, known by the brand name Levatol
- pindolol, known by the brand names Visken and (in Canada) Novo-Pindol and Syn-Pindolol
- propranolol, known by the brand names Inderal and (in Canada) Apo-Propranolol, Detensol, Novopranol, and pms Propranolol
- sotalol, known by the brand names Betapace and (in Canada) Sotacor
- timolol, known by the brand names Blocadren and (in Canada) Apo-Timol and Novo-Timol

What are the possible side effects?
- Low blood pressure, slow heart rate, congestive heart failure
- Tiredness and dizziness

What are the guidelines for taking beta blockers?

■ Tell your doctor if you have a history of heart disease, congestive heart failure, respiratory disorders such as bronchial asthma or allergies, kidney or liver disease, or diabetes.

■ If you need surgery, ask your doctor if he or she wants you to continue taking beta blockers until the day of your operation.

■ Call your doctor if you develop congestion, difficulty breathing, unexplained weight gain, distended neck veins, or swelling of the hands, ankles, or feet.

■ If you have diabetes, be aware that some commons signs of low blood sugar (such as a rapid heartbeat) are absent when taking beta blockers. However, you may still experience sweating, hunger, and tiredness. Also, know that your antidiabetic medication requirements may change, and you may need to have your prescription or diet modified.

■ Make sure your doctor or pharmacist knows all of the other medications you're currently taking, including nonprescription drugs. Some nonprescription medicines may block the blood pressure–lowering effects of the drug. Examples of these interacting drugs include cold and allergy remedies, anti-inflammatory drugs, and common pain killers.

■ Report excessive sweating, vomiting, or diarrhea. These conditions can predispose you to dizziness or low blood pressure. Also report difficulty breathing, wheezing, coughing, depression, dizziness, rash, fever, or swollen hands or feet.

■ If you're taking an extended-release form of the drug, be sure to swallow the capsule or tablet whole.

■ Minimize the risk of dizziness or fainting by rising slowly from a sitting or lying position. This is especially important during the first few days of therapy.

■ If you take one dose daily and forget to take it, take the missed dose within 8 hours of the scheduled administration time. If you take two or more doses a day, take a missed dose as soon as you remember, but never double the dose.

■ If you're taking propranolol or metoprolol, take your medication with food to increase absorption. Other beta blockers can be taken without regard to meals.

■ Check your pulse for 1 minute before taking the prescribed dose. If your pulse rate is below 60 beats per minute or above 100 beats per minute, call the doctor immediately. Don't take the drug until the doctor tells you to do so.

Be sure to tell your doctor or pharmacist about all other medications that you're currently taking, including nonprescription drugs.

- Weigh yourself at least once a week at the same time of day, on the same scale, and while wearing the same amount of clothing. Notify the doctor if you gain 3 pounds (1.4 kilograms) or more.
- Because beta blockers may cause dizziness, weakness, and fatigue, avoid overexertion or known sources of stress until your response to the drug has been established. Also avoid driving and other hazardous tasks that require sharp vision, mental alertness, and good coordination.
- Beta blockers may cause numbness, tingling, and coldness in the fingers and toes. To minimize these symptoms, avoid prolonged exposure to cold temperatures.
- Avoid alcohol, which can raise blood pressure.
- Stop smoking because tobacco can reduce the effectiveness of beta blockers.
- If side effects of beta blockers make you feel worse during therapy, don't stop taking the drug. Instead, report these effects to your doctor, who may switch you to another drug or adjust the dosage. Most of these side effects will go away over time.

DIURETICS

The kidneys are the most important organ involved in regulating fluid balance. After blood enters the kidneys, waste products are removed and water is reabsorbed back into the blood. The reabsorption of water is very important in conserving fluids.

Diuretics (commonly known as *water pills*) are drugs used to enhance the removal of water from the bloodstream. By decreasing the reabsorption of water, they can decrease the blood volume. When circulating volume decreases, blood pressure drops.

What are diuretics used for?
- To control high blood pressure
- To reduce fluid volume
- To treat swelling

What are some commonly used diuretics?

Loop diuretics

- bumetanide, known by the brand name Bumex
- ethacrynate sodium, known by the brand name Edecrin Sodium
- ethacrynic acid, known by the brand name Edecrin
- furosemide, known by the brand names Lasix and (in Canada) Furoside

Thiazide diuretics and thiazide-like diuretics

- bendroflumethiazide, known by the brand name Naturetin
- benzthiazide, known by the brand names Exna and Hydrex
- chlorothiazide, known by the brand names Diachlor, Diurigen, and Diuril
- chlorthalidone, known by the brand names Hygroton and (in Canada) Apo-Chlorthalidone and Novo-Thalidone
- hydrochlorothiazide, known by the brand names Esidrix and Hydro-DIURIL
- hydroflumethiazide, known by the brand name Saluron
- indapamide, known by the brand name Lozol
- methyclothiazide, known by the brand name Enduron
- metolazone, known by the brand names Diulo and Mykrox
- polythiazide, known by the brand name Renese
- quinethazone, known by the brand name Hydromox

Potassium-sparing diuretics

- amiloride, known by the brand name Midamor
- spironolactone, known by the brand name Aldactone
- triamterene, known by the brand name Dyrenium

What are the possible side effects?

Loop diuretics

- Decreased levels of potassium or other electrolytes
- Loss of appetite, nausea, stomach pain
- Dizziness
- Decreased blood pressure
- Dehydration

Thiazide diuretics and thiazide-like diuretics

- Decreased levels of potassium or other electrolytes
- Gout
- Kidney problems
- Elevated blood sugar levels

- Elevated triglyceride and cholesterol levels
- Loss of appetite
- Nausea, stomach pain, dizziness
- Decreased blood pressure, dehydration

Potassium-sparing diuretics
- Elevated potassium levels
- Nausea, vomiting, loss of appetite
- Headache, dizziness (occur less frequently)
- Breast enlargement or soreness

What are the guidelines for taking diuretics?

- If you have high blood pressure, expect to be taking diuretics for an extended period of time. It's important that you comply with therapy and return for all follow-up office visits. The doctor will want to periodically perform blood tests to detect early signs of drug toxicity.
- Tell your doctor if you have a history of gout. After starting therapy, tell the doctor if any symptoms of gout reappear.
- If you have diabetes, carefully monitor your blood and urine glucose (sugar) levels. You may need to check with your doctor about the need to adjust the dosage of your antidiabetic medication.
- Make sure your doctor or pharmacist knows all of the other medications you're currently taking, including nonprescription drugs. Some nonprescription medicines may block the blood pressure–lowering effects of the drug. Examples of these interacting drugs include cold and allergy remedies, anti-inflammatory drugs, and common pain killers.
- Don't discontinue this drug without first checking with your doctor. If side effects become intolerable, the doctor may prescribe another drug.
- Take a missed dose as soon as possible, but never double the dose.
- Watch for and immediately report any signs of infection (such as fever and sore throat) or swollen hands or feet.
- Report excessive sweating, vomiting, or diarrhea. These conditions can predispose you to dizziness or low blood pressure.
- Minimize the risk of dizziness or fainting by rising slowly from a sitting or lying position. This is especially important during the first few days of therapy.

If you have high blood pressure, expect to be taking diuretics for an extended period of time. It's important that you comply with therapy and return for all follow-up office visits. The doctor will want to periodically perform blood tests to detect early signs of drug toxicity.

NITRATES

People who suffer from angina pectoris experience periodic episodes of chest pain. This pain is caused by the inability of blood flow around the heart to keep up with the heart's demand for oxygen.

One of the oldest and most effective treatments for angina has been the use of rapid-acting vasodilators (drugs that relax the blood vessels) known as the *nitrates*. The most commonly used vasodilators, nitrates act in at least two ways. The first is to enhance the flow of blood around the heart by dilating the coronary circulation. The second is to reduce the heart's demand for oxygen by causing dilation of peripheral blood vessels. This dilation reduces the amount of work the heart has to perform in order to pump blood.

The choice of drug and form depends on the type of angina. For example, sublingual nitroglycerin and sublingual or chewable isosorbide dinitrate provide relief of acute anginal attacks. The long-acting nitrates and topical, transdermal, transmucosal, and extended-release oral nitroglycerin help prevent attacks.

What are nitrates used for?
- To produce rapid relief of anginal attacks
- To prevent anginal attacks
- To reduce the workload of the heart in emergency situations, such as congestive heart failure and heart attack

What are some commonly used nitrates?
- isosorbide dinitrate, known by the brand names Dilatrate-SR, Isordil, and Sorbitrate
- isosorbide mononitrate, known by the brand name Ismo
- nitroglycerin, known by the brand names Deponit, Nitro-Bid, Nitrodisc, Nitro-Dur, Nitrol, Nitrostat, and Transderm-Nitro
- pentaerythritol tetranitrate, known by the brand names Duotrate, Peritrate, and PETN

What are the possible side effects?
- Headache (sometimes throbbing), dizziness, weakness
- Rapid heart rate
- Burning sensation under the tongue, dry mouth
- Flushing

- Blurred vision
- Dizziness, palpitations, fainting

What are the guidelines for taking nitrates?

- Make sure your doctor knows all of the medications you're taking, including nonprescription medicines.
- Use oral tablets, topical ointments, and transdermal patches as prescribed, even if you aren't experiencing anginal pain. Taking the drug on schedule will help prevent pain. This drug isn't habit-forming.
- Call the doctor immediately if you develop symptoms of possible toxicity: blue lips, palms, or fingernails; fainting or extreme dizziness; a feeling of pressure in the head; difficulty breathing; weakness or fatigue; weak, rapid heartbeat; fever; or seizures.
- Store the drug in a cool, dark place in its original container. Keep the container tightly closed and replace the supply every 3 months.
- Avoid alcohol, which may lower blood pressure when taken with nitrates.
- Take oral tablets on an empty stomach 30 minutes before or 1 to 2 hours after meals. Unless they're chewable tablets, swallow them whole.
- Take a sublingual tablet as soon as you feel anginal pain. Wet the tablet with saliva, place it under your tongue, and then sit or lie down and relax. Allow the tablet to dissolve naturally and do not swallow until it has done so; then relax for 15 minutes after the pain subsides to prevent dizziness.
- If one tablet doesn't relieve the pain within 5 minutes, take a second one; if there's no relief within another 5 minutes, take a third tablet. If pain persists after another 5 minutes, call the doctor immediately and get to an emergency room. Never take more than three tablets.
- Take an additional dose of the short-acting oral or sublingual form 5 to 10 minutes before a stressful situation or strenuous exercise; the drug's effect will last up to 30 minutes.
- If the doctor has prescribed topical nitroglycerin ointment, you should spread it in a uniform, thin layer on any hairless area (without rubbing it in), and then cover it with plastic film to aid absorption and protect clothing. If you're using ointment applied to a strip of ruled paper, keep the paper on the skin to protect clothing and ensure that the ointment remains in place.
- If you're using the transdermal patch, apply it to any hairless area except the ends of your arms (near the wrists) or bottom of your legs (near the ankles) because absorption is poor at these sites. Also avoid

standing in front of microwave ovens because a radiation leak may heat the patch's aluminum backing and cause a burn.

CALCIUM CHANNEL BLOCKERS

Calcium is involved in many important physiologic processes, including normal cardiac and vascular muscle contractions. By blocking the entry of calcium into these types of muscle cells, calcium channel blockers can cause vasodilation (relaxing of the blood vessels), decrease the heart rate, and lower blood pressure.

Not all calcium channel blockers are alike. Some act primarily on the blood vessels to cause vasodilation and lower blood pressure; others act primarily on the heart to slow the heart rate and reduce contractility.

What are calcium channel blockers used for?
- To decrease the severity and frequency of anginal attacks
- To treat high blood pressure
- To limit neurologic damage after a stroke (nimodipine)
- To treat abnormal heart rhythms

Not all calcium channel blockers are alike. Some act primarily on the blood vessels to cause vasodilation and lower blood pressure; others act primarily on the heart to slow the heart rate and reduce contractility.

What are some commonly used calcium channel blockers?
- bepridil, known by the brand names Bepadin and Vascor
- diltiazem, known by the brand names Cardizem, Cardizem CD, Cardizem SR, and (in Canada) Novo-Diltazem
- felodipine, known by the brand names Plendil and (in Canada) Renedil
- isradipine, known by the brand name DynaCirc
- nicardipine, known by the brand name Cardene
- nifedipine, known by the brand names Adalat, Apo-Nifed, Novo-Nifedin, Procardia, and (in Canada) Nu-Nifed
- nimodipine, known by the brand name Nimotop
- verapamil, known by the brand names Calan, Calan SR, Isoptin, Isoptin SR, and (in Canada) Apo-Verap and Novo-Veramil

What are the possible side effects?
- Difficulty breathing, coughing, wheezing
- Dizziness, fainting, headache, tiredness

- Chest pain; irregular, rapid, or slow heartbeat; low blood pressure; swelling of the hands, ankles, or feet
- Constipation
- Skin flushing or rash

What are the guidelines for taking calcium channel blockers?

- Be sure to tell your doctor or pharmacist about all other medications you're currently taking, including nonprescription drugs. Some nonprescription medicines may block the blood pressure–lowering effects of the drug. Examples of these interacting drugs include cold and allergy remedies, anti-inflammatory drugs, and common pain killers.
- Don't discontinue this drug without first checking with your doctor. If side effects become intolerable, the doctor may prescribe another drug.
- Watch for and immediately report any signs of infection (such as fever and sore throat) or swollen hands or feet.
- Report excessive sweating, vomiting, or diarrhea. These conditions can predispose you to dizziness or low blood pressure.
- Minimize the risk of dizziness or fainting by rising slowly from a sitting or lying position. This is especially important during the first few days of therapy.
- Weigh yourself once a week at the same time of day, on the same scale, wearing the same amount of clothes. Notify the doctor if you gain 3 pounds (1.4 kilograms) or more.
- Measure your pulse rate for 1 minute before each dose, and notify the doctor if the rate is below 50 beats per minute.
- Swallow oral medication whole, without crushing or chewing it.
- Take a missed dose as soon as you remember, unless it's almost time for the next scheduled dose. In this case, omit the missed dose and resume your schedule with the next dose. Never double the dose.
- If you're also taking nitroglycerin or another nitrate for angina, continue taking the nitrate according to your doctor's advice.
- Take calcium channel blockers with food to prevent stomach upset.
- Avoid constipation by eating plenty of fruits and vegetables, or take a mild laxative if recommended by the doctor. This is especially important if you're taking verapamil.

DIGITALIS GLYCOSIDES

Digitalis glycosides are so named because they're derived from the dried leaves of the foxglove plant *Digitalis purpurea* or *Digitalis lanata*. The drugs produced from these plants have glycoside (sugar) components. Because they are used to treat heart ailments, many clinicians refer to them as *cardiac glycosides*. All the digitalis glycosides produce similar effects on the heart and blood vessels; however, they differ in their onset and duration of action.

What are digitalis glycosides used for?
- To increase the force of contraction in the failing heart
- To control certain abnormal heart rhythms, such as atrial flutter or fibrillation

What are some commonly used digitalis glycosides?
- digoxin, known by the brand names Lanoxicaps, Lanoxin, and (in Canada) Novodigoxin
- digitoxin, known by the brand names Crystodigin and (in Canada) Digitaline

What are the possible side effects?
- Abnormal heart rhythms, low blood pressure, heart failure
- Visual disturbances
- Nausea, vomiting, diarrhea

What are the guidelines for taking digitalis glycosides?
- There's only a small difference between the therapeutic and toxic blood levels of digitalis glycosides. Consequently, many patients treated with these agents develop toxic reactions. Early signs of toxicity include visual disturbances (such as the appearance of yellow-green halos around objects), loss of appetite, or nausea. If you experience any of these early signs of toxicity, call your doctor.
- Be sure to inform your doctor and pharmacist about any other drugs you're taking, to prevent unwanted interactions. Be especially careful if you're taking laxatives, antacids, cold or allergy medicines, or diet pills unless the doctor has recommended their use.
- Take this medication at the same time each day.

There's only a small difference between the therapeutic and toxic blood levels of digitalis glycosides. Consequently, many patients treated with these agents develop toxic reactions. Early signs of toxicity include visual disturbances, loss of appetite, or nausea. If you experience any of these early signs of toxicity, call your doctor.

- Measure your pulse rate for 1 minute before each dose. Call the doctor if the rate is below 60 beats per minute or over 100 beats per minute or if you notice skipped beats or new irregularities.
- Call the doctor if you have signs of fluid retention, such as lung congestion, shortness of breath, or swelling of the feet or ankles.
- Weigh yourself once a week on the same scale, at the same time of day, and wearing similar amounts of clothing. Notify the doctor if you gain 3 pounds (1.4 kilograms) or more.
- If your doctor also has prescribed a diuretic (water pill), remember to take a potassium supplement or to eat foods high in potassium.
- Watch for and immediately report early symptoms of toxicity, such as loss of appetite, nausea, diarrhea, or a bloated feeling. Other symptoms include weakness, blurred vision, and halos around lights.
- Remember to follow a low-salt diet if your doctor has recommended one.

INOTROPICS

The inotropics are drugs that provide emergency treatment of shock by increasing blood pressure and the heart's output of blood. If shock is caused by blood loss, the doctor will provide blood replacement before these drugs can be effective. Inotropics are usually used only during an emergency, when a drop in blood pressure is life-threatening.

What are inotropics used for?
- To increase myocardial contractility
- To increase blood pressure

What are some commonly used inotropics?
- amrinone, known by the brand name Inocor
- dobutamine, known by the brand name Dobutrex
- dopamine, known by the brand name Intropin
- epinephrine, known by the brand name Adrenaline
- isoproterenol, known by the brand name Isuprel
- norepinephrine, known by the brand name Levophed

What are the possible side effects?

- Local tissue damage at the infusion site
- Restlessness, nervousness, anxiety, fear, dizziness, vertigo, headache, insomnia
- Pallor, palpitations, flushing, heart rate disturbances, blood pressure changes, stroke, decreased circulation in the fingers and toes, chest pain
- Weakness, mild tremors
- Nausea, vomiting, diarrhea

What else should you know about inotropics?

- Expect to have your blood pressure and heart rate closely monitored during therapy.
- If you notice any pain at the infusion site, tell the nurse or doctor immediately.
- These drugs are usually used only in critical care areas of the hospital.

ANTIARRHYTHMICS

These drugs are used to treat arrhythmias (irregular heart rate or rhythm). There are many different types of antiarrhythmics, and the one that your doctor will choose for you is based on the type and severity of the arrhythmia that you have.

In most people, the heart beats about 70 to 80 times per minute when at rest. During periods of exercise or stress, the heart rate increases to meet the tissues' demands for more blood and oxygen. Under normal conditions, these increases are smooth and predictable.

Small variations in the heart rate are normal; an occasional skipped beat is not necessarily a sign of disease. However, when the heart repeatedly deviates from its normal pattern of rhythmic pumping, its ability to move blood through the vascular system decreases. If the heart's pumping ability decreases enough, blood flow to the brain decreases and the person faints. Under the worst conditions, the person may die.

What are antiarrhythmics used for?

There are many different types of arrhythmias, and not all of them are life-threatening or even dangerous. So the type of antiarrhythmic the doctor prescribes will depend on the type of arrhythmia, which could include some of the following:

- bradyarrhythmias, or persistent decreases in heart rate, where the heart beats more slowly than normal
- tachyarrhythmias, or persistent increases in heart rate, where the heart beats faster than normal
- fibrillation, which occurs when the heartbeat is so fast that no rhythmic pattern is present, and pumping stops.

What are some commonly used antiarrhythmics?

- amiodarone, known by the brand name Cordarone
- bretylium tosylate, known by the brand name Bretylol
- disopyramide, known by the brand names Norpace and (in Canada) Rythmodan
- flecainide, known by the brand name Tambocor
- lidocaine, known by the brand name Xylocaine
- mexiletine, known by the brand name Mexitil
- moricizine, known by the brand name Ethmozine
- procainamide, known by the brand names Promine and Pronestyl
- propafenone, known by the brand name Rythmol
- quinidine bisulfate, known by the brand name Biquin Durules (in Canada)
- quinidine gluconate, known by the brand names Duraquin, Quinaglute Dura-Tabs, Quinalan, and (in Canada) Quinate
- quinidine polygalacturonate, known by the brand name Cardioquin
- quinidine sulfate, known by the brand names CinQuin, Quine, Quinidex Extentabs, and Quinora
- sotalol, known by the brand names Betapace and (in Canada) Sotacor
- tocainide, known by the brand name Tonocard

What are the possible side effects?

- Dizziness, headache, light-headedness, confusion, restlessness, cold sweat, fainting
- New or worsened arrhythmias, low blood pressure, palpitations
- Ringing in the ears, excessive salivation, blurred vision
- Diarrhea, nausea, vomiting, loss of appetite, abdominal pains
- Blood abnormalities
- Rash, itching

Small variations in the heart rate are normal; an occasional skipped beat is not necessarily a sign of disease. However, when the heart repeatedly deviates from its normal pattern of rhythmic pumping, its ability to move blood through the vascular system decreases.

- Swelling of the feet or ankles
- Asthmatic attacks

What are the guidelines for taking antiarrhythmics?

- Report for regular checkups. The doctor will need to check your pulse rate, rhythm, and blood pressure. Periodic blood tests will be needed to see if your dosage is correct and to check for early signs of side effects.
- Make sure your doctor and pharmacist know about all of the drugs you're taking, including nonprescription drugs. Don't take any other medicines without checking with your doctor or pharmacist.
- Call your doctor if you feel palpitations or persistent changes in heart rate or rhythm. Take your pulse every morning before getting out of bed, and call the doctor if the rate drops below 60 beats per minute or exceeds 100 beats per minute.
- Watch for possible neurologic side effects (confusion, dizziness, and fatigue), especially if you're taking amiodarone or disopyramide. Call the doctor if such symptoms occur, and avoid driving and other hazardous activities that require coordination and alertness.
- Report suspected drug-related reactions, such as blurred vision, sensitivity to light, rash, difficulty breathing, cough, chest pain, fever, palpitation, dizziness, swelling, or weakness.
- If you're taking an extended-release form of the drug, be sure to swallow the tablet or capsule whole.

Anticoagulants

Following a traumatic injury to small blood vessels, human blood starts a process to repair the damage. The clotting process involves a complex chain of events that leads to the formation of a clot or plug that stops further bleeding. This type of clot is known as a *thrombus*. Under normal circumstances, the clot stops the bleeding and the body initiates a repair process to restore the vessel to normal. However, if the clot becomes dislodged within the vessel, it can travel in the bloodstream until it blocks a small blood vessel. Traveling clots are called *emboli*. Emboli can block the blood flow to a limb, the lungs, heart, or brain and produce devastating consequences.

Anticoagulants (commonly known as *blood thinners*) interfere with the blood's ability to form clots. They're useful in treating thromboembolic disorders and in preventing them in high-risk people.

What are anticoagulants used for?
- To help prevent and treat thromboembolic diseases, including pulmonary emboli and deep vein thrombosis
- To prevent clot formation in high-risk people, such as those suffering a heart attack or atrial fibrillation, those on prolonged bed rest, and those undergoing dialysis, cardiovascular surgery, or cardiopulmonary bypass procedures
- To treat serious blood clotting abnormalities, such as disseminated intravascular coagulation

What are some commonly used anticoagulants?
- dicumarol (generic)
- heparin calcium, known by the brand names Calciparine and (in Canada) Calcilean
- heparin sodium, known by the brand names Liquaemin and (in Canada) Hepalean
- warfarin, known by the brand names Coumadin, Panwarfin, and (in Canada) Warfilone Sodium

What are the possible side effects?
Heparin
- Hepatitis
- Bleeding
- Rash, itching
- Allergy
- Fever

Warfarin
- Nausea, cramps
- Bleeding
- Skin disorders
- Fever

What are the guidelines for taking anticoagulants?
- Tell your doctor about any recent surgery involving the eye, brain, or spinal cord. Patients who've had these types of surgery should avoid taking anticoagulants.

Anticoagulant alert

Both heparin and warfarin interact with a large number of other drugs. Typically, the result is an increased risk of bleeding, diminished anticoagulant action, or ulcerogenic effects.

Hazardous interactions

The risk of bleeding increases when heparin is given with dextrans, dipyridamole, piperacillin, or valproic acid. It also increases when heparin is given with aspirin, carbenicillin, cefamandole, chloroquine, hydroxychloroquine, moxalactam, nonsteroidal anti-inflammatory agents, or plicamycin. The drug's anticoagulant effect diminishes when used with antihistamines, digitalis glycosides, oral contraceptives, protamine, or tetracycline.

The risk of bleeding rises when warfarin is given with amiodarone, chloramphenicol, clofibrate, diflunisal, thyroid drugs, heparin, anabolic steroids, cimetidine, disulfiram, glucagon, inhalation anesthetics, metronidazole, quinidine, influenza vaccine, sulindac, sulfinpyrazone, or sulfonamides. The risk also rises with concurrent, prolonged use of Tylenol or other drugs containing acetaminophen. What's more, fatal hemorrhage can occur several weeks after cessation of barbiturate therapy unless the warfarin dosage is reduced.

The risk of ulcerogenic effects increases when warfarin is used with ethacrynic acid, indomethacin, mefenamic acid, oxyphenbutazone, phenylbutazone, or salicylates.

Decreased effectiveness

Warfarin's effectiveness decreases when carbamazepine, ethchlorvynol, griseofulvin, haloperidol, paraldehyde, or rifampin is given concurrently. Similarly, its effectiveness diminishes when given with laxatives or diuretics.

- Give your doctor a complete medical history. Patients with liver or kidney disease, alcoholism, high blood pressure, allergies, asthma, or stomach ulcers should use anticoagulants cautiously.
- You should understand that dosage adjustments are made following the results of blood tests. It is very important that you report for all follow-up blood tests, especially at the beginning of your treatment.
- Call the doctor immediately if you have bleeding gums, bruises, blotchy red spots on your skin, nosebleeds, bloody or tarry stools, or blood in your urine. Also call at once if you vomit blood or if your vomit looks like coffee grounds; this could be a sign of gastrointestinal bleeding.
- Take the prescribed dose of your anticoagulant at the same time each day.
- To minimize the severity of bleeding from your gums, use a soft-bristled toothbrush and floss gently with waxed floss. Be sure to tell your dentist that you're taking an anticoagulant.
- Shave with an electric razor instead of a blade.
- Avoid aspirin. Always check with your doctor before taking any nonprescription drugs because many of these drugs contain aspirin; also check the label before taking one. (See *Anticoagulant alert.*)

- Large doses of vitamin K can interfere with warfarin's anticoagulant action. Keep your intake of foods containing vitamin K consistent to prevent altered drug effects. Leafy green vegetables contain the highest amounts of vitamin K; fruits, cereals, dairy products, and meats supply lower amounts. Patients who have gone on certain fad diets (such as an all-lettuce diet) have experienced difficulties while taking warfarin.
- Avoid excessive alcohol consumption, which can increase the risk of bleeding.
- Wear a medical identification bracelet or carry a card that specifies the prescribed drug and its dosage.

THROMBOLYTICS

Thrombolytics have been nicknamed "clot busters" because they accelerate the natural body processes that break down blood clots.

Scientists have found that most heart attacks are caused by clots that block one of the main arteries supplying blood to the heart. When the artery is blocked by a clot, heart muscle becomes starved for oxygen and nutrients. If the clot stays in place, heart muscle can die, and the heart becomes severely damaged.

Thrombolytic drugs are given soon after heart attack symptoms begin. When they reach the blocked blood vessel, they cause it to rapidly dissolve, restoring blood flow to the heart muscle.

What are thrombolytics used for?
- To dissolve clots that cause heart attacks
- To dissolve clots in the lungs that cause pulmonary emboli
- To dissolve clots that form in intravenous access devices
- To treat leg clots (deep vein thrombosis)

What are some commonly used thrombolytics?
- alteplase, commonly known as tissue plasminogen activator and t-PA, and known by the brand name Activase
- anistreplase, known by the brand name Eminase
- streptokinase, known by the brand names Kabikinase and Streptase
- urokinase, known by the brand name Abbokinase

What are the possible side effects?

- Bleeding
- Low blood pressure, heart rhythm disturbances
- Nausea, vomiting
- Allergy, rash

Thrombolytic treatment should begin as soon as possible after symptoms of a heart attack begin. These drugs are less effective if given 6 hours or more after the onset of symptoms.

What else should you know about thrombolytics?

- Thrombolytic treatment should begin as soon as possible after the symptoms of a heart attack begin. These drugs are less effective if given 6 hours or more after the onset of symptoms. The goal of therapy is to reduce the damage caused by the attack and ultimately to keep the patient from dying.
- The most common side effect is bleeding, usually from puncture sites (where blood samples are drawn or intravenous lines are placed). Occasionally, serious bleeding can develop from the nose or gastrointestinal tract or into the brain. If you notice any unusual bleeding or discoloration of stools, call the nurse or doctor immediately.
- Thrombolytics may cause mild allergic reactions; serious reactions are rare. Fever may also occur, but it is easily treated.
- Disturbances in heart rhythm may occur, but they generally signal that the clot has dissolved.
- You should understand the seriousness of your condition. Doctors and nurses will closely monitor blood studies and your electrocardiogram for several days after you're admitted to the hospital.
- Tell the doctor about any side effects, such as dizziness, shortness of breath, wheezing, a feeling of tightness and pressure in the chest, and swelling of the face, hands, or feet.
- Watch for signs of bleeding because you'll be taking anticoagulants (blood thinners) during your hospital stay. Use a soft-bristled toothbrush and waxed dental floss to avoid bleeding gums.
- Use an electric razor instead of a blade for shaving. Take extra care not to bump or bruise yourself.
- Keep all follow-up appointments with your doctor.
- If you continue taking anticoagulants at home, report for all blood tests as needed. Close monitoring is necessary to properly adjust the dosage.

ANTIADRENERGICS

The adrenergic nervous system, sometimes called the *sympathetic nervous system,* is important for regulation of heart rate and blood pressure. Drugs that inhibit the effects of this system are useful in treating patients with moderate to severe high blood pressure.

What are antiadrenergics used for?

- To treat moderate to severe high blood pressure
- To treat symptoms accompanying benign enlargement of the prostate gland in men (terazosin)

What are some commonly used antiadrenergics?

- clonidine, known by the brand names Catapres and Catapres-TTS
- guanadrel, known by the brand name Hylorel
- guanethidine, known by the brand names Ismelin and (in Canada) Apo-Guanethidine
- methyldopa, known by the brand names Aldomet and (in Canada) Apo-Methyldopa and Novomedopa
- prazosin, known by the brand name Minipress
- reserpine, known by the brand names Serpalan and (in Canada) Serpasil and Novoreserpine
- terazosin, known by the brand name Hytrin

What are the possible side effects?

Clonidine
- Dizziness, weakness, fainting, slow heart rate, heart rhythm disturbances
- Nasal congestion

Guanadrel and guanethidine
- Dizziness, weakness, fainting, slow heart rate, heart rhythm disturbances
- Nasal congestion
- Diarrhea
- Swelling of the feet or ankles
- Weight gain
- Sexual dysfunction

Methyldopa
- Blood disorders
- Tiredness, dizziness, decreased mental acuity
- Dry mouth
- Nasal congestion

Prazosin and terazosin
- Dizziness and fainting, especially at the start of therapy ("first-dose" effect)
- Weakness
- Rapid heart rate
- Nasal congestion

Reserpine
- Fatigue, drowsiness, mental depression

What are the guidelines for taking antiadrenergics?

- Remember to take your medication regularly, even when you're feeling better. Most side effects will diminish within 4 to 6 weeks; if they persist, contact the doctor. Don't discontinue the drug without the doctor's approval.
- To minimize dizziness, rise slowly from a lying or standing position, avoid prolonged standing in one position, and avoid alcohol, hot showers, and hot baths. Lie down or place your head between your knees if you feel dizzy, weak, or faint.
- These drugs may cause drowsiness and nasal congestion.
- To relieve dry mouth, use sugarless hard candy, ice chips, or chewing gum, or rinse your mouth with water. Remember to use a soft-bristled toothbrush and waxed dental floss. If you wear dentures, remove them and rinse them two or three times a day to keep the gums moist, but avoid mouthwashes containing alcohol because they can worsen mouth dryness.
- Tell your dentist about your medication regimen because dry mouth can promote tooth decay.
- Watch for signs of fluid retention, such as swollen ankles or feet, and weigh yourself daily at the same time and on the same scale. Notify your doctor if you gain 3 pounds (1.4 kilograms) or more.
- Be sure to tell your doctor or pharmacist about all other medications you're currently taking, including nonprescription drugs. Some nonprescription medicines may block the blood pressure–lowering effects of the drug. Examples of these interacting drugs include cold

and allergy remedies, anti-inflammatory drugs, and common pain killers.

- Take a missed dose as soon as possible, but never double the dose. If it's almost time for your next dose, skip the missed dose and resume your regular dosage schedule.
- Because food interferes with absorption, take the drug on an empty stomach. Or take it 1 hour before or 2 hours after meals.
- Watch for and immediately report any signs of infection (such as fever and sore throat) or swollen hands or feet.
- Report excessive sweating, vomiting, or diarrhea. These conditions can predispose you to dizziness or low blood pressure.

SURGERIES

HEART TRANSPLANT

The first heart transplant in the United States was performed in 1968. In this complex procedure, a diseased heart is replaced with a donated healthy heart. (Alternatively, the diseased heart may be replaced with an artificial heart — a more controversial procedure.) The heart donor must be certified as brain dead and screened for heart abnormalities and terminal illnesses. Preferably, male donors should be younger than age 35 and female donors younger than age 45.

Because of improvements in technique and drugs that help to prevent rejection, the number of heart transplants performed is steadily increasing. The use of this procedure is limited largely by its high cost and the scarcity of donor hearts.

Transplantation may be the only means available to prolong a person's life, but it is by no means a certain cure.

Why is this surgery done?
Heart transplantation is done to restore the function of the heart in people with very severe heart disease after more conservative medical or surgical therapies have failed. Candidates for heart transplantation must meet several strict criteria, including previous adherence to medical therapy and emotional stability.

Most candidates for this surgery have severe coronary artery disease with widespread left ventricular dysfunction caused by a heart attack and its complications. However, other serious heart conditions can cause a person to need a heart transplant.

When shouldn't this surgery be done?

Heart transplants should not be performed on people who have irreversible high blood pressure resulting from disease affecting blood vessels of the lungs, severe peptic ulcers, unresolved blood clots in the lung, acute infection, cancer, severe liver or kidney dysfunction, or insulin-dependent diabetes. Heart transplants also may not be advisable for elderly or malnourished people or for those with a mental disability.

What happens before the surgery?

- A nurse or doctor will discuss the procedure with the person undergoing it and the family, including possible complications and its impact on their lives.
- The nurse or doctor will explain that a transplant requires a prolonged recovery period, which may cause changes in family functioning.
- The person and family are encouraged to ask questions, and are referred for psychological counseling as necessary.
- The person and family are informed that a heart transplant doesn't guarantee a life free from medical problems and that it requires lifelong follow-up care.
- The person is told what to expect before surgery, including food and fluid restrictions and the need for a breathing tube and assistance with breathing. The person and family are prepared for the sights and sounds of the recovery room and intensive care unit. If possible, they are given a tour of these facilities and an opportunity to meet the staff.
- Procedures to prevent infection and the tests used to detect rejection and other complications are discussed. Drugs that will be used to combat rejection will be explained.
- The person or a responsible family member will sign a consent form.

What happens during the surgery?

The two methods of heart transplantation are orthotopic and heterotopic transplantation. In *orthotopic transplantation,* the recipient's

Heart transplants should not be performed on people who have irreversible high blood pressure resulting from disease affecting blood vessels of the lungs, severe peptic ulcers, unresolved blood clots in the lung, acute infection, cancer, severe liver or kidney dysfunction, or insulin-dependent diabetes.

heart is removed and the donor heart is implanted in its place. In *heterotopic transplantation,* the recipient's heart is left in place and the donor heart is positioned to the right of it. Currently, the orthotopic approach is preferred.

A specialized surgeon performs the heart transplant while the person is under general anesthesia. The donor heart must continue beating when it is removed from the brain-dead donor because it can sustain severe physiologic damage after 20 to 30 minutes without oxygen. Drug therapy to prevent or delay rejection of the donor heart begins before surgery and continues after the procedure.

What are the possible complications?

Serious postoperative complications of heart transplantation include infection and rejection; most transplant recipients can expect to experience one or both of these complications. Rejection, caused by the person's immune response to a foreign substance (the donor heart), usually occurs within the first 6 weeks after surgery. It's treated with potent drugs, sometimes in massive doses. However, the resulting depression of the immune system leaves the person vulnerable to potentially life-threatening infection.

Other complications resemble those associated with any open-heart surgery. Among them are impaired blood flow to the kidneys, stroke, and such lung complications as a blood clot, pneumonia, and failure to wean from a ventilator. Psychological problems also are common after a heart transplant; they include depression, mood changes, increased stress, difficulty returning to work, changes in body image, and problems adhering to the treatment plan. Such complications may occur during initial hospitalization or later during recovery.

What happens after the surgery?

- Precautions to prevent infection are implemented for 1 to 2 weeks.
- The person receives drugs to prevent rejection of the heart. These drugs typically mask obvious signs of infection; therefore, subtle signs of infection such as fever are carefully noted. To prevent infection, antibiotics may be administered, and sterile technique is maintained when the incision and drainage sites are cared for.
- A nurse will check the person's blood pressure, temperature, pulse, and respirations every 15 minutes until his or her condition stabilizes. After that, the nurse will monitor the person as needed.

SELF-HELP

How to care for yourself after a heart transplant

After you've been discharged from the hospital, follow these important guidelines.

Take special precautions
- The doctor will schedule frequent (weekly to monthly) heart biopsies to check for signs of rejection. Make sure you keep appointments to avoid being hospitalized again.
- Immediately report to your doctor any signs of rejection (fever, weight gain, shortness of breath, drowsiness, weakness) or infection (chest pain, fever, sore throat, or redness, swelling, or drainage at the incision site).
- Make sure you know the dosage, schedule, and possible side effects of all drugs prescribed by your doctor.
- Follow the diet prescribed by your doctor, especially noting salt and fat restrictions.

Other instructions
- Maintain a balance between activity and rest. Try to sleep at least 8 hours a night, to rest briefly each afternoon, and to take frequent breaks during tiring physical activity.
- Follow your doctor's instructions regarding climbing stairs, engaging in sexual activity, taking baths and showers, and doing light housework and other chores. Avoid lifting heavy objects (more than 20 pounds, or 9 kilograms), driving, and strenuous activities—such as mowing the lawn or vacuuming—until the doctor approves.
- Follow the exercise program your doctor has prescribed.
- Ask your doctor about support groups and counseling services to deal with any psychological problems you may have, such as depression, mood swings, and overeating.

- A nurse will monitor the person's electrocardiogram for disturbances in heart rate and rhythm and will notify the doctor if there are any abnormalities.
- Oxygen levels are assessed by listening to the lungs during breathing and observing movement of the chest. Oxygen and carbon dioxide levels in arterial blood are checked every 2 to 4 hours, and the settings on the ventilator are adjusted as needed to maintain prescribed oxygen levels.
- Drainage in tubes placed in the chest will be carefully observed for hemorrhage, excessive drainage, or sudden decrease or cessation of drainage.
- The person will receive pain medications as prescribed by the doctor. (See *How to care for yourself after a heart transplant.*)
- The person will be observed closely for symptoms of stroke.
- After weaning the person from the ventilator and removing the breathing tube, a nurse will begin chest physiotherapy, encouraging the person to cough, turn frequently, and breathe deeply. The nurse will also encourage range-of-motion exercises, to improve circulation and prevent the complications of prolonged bed rest.

VENTRICULAR ASSIST DEVICE

A temporary life-sustaining treatment for heart failure, the ventricular assist device is used to decrease the heart's workload while maintaining normal blood pressure and cardiac output. Ventricular assistance allows the heart to rest and recover adequate ventricular function and is considered a bridge to heart transplantation or implantation of a mechanical or artificial heart.

Used most commonly to assist the left ventricle, this device may also be used to assist the right ventricle or both ventricles. It works by diverting blood flow from the diseased chamber into a pump and then returning it to the blood vessel that leaves the heart (the aorta in the case of a left ventricular assist device or the pulmonary artery in the case of a right ventricular assist device).

Ventricular assist devices have much in common with the artificial heart. The main differences are that ventricular assist devices help the heart rather than replace it and are used temporarily rather than permanently. Because of these differences, ventricular assist devices don't have to be as compact as an artificial heart. Nevertheless, recent advances in technology have reduced their size.

Ventricular assist devices are inserted to temporarily reduce the ventricle's workload, promote heart rest, and improve the heart's ability to contract.

Why is this treatment done?

Ventricular assist devices are inserted to temporarily reduce the ventricle's workload, promote heart rest, and improve the heart's ability to contract. Candidates for a ventricular assist device include people with inadequate blood flow from the heart after a massive heart attack; people who cannot be weaned from heart-lung bypass despite intravenous fluids, drug therapy, or insertion of balloon pump in the aorta; and people with inflammation of the walls of the heart who have inadequate blood flow from the heart that does not respond to conventional treatment. Ventricular assist devices are sometimes used for people awaiting a heart transplant who have also been unresponsive to other treatments, including intravenous fluids and drugs. They may also be used for people who reject a heart transplant and for people undergoing high-risk procedures to clean out the coronary arteries (such as those whose heart disease is so severe that they are not candidates for bypass grafting).

When shouldn't this treatment be done?

People who are poor candidates for a ventricular assist device include those with severe kidney failure; severe vascular disease of the brain, lung disease, or liver disease; cancer that has spread; or significant blood disorders. Another option for these people may be replacement of the heart muscle. Other situations in which the treatment should not be done include a body surface area of less than 1 square meter or difficulty inserting the catheter.

What happens before the treatment?

- A doctor or nurse will explain the procedure, including its risks, and will answer any questions the person or the family may have. Informed consent is obtained.
- Food and fluids are restricted before surgery and heart function is monitored continuously, using an electrocardiograph and arterial catheters.
- If time allows, a nurse will shave the person's chest and scrub it with an antiseptic solution.
- A nurse will place an air mattress or a sheepskin on the person's bed to help position the person after surgery and prevent skin breakdown.

What happens during the treatment?

Insertion of a ventricular assist device is usually performed in the operating room. With the person under general anesthesia, the surgeon makes an incision in the chest, then positions the catheters in the heart and the appropriate artery. After suturing the catheters in place, the surgeon connects them to tubing attached to the pump head of the ventricular assist device. Usually, the pump itself remains outside the body, and the synthetic tubing enters the chest through the incision. Finally, the surgeon turns on and adjusts the pump, checks that it is functioning properly and that the sutures aren't leaking, and applies a bandage.

What are the possible complications?

Insertion of a ventricular assist device carries a high risk of complications. Hemorrhage is a common surgical complication; clotting disorders result from prolonged heart-lung bypass. Other complications include partial paralysis of the diaphragm, acute respiratory failure, kidney failure, multisystem organ failure, and failure of the ventricular assist device. The device can damage blood cells, causing blockage of a blood vessel that carries blood to the heart or a stroke. If the ventricular assist device hasn't improved ventricular function in 96 hours, a heart transplant may be considered.

What happens after the treatment?

▪ The person returns to the intensive care unit with the ventricular assist device in place.

▪ The person will be sleepy from the anesthetic when he or she arrives in the intensive care unit. As the anesthetic wears off, pain medication will be administered as prescribed.

▪ While the device is in place, the person is kept immobilized to prevent the breathing tube from coming out and to avoid contaminating or disconnecting the device.

▪ A nurse will carefully observe the person for signs of bleeding or ineffective pumping of the device.

▪ Blood thinners are administered, as prescribed, to prevent clot formation. Blood samples will be taken every 4 hours to monitor the effects of the blood thinners, and the doctor will be notified of abnormal results.

▪ The person is carefully observed for signs of infection.

▪ Oxygen levels, kidney function, and neurologic status are monitored.

▪ If the person receives the ventricular assist device as a bridge to transplantation, he or she will undergo the transplant when a donor heart becomes available.

▪ The person not awaiting a heart transplant will be weaned from the ventricular assist device when he or she has been stabilized.

▪ Weaning from the device can begin by turning the device off for a few minutes once a day to evaluate ventricular function.

▪ After being weaned from the device, the person usually receives support with drug therapy or a balloon pump inserted into the aorta.

CORONARY ARTERY BYPASS GRAFTING

A surgical procedure, coronary artery bypass grafting establishes a shunt (a passage between two blood vessels) to circumvent a blocked coronary artery. The number of obstructions bypassed varies from one to five or more.

The bypasses are made of grafts from the person's own body, usually from a segment of the saphenous vein or the internal mammary artery; they permit blood flow from a major artery to the area past the coronary artery blockage, ultimately restoring blood flow to the heart muscle. The internal mammary approach has recently become common.

Coronary artery bypass graft techniques vary according to the person's condition and the number of arteries being bypassed. During the procedure, the person must be placed on a heart-lung machine because the heart must be immobilized for surgical manipulation. In people with left main coronary artery blockage exceeding 50% and those with three-vessel coronary artery disease and decreased left ventricular function, coronary artery bypass grafting has been shown to provide relief of symptoms and longer survival than does medical therapy.

Coronary artery bypass grafting improves blood flow to the heart and relieves anginal pain.

Why is this surgery done?

Coronary artery bypass grafting improves blood flow to the heart and relieves anginal pain.

What happens before the surgery?

- The surgeon explains the procedure and the complex equipment and procedures used in the intensive care or recovery unit. If possible, a tour will be given of these facilities.
- The person is told that he or she will awaken from surgery with a breathing tube in place (which will make speaking impossible) and will be connected to a mechanical ventilator. The person is also told that he or she will be connected to a heart monitor and other monitoring equipment and have a tube that goes from the nose to the stomach, in addition to a urinary catheter. This equipment will cause little discomfort and will be removed as soon as possible.
- The person or a responsible family member signs a consent form.
- The evening before surgery, the person showers with an antiseptic soap and is shaved from chin to toes.
- Food and fluids are restricted after midnight, and a sedative is given at bedtime if ordered by the doctor. On the morning of surgery, a sedative is provided, as ordered, to help the person relax.
- Heart monitoring begins before surgery.

What happens during the surgery?

Surgery begins with a series of incisions in the person's thigh or calf to remove a segment of the saphenous vein for grafting or, more commonly, in the chest to remove a segment of the internal mammary artery.

When the grafts are obtained, the surgeon initiates heart-lung bypass, which cools the body's temperature to 92° F (33° C) to reduce the heart's need for oxygen. To further reduce the heart's oxygen demands during surgery and to protect the heart, the surgeon stops the electrical conductivity of the heart and lowers the temperature of the heart by injecting a cold solution (potassium-enriched normal saline solution) into the aortic root and coronary arteries.

After the person is fully prepared, the surgeon sutures the grafts in place, discontinues the heart-lung bypass, implants pacing electrodes, inserts a chest tube, and closes the incision. Finally, a sterile dressing is applied.

What are the possible complications?

Coronary artery bypass grafting relieves anginal pain in over 90% of people, and its long-term effectiveness is well established. However, such problems as graft closure and development of blockages in other coronary arteries sometimes call for repeat surgery. Approximately 5% to 10% of people develop graft closure within 1 year, and about 60% develop atherosclerotic disease of saphenous vein grafts within 10 years. Internal mammary bypass grafts remain open much longer, sometimes indefinitely.

Other potential complications include abnormal heart rhythms, high or low blood pressure, blood clots that may lead to a stroke, heart attack, and infections. The person also may experience depression, possibly weeks after discharge.

People at higher risk for complications after coronary artery bypass grafting include heavy smokers and those with serious lung problems, kidney or metabolic disorders, or significantly reduced blood supply to the brain (as in carotid artery stenosis), which increases the risk of stroke during surgery. People receiving blood thinners must be identified before surgery.

What happens after the surgery?

■ Vital signs and other important parameters are checked and recorded frequently until the person's condition stabilizes. The electro-

SELF-HELP

Recovering from a coronary artery bypass graft

After you've been discharged from the hospital, follow these important guidelines.

Take special precautions
- Know the dosage, schedule, and possible side effects of all prescribed medications.
- Follow the diet prescribed by your doctor, especially any salt and cholesterol restrictions. Adhering to your diet can help reduce the risk of a recurring arterial blockage.
- Avoid lifting heavy objects (more than 20 pounds, or 9 kilograms), driving a car, or doing strenuous work (such as mowing the lawn or vacuuming) until the doctor approves. Follow the exercise program prescribed by your doctor.

Know when to call your doctor
- Immediately notify the doctor if you develop any signs of infection (fever, redness, swelling, or drainage from leg or chest incisions) or possible recurring arterial blockages (chest pain, dizziness, shortness of breath, or prolonged recovery time from exercise).
- Also report to your doctor any muscle and joint pain or weakness.

Other points to remember
- You may feel depressed after the surgery. This depression may begin several weeks after discharge from the hospital. Be aware that this is a normal reaction and should subside quickly.
- Maintain a balance between activity and rest. Try to sleep at least 8 hours a night, to schedule a short rest period for each afternoon, and to rest frequently during tiring physical activity. Follow your doctor's instructions regarding climbing stairs, engaging in sexual activity, taking baths and showers, and doing light chores.
- Contact a local chapter of the Mended Hearts Club and the American Heart Association for additional information and support.

cardiogram is monitored for disturbances in heart rate and rhythm, and abnormalities are reported to the doctor.
- Heart sounds are monitored and oxygenation is evaluated by listening to the person's lungs and observing his or her color and chest movement during breathing. The doctor is notified of any abnormalities.
- Oxygen and carbon dioxide levels in arterial blood are measured every 2 to 4 hours, and settings on the ventilator are adjusted as needed to maintain values within prescribed limits.
- Within 6 to 24 hours after the procedure, the person will begin taking a daily dose of aspirin to reduce the incidence of clot formation in the saphenous vein graft.
- Chest tube drainage is checked regularly for hemorrhage, excessive drainage, and sudden decrease or cessation of drainage.
- Pain medication is administered as ordered by the doctor.

- Throughout recovery, the person is carefully assessed for signs and symptoms of stroke, blood clot to the lung, and impaired blood flow to the kidneys. (See *Recovering from a coronary artery bypass graft.*)
- After the person is weaned from the ventilator and the breathing tube is removed, chest physiotherapy will be initiated. The person will be encouraged to cough, turn frequently, and breathe deeply. Exercises to improve circulation and prevent complications of prolonged bed rest will also be encouraged.

HEART VALVE REPLACEMENT

Heart valve replacement removes a diseased or dysfunctional heart valve and replaces it with a prosthesis (artificial valve). This procedure is often necessary in severe valvular disease when a heart valve cannot open fully, preventing the passage of blood from one heart chamber to another (valvular stenosis), or when the valve cannot fully close, allowing backflow of blood into a heart chamber (valvular insufficiency). Valvular heart disease most commonly affects the mitral and aortic valves (valves on the left side of the heart) because of the high pressure generated by the left ventricle.

Why is this surgery done?

Heart valve replacement is done to improve blood circulation in severe valvular disease. Mitral valve replacement may be required for mitral stenosis and mitral insufficiency; aortic valve replacement for aortic stenosis and aortic insufficiency.

What happens before the surgery?

- The procedure is explained to the person and family. The person is told that he or she will awaken from surgery in the intensive care unit or recovery room. If possible, the doctor will arrange a tour of this unit so that the person will not be unduly frightened by the surroundings after surgery.
- The person is told that he or she will be connected to a heart monitor and have intravenous feeding tubes and tubes placed in arteries to monitor heart and lung function. The person will breathe through a tube that's connected to a mechanical ventilator and will have a tube in the chest.

- Monitoring of the person's heart begins before surgery.
- Necessary laboratory studies and blood typing and crossmatching will be done.
- The person signs a consent form.

What happens during the surgery?

Heart valve replacement requires open-heart surgery with heart-lung bypass and is performed by a surgeon who specializes in cardiology. After initiating heart-lung bypass, the surgeon exposes and removes the diseased heart valve, then sutures the prosthetic valve in correct position. When the new valve is securely in place, the surgeon disconnects the person from heart-lung bypass, restarts the heart, inserts a tube in the chest and between the lungs, closes the incision, and applies a sterile dressing.

What are the possible complications?

Valve replacement surgery carries a low mortality rate but can cause serious complications. Hemorrhage may result from the surgery, blood thinner therapy, or a coagulation disorder from heart-lung bypass during surgery. Stroke may result from clot formation due to turbulent blood flow through the prosthetic valve or from poor circulation to the brain during heart-lung bypass. Infection can develop within days of surgery or months later. Valve dysfunction or failure may occur as the prosthetic device wears out. Other complications include a blood clot to the lung and impaired blood flow to the kidneys.

What happens after the surgery?

- Vital signs are checked and recorded every 15 minutes and as needed until the person's condition stabilizes.
- Heart sounds are checked frequently; distant heart sounds or new murmurs, which may indicate prosthetic valve failure, are reported to the doctor.
- The electrocardiogram is monitored for disturbances in heart rate and rhythm. The doctor is notified of any abnormalities.
- Oxygenation is monitored by listening to the lungs and observing movement of the chest during breathing. Abnormalities are reported to the doctor.
- Oxygen and carbon dioxide levels in the arterial blood are checked every 2 to 4 hours, and the ventilator is adjusted as necessary.

SELF-HELP

Recovering from a heart valve replacement

After you've been discharged from the hospital, follow these important guidelines.

Know when to call your doctor
■ Follow instructions regarding care of your incision. Immediately report chest pain; fever; or redness, swelling, or drainage at the incision site.
■ Notify the doctor if you have symptoms of possible valve problems: fatigue, shortness of breath, palpitations, and dizziness.
■ Also report the following symptoms to your doctor: fever, muscle and joint pain, weakness, and chest discomfort.

Balance activity and rest
■ Maintain a balance between activity and rest. Try to sleep at least 8 hours a night, to schedule a short rest period each afternoon, and to rest frequently during tiring physical activity.
■ Follow your doctor's instructions regarding climbing stairs, engaging in sexual activity, taking baths and showers, and doing light housework and other chores. Avoid lifting heavy objects (more than 20 pounds, or 9 kilograms), driving a car, or doing strenuous work (such as mowing the lawn or vacuuming) until your doctor approves.
■ Follow the exercise program prescribed by your doctor.

Other instructions
■ Know the dosage, schedule, and possible side effects of all prescribed drugs. Wear a medical identification bracelet and carry a card with information and instructions about your blood thinner and antibiotic therapy.
■ Follow the prescribed diet, especially salt and fat restrictions.
■ Be aware that you may feel depressed after you're discharged from the hospital. This depression is usually temporary.
■ Inform your dentist or any other doctors about your prosthetic heart valve before undergoing any surgical procedures because you'll usually need to take antibiotics beforehand. Such procedures, including dental work, are usually delayed for 6 months after surgery.
■ Be sure to keep all follow-up medical appointments.

■ Drainage in the tubes placed in the chest will be carefully observed for hemorrhage, excessive drainage, or a sudden decrease or cessation in drainage.

■ Pain medication will be administered as prescribed by the doctor.

■ The person will be observed carefully for complications throughout the recovery period. (See *Recovering from a heart valve replacement.*)

■ After the person is weaned from the ventilator and the breathing tube is removed, health care providers initiate chest physiotherapy and encourage the person to cough, turn frequently, and do deep-breathing exercises. His or her activities will gradually be increased.

HEART SURGERY FOR CONGENITAL DEFECTS

Congenital heart defects vary in severity. Mild defects allow children to grow normally without surgical treatment. However, most congenital heart defects eventually require surgical repair, usually during infancy or childhood. The type of corrective surgery and its timing depend on the type and extent of the defect. Recent advances in technology allow certain small congenital heart defects to be repaired in a cardiac catheterization lab instead of an operating room.

Congenital heart defects are classified as acyanotic or cyanotic. In children with acyanotic defects, unoxygenated blood (blood without oxygen) does not enter the circulation; in those with cyanotic defects, unoxygenated blood does enter the bloodstream. The prognosis for repair of acyanotic defects is excellent; the prognosis for cyanotic defects is good but depends on the size of the defect and prompt detection of the problem. (See *Common congenital heart defects*.)

Why is this surgery done?

Heart surgery for congenital defects is done to improve blood flow and subsequent oxygenation of the body. Surgical correction is recommended for congenital heart defects that cause inadequate oxygenation, failure to thrive, and poor quality of life; sometimes it's recommended for defects that don't cause symptoms. For example, coarctation of the aorta requires surgical correction because it causes persistent high blood pressure with a risk of further complications, such as hemorrhage into the brain, aortic aneurysm, and inflammation of the lining of the aortic and mitral valves.

What happens before the surgery?

- Unless the congenital heart defect is completely nonthreatening, the infant should be examined every 1 to 2 weeks for the first 6 weeks of life to monitor for complications such as congestive heart failure.
- Before surgical repair of a congenital heart defect, the child will have a thorough diagnostic evaluation, including a physical exam, a detailed family history, and diagnostic tests (chest X-ray, electrocardiogram, echocardiogram—an ultrasound test that shows the size, shape, and motion of various heart structures—and usually cardiac catheterization).

Common congenital heart defects

DEFECT	DESCRIPTION
Ventricular septal defect	One or more abnormal openings in the ventricular septum (the wall that separates the ventricles) allows shunting of blood from the left to the right ventricle. This defect results from incomplete closure of the ventricular septum by the eighth week in the womb; it varies in size from a pinhole to absence of the entire septum. This defect causes recirculation of some oxygenated blood through the lungs, which may lead to congestive heart failure.
Atrial septal defect	One or more openings between the left and right atria allows left-to-right shunting of blood between the chambers. This defect results from delayed or incomplete closure of the wall separating the atria. Small defects usually cause no symptoms and may be undetected in children; they may lead to congestive heart failure and vascular disease of the lungs in adults.
Patent ductus arteriosus	An abnormal opening between the pulmonary artery bifurcation and the descending aorta allows left-to-right shunting of blood from the aorta to the pulmonary artery, resulting in recirculation of oxygenated blood through the lungs. This defect is caused by failure of the ductus to close after birth; it may produce no symptoms initially but eventually can cause congestive heart failure, vascular disease of the lungs, and infection of the lining of the heart.
Coarctation of the aorta	The aorta is constricted, usually below the left subclavian artery near the junction of the ligamentum arteriosum and pulmonary artery. The defect may result from spasm and constriction of smooth muscle in ductus arteriosus during normal closure or from abnormal development of the aortic arch.
Tetralogy of Fallot	A complex of four defects: ventricular septal defect, overriding aorta, pulmonary stenosis, and right ventricular hypertrophy. Blood shunts from right to left through the ventricular septal defect, permitting mixing of unoxygenated and oxygenated blood and causing cyanosis. The defect is caused by incomplete development of the ventricular septum and pulmonary outflow tract.
Transposition of the great arteries	The normal position of the great arteries is reversed; the aorta arises from the right ventricle and the pulmonary artery from the left ventricle, producing two noncommunicating circulatory systems. Unoxygenated blood flows through the right atrium and ventricle and out the aorta to the systemic circulation; oxygenated blood circulates through the left side of the heart and back to the lungs. This defect results from faulty development of the embryo.

■ Careful explanations of all treatments and diagnostic procedures are provided to the child and parents.

■ The child and parents are prepared for the sights and sounds of the intensive care unit. They're told to expect intravenous lines, monitoring equipment, and breathing and chest tubes. They're encouraged to ask questions and express their concerns. If possible, they'll meet the unit's staff.

■ The child will be prepared to use an alternative method of communication (pointing to pictures, using a writing pad) because he or she won't be able to talk when the breathing tube is in place.

- The child can have nothing to eat or drink for 6 to 8 hours before surgery.
- The parents will sign a consent form.

What happens during the surgery?

After determining the type of surgery needed, based on the type, size, and location of the defect, a specialized surgeon performs the procedure. These procedures require general anesthesia and intensive care afterward. The following brief descriptions review treatments of the most common congenital heart defects.

Small ventricular septal defects often close spontaneously. Surgical correction of medium to large ventricular septal defects involves closing the septal defect by suturing it or by covering it with a Dacron patch. This surgery requires a heart-lung bypass.

Surgical correction of an atrial septal defect usually occurs during the preschool years. Again, depending on its size, the defect is closed by sutures or by placement of a Dacron patch. This surgery requires heart-lung bypass.

Surgical correction of patent ductus arteriosus is performed between ages 1 and 2. The surgeon cuts into the wall of the chest, divides the ductus in two, and ties off the divided ends.

Surgical repair of coarctation of the aorta is performed in all infants with symptoms and in children without symptoms at age 4. This surgery involves an incision in the wall of the chest with removal of the defect and reconnection of the ends of the aorta.

Because tetralogy of Fallot causes numerous clinical problems, surgical management depends on the child's signs and symptoms; its purpose is to enhance lung circulation and improve oxygenation. Corrective surgery to relieve the narrowing in the pulmonary artery and close the defect in the wall between the ventricles can be performed on an infant or older child.

For transposition of the great arteries, the current trend is to perform surgical repair before age 12 months. Surgery attempts to redirect venous blood flow to the appropriate ventricle.

What are the possible complications?

Surgical repair of heart defects can cause severe complications, including shock, congestive heart failure, lack of oxygen in the blood, excess carbon dioxide in the blood, irregular heartbeat, stroke, kidney damage, blood clot to the lung, low blood pressure, hemorrhage, and cardiac arrest. As in any surgical procedure, infection poses a constant threat. Infants are also particularly susceptible to alterations in temperature regulation after such surgery.

What happens after the surgery?

- The child awakening from anesthesia will be anxious when confronted with the tubes, monitors, and alarms of the intensive care unit. To help decrease anxiety, the child will be addressed in a soft, soothing voice and touched gently. Parents will be encouraged to visit as often as possible.
- Vital signs are monitored every 15 minutes until they are stable, then as frequently as ordered by the doctor. Heart sounds are monitored and the doctor is notified of any abnormalities.
- Oxygenation is monitored by observing the child's color, listening to the lungs, and watching movement of the chest during breathing. The oxygen and carbon dioxide levels in arterial blood are checked every 2 to 4 hours, and the settings on the ventilator are adjusted as needed.
- The electrocardiogram is monitored for changes in heart rate and rhythm. Abnormalities are reported to the doctor.
- The child will be monitored closely for hemorrhage and excessive or insufficient drainage coming from the tubes in the chest.
- Pain medications will be administered as ordered by the doctor.
- The child will be observed closely for complications, including stroke, blood clot to the lung, and reduced blood flow to the kidneys. (See *Caring for a child after defect repair.*)
- When the child is weaned from the ventilator and the breathing tube is removed, chest physiotherapy will be started. The child will be encouraged to cough, turn, and deep-breathe frequently. Exercises to improve circulation and prevent the complications of prolonged bed rest will also be initiated.

BLOOD VESSEL REPAIR

Blood vessel repair, performed to improve circulation, includes procedures that bypass obstructions or that replace, remove, or reinforce portions of a diseased blood vessel. This surgery can be an emergency procedure—for example, for life-threatening dissecting or ruptured aortic aneurysm or limb-threatening acute arterial occlusion.

 ADVICE FOR CAREGIVERS

Caring for a child after defect repair

After your child has been discharged from the hospital, follow these important guidelines.

Be gentle but diligent
- Relate to your child in a loving, consistent manner, and offer him or her opportunities to express feelings and concerns through conversation and play.
- Follow your doctor's instructions about the child's need for rest and activity restrictions.
- Make sure that the child eats a balanced diet.
- Know the dosage, schedule, administration route, and possible side effects of all prescribed medications.

Other precautions
- Inform all health care providers about the heart surgery before any dental or other surgical procedure because antibiotic therapy is usually needed.
- Avoid exposing the child to infection during flu season and other viral epidemics. He or she may need preventive antibiotics and a flu vaccine.
- Notify the doctor immediately if the child develops chest pain, fever, muscle or joint pain, or weakness.
- Make certain that the child has regular checkups to monitor his or her health status.

Why is this surgery done?

Blood vessel repair is done to restore the opening in a blood vessel. It may be used to treat blood vessels damaged by cholesterol deposits or blood clots (as in aortic aneurysm or arterial occlusive disease), vascular trauma, infections, or birth defects. Blood vessel surgery may also be used for people with obstructions that severely compromise circulation or for people whose vascular disease does not respond to drugs or such nonsurgical treatments as balloon catheterization.

When shouldn't this surgery be done?

People who should not undergo blood vessel surgery include those whose underlying disease makes surgery too risky and those whose disease is too mild to warrant surgery. The latter group may benefit from procedures that clean out the arteries or laser surgery.

What happens before the surgery?

- If the person requires emergency surgery, the procedure and its possible complications are briefly explained, if possible.
- The person will be told that an intravenous line will be in place to provide access for fluid and drugs, that electrodes will be placed on the chest to allow for continuous heart monitoring, and that a catheter will be placed in an artery to provide continuous blood pressure monitoring.
- A urinary catheter may be inserted to allow accurate measurement of urine output.
- A breathing tube will be inserted and the person will be placed on a ventilator. Vital signs will be checked regularly.
- A complete blood vessel assessment will be performed the day before nonemergency surgery.
- Food and fluids must be restricted for at least 12 hours before surgery. The person will probably receive a sedative to help him or her relax and sleep the night before surgery.
- The person will sign a consent form.

What happens during the surgery?

The specific surgical procedure used depends on the type, location, and extent of blood vessel blockage or damage. Types of surgery include removal of a weakened area of an artery (aneurysm resection), bypass grafting for blocked arteries, removal of cholesterol deposits from the carotid arteries, removal of a blood clot, and vein stripping for varicosities.

These procedures are performed under general anesthesia; some may necessitate use of heart-lung bypass.

What are the possible complications?

All blood vessel surgeries may cause serious complications, such as vessel trauma, blood clots, hemorrhage, and infection. Lung complications such as pneumonia may result from immobility or the breathing tube. Grafting procedures carry added risks: The graft may occlude, narrow, dilate, or rupture.

What happens after the surgery?

- Vital signs are checked and recorded every 15 minutes until the person's condition stabilizes and every 30 to 60 minutes thereafter.
- The person's electrocardiogram is monitored for abnormalities of heart rate or rhythm.
- The person's bandage is checked regularly for excessive bleeding.
- Pain medication is administered as prescribed by the doctor.
- Throughout the recovery period, the person will be assessed frequently for signs of complications. Fever, cough, congestion, or shortness of breath may indicate lung infection. Low urine output may point to kidney problems. Severe pain and bluish discoloration in a limb may indicate a blockage. Low blood pressure, restlessness, confusion, shallow breathing, abdominal pain, and increased abdominal girth may signal hemorrhage. The doctor will be notified immediately of any of these signs.
- The incision site will be checked frequently for drainage and signs of infection.
- The person will be weaned from the ventilator as his or her condition improves. To promote good lung hygiene, the person will be encouraged to cough, turn frequently, and do deep-breathing exercises.
- Exercises to improve circulation and prevent the complications of prolonged bed rest will be encouraged. (See *Recovering from blood vessel repair*.)

SELF-HELP

Recovering from blood vessel repair

After you've been discharged from the hospital, follow these important guidelines.

Know when to call your doctor
Know that your doctor may suggest that you check your pulse in the affected arm or leg before rising from bed each morning. If you can't do this yourself, a family member will be taught to do it. Notify the doctor if you can't feel the pulse or if the arm or leg is cold, pale, or painful.

Other measures
- Take your medications as prescribed by your doctor. Make sure you understand the schedule and the expected side effects of all prescribed medications.
- Keep all scheduled follow-up appointments with your doctor.

PERMANENT PACEMAKERS

Permanent heart pacemakers may be required to maintain an effective heart rate after an abnormal heart rhythm has been corrected and adequate pumping function has been established. Technological improvements—for example, advances that make pacemakers more effective and small, lightweight pulse generators that contain batteries that last 7 to 10 years—have greatly extended the use of permanent pacemakers.

Permanent pacemakers consist of a pulse generator implanted under the skin that contains the battery and the electronic circuitry and a pacemaker catheter with a lead on the end. The catheter carries the impulses from the pulse generator to the heart and returns messages from the heart to the pulse generator. The lead with an electrode on its tip is in contact with heart tissue; it delivers the impulse and senses the activity of the heart. Pacemaker leads can be placed in the atria, ventricles, or both chambers of the heart. Having leads in contact with the atria and ventricle provides the closest simulation of normal heart function.

Permanent pacemaker modes

Permanent pacemakers can function in either a fixed (asynchronous) mode or a demand (synchronous) mode. A *fixed mode* releases the impulse at a preset rate regardless of the heart's activity. A *demand mode* senses the heart's electrical activity and inhibits firing of the pulse generator as long as the heart rate exceeds a rate programmed in the permanent pacemaker. Most pacemakers are programmed in the demand mode to avoid interfering with the heart's normal activity.

One of the newest advances in permanent pacemaker design is the ability to adjust the heart rate in response to the person's physical activity (unlike conventional pacemakers, which pace at a preset rate regardless of the person's activity). This function more closely simulates the normal function of the heart. For example, the heart rate accelerates with activity to meet the body's increased need for oxygen. Conversely, the heart rate decreases during sleep.

Early pacemakers required the person to avoid microwave ovens, which interfered with pacemaker function. Now, a metal covering protects the circuitry in the permanent pacemaker pulse generator, so exposure to microwaves is no longer hazardous. However, some dangers remain. For example, during surgery, people must be closely monitored if electrocautery will be used. Radiation therapy can have a cumulative effect on the pulse generator's circuitry, causing pacemaker failure. The pacemaker should be covered with a lead shield during radiation therapy and checked for proper function afterward.

A permanent pacemaker will last several years, depending on how it is programmed and how often the heart paces on its own. The more often the pacemaker must initiate a heartbeat, the sooner the battery will become depleted. The usual life expectancy of a lithium battery is 7 to 10 years.

Most permanent pacemakers can now be reprogrammed by a doctor or another specially trained person if pacemaker problems arise after implantation. A magnetic device supplied by the manufacturer is placed on the skin over the location of the pulse generator; using certain commands, the device can reprogram the pacemaker mode, the rate, the sensitivity, and other variables.

Why is this surgery done?

Permanent pacemakers are implanted to provide electrical impulses to the heart at a rate that's adequate to maintain normal cardiac output. Candidates for permanent pacemakers include people with persistent abnormal heart rates and rhythms.

What happens before the surgery?

- The person is taught about pacemaker insertion, including the reason for the pacemaker and what the pacemaker does. He or she is shown a sample pacemaker unit; learns the type of anesthesia to be used; and is told what to expect in the operating room, in the recovery area, and on return to the room after the pacemaker has been inserted.
- An electrocardiogram is taken.
- Vital signs are recorded.
- The person signs a consent form.
- The surgical site is shaved, if necessary, and cleaned with an antiseptic solution.
- An intravenous line is inserted in case emergency medications are needed.
- A sedative is given before surgery as prescribed by the doctor.

What happens during the surgery?

Permanent pacemakers are inserted by a surgeon or cardiologist in an operating room. Local anesthesia is generally used, but other forms of

SELF-HELP

Living with a permanent pacemaker

Once you've been discharged from the hospital after receiving a permanent pacemaker, follow these important guidelines.

Take special precautions
- Be alert for signs or symptoms of infection (fever, redness, swelling, or drainage) at the incision or insertion site.
- Inform any dentists or doctors that you have a permanent pacemaker.
- Take your resting pulse daily as instructed, and notify your doctor of any abnormalities.

Other instructions
- Keep all follow-up appointments with your doctor.
- Follow your doctor's instructions regarding use of the telephone to monitor pacemaker function.
- Carry an identification card that lists pacemaker data as well as the date of implantation and your doctor's name.

anesthesia may be used, depending on the person and the route of pacemaker insertion.

The surgeon may implant the leads by directly penetrating the chest wall and attaching the lead to the external surface of the heart. This approach provides stability for the leads but requires surgery under general anesthesia; therefore, it is used during open-heart surgery. More commonly, the surgeon inserts the leads through a vein into the right side of the heart. The surgeon attaches the leadwires to the pulse generator, which he or she implants in a pocket under the skin below the clavicle (most common) or in a pocket under the skin of the abdomen. The surgeon then programs and tests the pulse generator and closes the incision.

What are the possible complications?

Complications of permanent pacemaker insertion include infection, abnormal heart rhythms, and displacement of the leadwires. When the surgeon implants the leads directly in the chest wall, the person is at risk for complications associated with chest surgery and general anesthesia (such as pneumonia). If he or she inserts the leads through a vein, blood clots may form.

Other complications are related to the pacemaker (for example, battery failure, a displaced electrode, or pacemaker-induced abnormal heart rhythms). For more details on complications, see "Temporary Pacemakers," page 55.

What happens after the surgery?

- The person's electrocardiogram, vital signs, and level of consciousness are monitored for at least the first 24 hours after pacemaker insertion.
- The bandage is checked for bleeding and changed.
- Pain medications are administered as prescribed by the doctor.
- The doctor or nurse provides instructions regarding restricted activities. The person may be told to limit the use of the involved extremity for the first 24 to 72 hours. (See *Living with a permanent pacemaker.*)
- The person and the electrocardiogram are monitored for signs of pacemaker malfunction or failure.
- Antibiotics are administered for 24 to 48 hours, as prescribed by the doctor.

IMPLANTABLE CARDIOVERTER-DEFIBRILLATOR

The implantable cardioverter-defibrillator is a surgically implanted device used to treat life-threatening irregularities in the heartbeat. It consists of a set of leads and a pulse generator. The defibrillator monitors the heartbeat. When it detects a life-threatening abnormality, it delivers an electric shock directly to the heart within 10 to 35 seconds to reestablish a normal heartbeat. If this shock fails to convert the person's heartbeat, the device will recycle and deliver up to four more shocks, depending on the specific model.

The implantable cardioverter-defibrillator generator weighs less than ½ pound (0.2 kilogram) and has a battery life of 3 to 5 years, with the ability to deliver 200 to 300 shocks.

Why is this procedure done?
The implantable cardioverter-defibrillator is used to detect and terminate sustained, life-threatening abnormal heartbeats originating in the ventricle. It is also an appropriate treatment for survivors of sudden cardiac arrest not related to a heart attack. Because implantation of the device requires open-heart surgery, it's usually reserved for people who don't respond to or can't tolerate conventional drug therapy and for people with a life expectancy of at least 1 year. In people with severe left ventricular disease (especially those for whom drug therapy is less effective in reducing mortality), the implantable cardioverter-defibrillator may be considered earlier.

When shouldn't this procedure be done?
The implantable cardioverter-defibrillator should not be used for people who have fainting spells that are not the result of a documented life-threatening heart rhythm disturbance originating in the ventricle or for the treatment of slow heart rates. The device should not be implanted during an emergency.

What happens before the procedure?
- The procedure is explained to the person.
- The person will sign a consent form.

What happens during the procedure?

The implantation procedure, typically combined with coronary artery bypass graft surgery, is performed under general anesthesia. The Ventak defibrillator has four leads. Two leads end in coil electrodes that the surgeon places on or in the left ventricle, and two end in patch electrodes that the surgeon places over the left and right ventricles. These two are connected to the pulse generator, which is implanted in the abdomen.

The implantable cardioverter-defibrillator continuously monitors heart rate through a system of rate-sensing leads. When the device detects life-threatening ventricular rhythms, the capacitor-charging cycle begins, and the cardioverter-defibrillator delivers either a low-energy cardioversion shock or high-energy defibrillation shock. Because most devices deliver shocks based on heart rate, care must be taken to set the implantable cardioverter-defibrillator detection rate above the person's exercise heart rate.

What are the possible complications?

People requiring cardioverter-defibrillator implantation are subject to the same risks as those associated with open-heart surgery. In addition, death—caused by the inability to terminate a life-threatening ventricular rhythm induced during surgery to test the device—is an uncommon but potential risk of this procedure. Infection in the area around the device is especially serious and may occur during hospitalization or several months later. The device also may erode through the skin.

People may also develop device-related complications. For example, the cardioverter-defibrillator may deliver inappropriate shocks for non-life-threatening heart rhythm abnormalities, or it may interact adversely with permanent pacemakers. Lead or patch dislodgment may cause oversensing from random noise, or undersensing because of loss of the signal from the heart by the cardioverter-defibrillator. The device may fail to terminate a ventricular rhythm. External defibrillation may be more difficult because patches electrically "shield" the heart muscle.

What happens after the procedure?

- The person is monitored for abnormal heart rhythms and appropriate functioning of the device.
- The person is observed for signs of infection.

SELF-HELP

Living with a cardioverter-defibrillator

Once you've been discharged from the hospital after receiving a cardioverter-defibrillator, follow these important guidelines.

Restrict your activities

Follow your doctor's instructions regarding activity restrictions. Typically, you should avoid activities that involve rough, physical contact or that would be dangerous if you lost consciousness (for example, driving a car or operating heavy machinery).

Know when to call your doctor

- Notify the doctor after you receive a shock. If you receive multiple shocks within a short time, go to a hospital emergency room.
- If you notice signs of infection, inform your doctor immediately.

Other instructions

- Keep a diary of symptoms and related events.
- Avoid exposure to strong magnetic fields (such as power plants or large running engines) because they may inactivate your cardioverter-defibrillator.
- The device will trigger the metal detector at an airport, but this will not cause it to discharge. Most people who show their identification card to airport personnel are permitted to bypass the security checkpoint. A person who has a cardioverter-defibrillator should never be frisked with magnets.
- Keep follow-up appointments with your doctor, as scheduled, to maintain proper function of the device.
- Your family should initiate CPR if you become unconscious and do not have a pulse.

- The person is scheduled to have the device tested and to have exercise testing before returning home. Drug therapy may be prescribed to limit the frequency of shocks or to treat other abnormal heart rhythms.
- The person is taught how the device functions, how to take care of the incision, and about signs of infection before returning home. (See *Living with a cardioverter-defibrillator.*)
- A follow-up appointment is scheduled with the doctor.
- The person's family will be encouraged to have CPR training.
- The sensation of a shock, commonly described as a "punch" or "kick" in the chest, is explained to the person. Because detection of a heartbeat disturbance and delivery of therapy may take up to 30 seconds, the person may become dizzy or light-headed and even lose consciousness before a shock is delivered. The person is also told that a family member touching him or her at the time of shock delivery may experience a mild tingling sensation, which is not harmful.
- The person should wear a medical identification bracelet or carry an identification card. He or she will receive a temporary card before leaving the hospital and will receive a permanent card in 4 to 8 weeks.

RESECTION OF THE HEART'S INNER LINING

Also known as *endocardial resection,* this is an open-heart surgical procedure in which scar tissue from the endocardium (the inner lining of the left ventricle) is removed to permanently cure a person with recurrent sustained ventricular tachycardia, a life-threatening heart rhythm.

Why is this surgery done?

This procedure is done to remove or destroy diseased areas of the heart that are the site of origin for sustained, life-threatening ventricular rhythms that do not respond to other therapies. It is most successful in people with a fast heart rate that can be traced to a discrete left ventricular aneurysm (weakening in the wall of the heart).

What happens before the surgery?

- The procedure and what to expect afterward is explained to the person and the family.
- The person signs a consent form.

What happens during the surgery?

Under general anesthesia, an incision is made in the chest to visualize the heart. After the focus of the abnormal heart rhythm is identified, a 2- to 3-millimeter thickness of subendocardial scar tissue is removed from healthy heart. This resection usually includes the full extent of visible scar tissue. Border zones of diseased endocardium may be treated by cryoablation, in which a special probe is used to freeze the area surrounding the resection site. This helps to further interrupt the pathway of the abnormal heart rhythm without producing structural damage to the heart.

What are the possible complications?

Associated complications vary greatly, depending on the person's underlying heart function. Also, because this procedure requires open-heart surgery, the person is at risk for the complications associated with bypass surgery: hemorrhage, infection, stroke, and shock.

What happens after the surgery?

- The person recovers in the intensive care unit.
- The person's electrocardiogram is monitored for disturbances in rate and rhythm, and the doctor is notified of any abnormality.
- The person is observed carefully for signs of complications.
- The bandage will be changed using sterile technique.
- The person will be encouraged to cough, turn frequently, and do deep-breathing exercises.
- Before leaving the hospital, the person will be tested to make certain that the surgery was effective. If the abnormal heart rhythm recurs, appropriate therapy (drug or implantable cardioverter-defibrillator) will be initiated.

REMOVAL OF PLAQUE FROM THE CAROTID ARTERY

This surgical procedure, also known as *carotid endarterectomy,* involves removal of plaque (cholesterol-containing deposits) from the carotid arteries to improve blood flow to the brain. Because carotid blockage commonly leads to stroke, this procedure may be considered a preventive treatment for stroke. However, it carries significant surgical risks, so the risks must be carefully weighed against the benefits.

Why is this surgery done?

Plaque is surgically removed from the carotid artery to improve blood flow to the brain and alleviate symptoms of reduced blood flow. The procedure is performed to prevent total blockage of the carotid artery, to remove a potential source of blood clots, and to prevent stroke.

This procedure is performed on people who have experienced a stroke or reversible symptoms of reduced blood flow to the brain, such as fainting and dizziness. People who have both coronary artery disease and carotid artery disease may have both conditions repaired at the same time if they are otherwise medically stable.

When shouldn't this surgery be done?

This procedure should not be performed on people with uncontrolled high blood pressure, those with an acute blockage of the ca-

SELF-HELP

Caring for yourself after plaque removal

Once you've been discharged from the hospital after surgery, follow these important guidelines.

Adjust your lifestyle
Follow your doctor's instructions regarding lifestyle changes that may reduce the risk of the condition recurring. These changes may include stopping smoking, reducing fat in your diet, and controlling your weight.

Other instructions
- Use home health care agencies for follow-up care, if recommended by your doctor.
- Make sure you know the dose, schedule, and side effects of all drugs prescribed by your doctor.
- Immediately report any new symptoms, such as fainting or dizziness, to your doctor.
- Keep scheduled follow-up appointments with your doctor.

rotid artery causing severe brain damage and permanent partial paralysis, and people who are in generally poor health. Such people are treated instead with medical therapy, such as blood thinners.

What happens before the surgery?

- A doctor or nurse will explain the procedure, related diagnostic tests, and what will happen after the surgery to you and your family.
- Causes of the disease will also be explained so that you can make lifestyle changes to reduce the likelihood that plaque buildup will recur after surgery.
- A catheter is placed in an artery of your arm to monitor oxygen and carbon dioxide levels in the blood and blood pressure.
- You'll receive an electrocardiogram and an electroencephalogram (a test that records brain waves).
- You'll be told that a nurse will routinely check your level of consciousness, orientation, extremity strength, speech, and fine hand movements every hour, and that this is not an indication that you're not doing well.

What happens during the surgery?

During this procedure, light general anesthesia may be used to allow accurate monitoring of brain waves by electroencephalography during the surgery.

The surgeon makes an incision in the neck so that all branches of the carotid artery can be seen, then clamps the carotid arteries and, if blood flow to the brain is inadequate, constructs a shunt that permits blood flow past the obstruction. Shunts provide temporary bypass routes for blood flow to ensure adequate brain circulation during surgery.

The surgeon administers blood thinners to prevent blood clots from forming, then removes the plaque from the diseased artery. The artery is patched with a vein taken from another area of the person's body or with prosthetic material and then is closed. If a shunt was used, it is removed before the surgery is completed.

What are the possible complications?

The most common problem after removal of plaque from the carotid artery is fluctuating blood pressure, especially transient high blood pressure. Breathing difficulties after surgery can result from a collection of blood around the windpipe. Wound complications such as infection may also occur.

Rare complications include vocal cord paralysis and a sudden increase in blood flow to the brain, which can lead to headaches, seizures, and bleeding into the brain.

The most serious complication of the procedure is stroke, which is thought to result from pieces of plaque moving to the brain.

What happens after the surgery?
- Your vital signs are checked every 15 minutes for the first hour after surgery until your condition is stable. (See *Caring for yourself after plaque removal.*)
- Every hour for the first 24 hours, your extremity strength, fine hand movements, speech, visual acuity, and orientation are assessed.
- Fluid intake and urine output are monitored hourly for the first 24 hours.
- Your electrocardiogram is monitored for the first 24 hours.

OTHER TREATMENTS

TEMPORARY PACEMAKERS

A temporary pacemaker is an electrical device that provides short-term artificial stimulation to the heart. It is frequently used during emergency situations that require immediate heart pacing; it can be lifesaving for a person with an unstable heart rhythm that is interfering with blood circulation.

A temporary pacemaker has three components: the pulse generator, the leadwire, and the leads. Unlike a permanent pacemaker, a temporary pacemaker has an external pulse generator that the person may wear on the chest, waist, or upper arm or that may be hung at the bedside. The pulse generator produces the electrical impulses and contains the power source (a lithium or alkaline battery) and the electronic circuitry. The leadwire is the avenue by which the electrical impulse initiated by the pulse generator travels to the heart and by which the heart's activity is communicated back to the pulse generator. The leadwire is contained in insulated materials.

Electrical safety precautions must be observed when a person has a temporary pacemaker because the pacing wire provides a direct route to the heart for any stray electric current. Electrical equipment must be kept to a minimum and must be properly grounded. Family members must avoid simultaneous contact with the person and electrical equipment.

Temporary pacemaker modes

Temporary pacemakers can function in either a fixed (asynchronous) mode or a demand (synchronous) mode. A *fixed mode* releases the impulse at a preset rate regardless of the heart's activity. A *demand mode* senses the heart's activity and inhibits firing of the pulse generator as long as the heart rate exceeds the rate set on the temporary pacemaker.

Electrical safety precautions must be observed when a person has a temporary pacemaker because the pacing wire provides a direct route to the heart for any stray electric current. Electrical equipment must be kept to a minimum and must be properly grounded. Family members must avoid simultaneous contact with the person and electrical equipment.

Why is this procedure done?

Temporary pacemakers are inserted for the following reasons:
- to initiate an artificial electrical impulse to the heart when the heart rate is too slow or when the normal impulse encounters a conduction disturbance that does not allow an adequately pumping heart to meet the body's requirements
- to prevent abnormal impulse formation or conduction disturbances that can result from a heart attack, heart surgery, toxic reactions to drugs, or metabolism abnormalities
- to interrupt very rapid heartbeats that are unresponsive to drug therapy (less common use).

What happens before the procedure?

- The procedure is explained to the person and family.
- The person or a family member signs a consent form.
- Sedatives are administered as ordered by the doctor.
- An intravenous line is inserted in case emergency medications are necessary.
- Vital signs and an electrocardiogram are taken.

What happens during the procedure?

Temporary pacemakers are usually inserted by a cardiologist. A nurse customarily will assist during the procedure, and additional staff members may be present as needed.

Temporary pacing can be accomplished using several methods. Insertion of a catheter through a vein to the right ventricle of the heart is the most common approach. The tip of the catheter is put in contact with the inner layer of the heart.

Temporary epicardial pacing is commonly accomplished through an incision in the chest. The pacing electrodes are placed on the epicardial (outer) layer of the heart. This type of pacemaker is commonly used during and for the first few days after open-heart surgery. Typically, the pacing electrodes are sutured to the outer layer of the heart, brought out through the chest wall incision, and attached to a pulse generator or capped until they are needed.

External pacing is done from the outside of the body. Pacing electrodes are placed on the person's chest and back. From an external power source, small amounts of electricity are delivered through the electrodes to the heart. External pacing is used for emergency situations (while the person awaits insertion of a transvenous temporary pacemaker) or as backup for a permanent pacemaker during battery replacement.

Following lead placement, the temporary leads are connected to the external pulse generator. The catheter may be sutured in place, and a bandage is applied to the insertion site.

What are the possible complications?

Various types of abnormal heart rhythms may result as a complication of temporary pacing. Clot formation can result from the presence of the catheter or from inactivity. Rarely, the ventricle may be punctured as a result of insertion or movement of the catheter. Infection of the membrane surrounding the heart may also result from the use of a temporary pacemaker. Hiccups or abdominal twitching can result from placement of the pacing catheter against a thin-walled right ventricle or from rupture of the ventricle, which leads to electrical stimulation of the diaphragm.

Possible complications at the insertion site include infection, inflammation of the vein, blood vessel blockage, hemorrhage, and allergic reactions to the local anesthetic.

Also, a temporary pacemaker can malfunction because the pacing electrode tip is in the wrong position.

What happens after the procedure?

- Pain medication is administered as prescribed by the doctor.
- If the catheter was inserted through an artery in the arm or leg, the extremity will be immobilized.
- The person's electrocardiogram will be monitored.

- Pacemaker batteries will be checked and changed if necessary.
- The person will be observed closely for signs and symptoms of pacemaker malfunction—for example, a change in pulse rate, fatigue, shortness of breath, pain, or dizziness. The doctor will be notified if these symptoms occur.
- The insertion site will be observed daily for signs of infection, and a clean bandage will be applied.
- If the catheter was not sutured, it will be taped securely to avoid dislodgment.
- Circulation in the extremity below the catheter insertion site will be assessed by checking the pulse rate and the color, temperature, and sensation of the extremity.

*T*HERAPEUTIC REMOVAL OF BLOOD

In this procedure (also known as *phlebotomy*), blood is directly removed from a person's body. This therapy, one of the earliest known medical treatments, has historically been known as *bleeding*. For centuries, the widespread use of crude blood-letting techniques was more detrimental than therapeutic. However, the removal of a safe volume of blood (less than 15% of the total) remains the treatment of choice for several disorders.

For centuries, the widespread use of crude blood-letting techniques was more detrimental than therapeutic. However, the removal of a safe volume of blood (less than 15% of the total) remains the treatment of choice for several disorders.

Why is this treatment done?
Blood is removed to reduce the number of red blood cells, to decrease blood viscosity (thickness), and to reduce iron levels in the blood. Repeated blood removal is the treatment of choice to reduce excess iron and maintain safe iron levels in the blood. The disorder known as *hemochromatosis* is the most common form of iron overload in the United States.

Blood removal is also recommended for treatment of increased blood viscosity caused by the excessive production of red blood cells. The most common disorder in which this occurs is polycythemia vera, which results in uncontrolled production of white blood cells, platelets, and red blood cells. Blood removal may also be appropriate for people with severe lung disease, congenital heart disease that results in reduced oxygen levels in the blood, and other blood diseases.

When shouldn't this treatment be done?

Aggressive removal of blood should not be performed in elderly people and those with chronic lung disease. For these people, removal of lesser blood volumes over a longer period of time is recommended.

What happens before the treatment?

- Care is taken to make sure that the person is well rested and has a clear understanding of the procedure to be performed.
- The person should eat a balanced meal and drink extra fluids a few hours before blood removal unless this is prohibited by his or her medical condition.
- The person signs a consent form that includes a description of potential complications.
- Beforehand, the person performing the procedure will verify that the amount of blood to be removed does not exceed a safe amount (less than 15% of total blood volume).
- Vital signs will be taken and recorded, and the blood count will be tested immediately before each removal of blood.

What happens during the treatment?

Blood is removed by a qualified staff member in the blood bank, on the nursing unit, or in the outpatient clinic. The procedure is performed under sterile conditions. Skin preparation should include the use of an effective antiseptic.

For small people or those at high risk for side effects, intravenous solutions may be infused before or during blood removal. The volume of blood being removed should be continuously monitored to ensure adequate flow and avoid removal of an excessive amount.

What are the possible complications?

The most common complications of therapeutic blood removal are slow pulse rate, low blood pressure, fainting, seizures, local discomfort, and a bruise where the needle was inserted. People with active heart and lung disease may take longer to recover from such effects and therefore should be monitored closely.

What happens after the treatment?

- A pressure dressing is placed where the needle was inserted, and the person is instructed to leave it in place for 2 to 3 hours.

Recovering from blood removal

Once you've been discharged from the hospital after therapeutic removal of blood, follow these important guidelines:

- Don't drink alcohol or perform prolonged or strenuous physical exercise until after eating a balanced meal.
- Because of the potential risk of dizziness, don't drive, operate heavy equipment, or work in other hazardous situations for several hours after removal of blood.
- Keep all follow-up appointments with your doctor, as scheduled.

■ Vital signs are taken and recorded before allowing the person to sit up. Liquids and a high-carbohydrate snack are recommended before the person is sent home. (See *Recovering from blood removal*.)

COMPRESSION OF VEINS WITH INFLATABLE CUFFS

This procedure (also known as *intermittent pneumatic compression*) involves wrapping knee-high or thigh-high cuffs around the legs to prevent blood clots. Connected to a pump, the cuffs intermittently inflate and deflate, gently compressing the legs. This inflation and deflation mimics the normal pumping action of the heart, thus reducing pooling of venous blood and enhancing the return of venous blood to the heart.

Why is this treatment done?

Inflatable cuffs are used to prevent blood clots, to enhance blood flow in the veins, and to decrease lymphedema (swelling of the extremities due to a blockage of the lymph system). They're used for any person at risk for developing blood clots, especially immobile people and people who have had surgery. In addition, if the veins become stretched from pooling, small tears can develop in their inner walls, providing a site for clot formation.

Use of the inflatable cuffs enhances clot-dissolving activity; in people who have had surgery, it restores this activity, which usually decreases for 72 hours after surgery, to levels that existed before surgery.

Compression boot devices are used by professional sports teams to decrease swelling after acute musculoskeletal injury. The compression reduces the buildup of fluid and decreases pain. Within 24 hours, mobility is enhanced because of the decreased swelling. Boot devices can also be used to treat lymphedema from fluid build-up; however, different compression times and pressures are used.

When shouldn't this treatment be done?

Vein compression with inflatable cuffs should not be performed on people with evidence of reduced blood flow to the leg due to peripheral vascular disease or on people with blood clots or thrombophlebitis. It's not recommended for people who have been on prolonged bed rest without preventive therapy for blood clots unless tests have ruled out clot formation. The procedure is also not recommended for people with congestive heart failure because it can produce fluid overload in sensitive people.

If the cuffs cannot be placed on the legs, they may be applied to the arms; such use will not relieve pressure in the veins of the legs but will produce a clot-dissolving effect.

What happens before the treatment?
- People at risk for developing blood clots are identified.
- The person will be informed about the procedure, including its purpose and the sensations to be expected.

What happens during the treatment?
- The nurse wraps the inflatable cuffs from the ankle to the knee or thigh on each leg and then connects them to a pump. One cuff inflates fully and then deflates. Then the second cuff inflates and deflates.
- To prevent blood clots in deep veins, cuffs are applied to the legs as soon as the immobility risk factor becomes evident. For people who are having surgery, the cuffs are applied before anesthesia.
- The cuffs remain in place and therapy continues until the person is fully ambulatory and the risk of blood clots has diminished.
- The person's skin color, temperature, sensation, and ability to move the extremity are monitored.
- Therapy to prevent blood clots is maintained until the person is no longer at risk, usually until he or she is fully mobile.
- When the person must leave the nursing unit for diagnostic or therapeutic procedures, the cuffs should travel with him or her and therapy should be maintained in the new location.
- If compression therapy is interrupted for more than 1 hour, it should be discontinued until a test can be performed to rule out the formation of a clot during the interruption.
- The person will be encouraged to walk with the cuffs in place. The hoses can be disconnected and the cuffs can remain around the calves while the person is walking.
- The cuffs are removed daily to inspect the skin and provide skin care. (See *Using inflatable cuffs at home.*)

 SELF-HELP

Using inflatable cuffs at home

After you've been discharged from the hospital with inflatable cuffs, keep in mind the following.

Use cuffs correctly
- Don't interrupt therapy for more than 1 hour at a time when you're using the inflatable cuffs, to prevent formation of blood clots.
- You can leave the cuffs wrapped around your legs while walking; the hoses connecting the cuffs to the pump can simply be disconnected.

Other points to remember
- This treatment is easy to use and ideal for home use. Insurance companies permit reimbursement of expenses for home use.
- Home therapy is well suited for people recovering from surgery who won't be fully mobile at discharge and are at high risk for blood clot formation. It can also be used for cancer patients with chronic swelling of the arms or legs.

What are the possible complications?

During this therapy, some people find the cuffs hot and uncomfortable, but the use of fabric cuffs and cuffs that wrap only around the calves now minimizes such discomfort.

SCLEROTHERAPY FOR ESOPHAGEAL VARICES

Endoscopic sclerotherapy is used to treat swollen veins (varices) of the esophagus. Usually performed after a bleeding of the veins, the procedure involves injecting the veins with a sclerosant, a strongly irritating solution, which causes clot formation and stops the bleeding. Injection into the area beside the distended vein produces thickening and swelling that compresses the blood vessel, also halting the bleeding. Eradicating the distended blood vessel stops the bleeding and prevents rebleeding.

This procedure was first done in the late 1930s. From 1940 to 1970, it periodically gained and lost popularity as surgical procedures overshadowed it. Recent improvements in equipment and technique, combined with recognition of the shortcomings of some surgical procedures, have once again made sclerotherapy the initial treatment of choice in most hospitals.

After the initial treatment to control an acute bleeding episode, the person is usually scheduled for elective additional treatments. They are usually scheduled at intervals of a few weeks, depending on the risk level and healing rate of the person. Preventive sclerotherapy is aimed at preventing rebleeding.

A similar procedure has been used successfully in treating leg varicosities and hemorrhoids.

Why is this treatment done?

Endoscopic sclerotherapy is done to eradicate distended esophageal veins and to decrease the frequency and severity of bleeding. This procedure is the current treatment of choice to control hemorrhage from distended esophageal veins, a life-threatening condition. It is also used to prevent recurrence of bleeding.

When shouldn't this treatment be done?

Endoscopic sclerotherapy cannot be performed on an uncooperative person because any unscheduled movement could result in tearing of the vein or perforation of the esophagus with resulting hemorrhage.

What happens before the treatment?

- A doctor or nurse will discuss the procedure with the person.
- A nurse will record the person's vital signs and other pertinent data, and then insert an intravenous line for administering fluid or blood replacement.
- The person is instructed to lie still to prevent injury.
- The person receives a sedative but remains awake.

What happens during the treatment?

The procedure is performed by a doctor through an instrument that allows him or her to see inside the esophagus. After passing the instrument through the mouth to the esophagus, the doctor locates and identifies the branches of the blood vessels at or just above the junction of the stomach and the esophagus. If a bleeding vein is identified, a sclerosant is injected into the distended vein or the surrounding area. The needle is then withdrawn from the vein, and this injection procedure is repeated at various locations to eradicate all distended veins. The doctor will determine the number of injections and the volume of sclerosant used during each treatment.

What are the possible complications?

Endoscopic sclerotherapy is associated with a 20% to 40% incidence of complications and a mortality rate of 1% to 2%. Transient chest pain, difficulty swallowing, and fever commonly occur within the first 24 hours after the procedure. Allergic reactions to the sclerosant are also possible.

Ulceration at the injection site may occur in as many as 94% of people. However, ulceration is typically regarded as a stage of vein eradication, not a complication.

Lung complications can occur as well as traumatic esophageal perforation and hemorrhage. Tightening of the esophagus develops in 2% to 10% of people and usually responds to conservative dilatation treatment.

Infection occurs in 5% to 50% of people, but preventive therapy with antibiotics is not considered necessary except for people with prosthetic heart valves.

Recovering from sclerotherapy

Once you're discharged from the hospital after sclerotherapy for esophageal varices, make sure you follow these important guidelines:

- Report any fever, bleeding, breathing problems, chest pain, or difficulty swallowing to your doctor immediately.
- Use mild pain relievers, if prescribed by your doctor, for transient, mild chest pain.
- Follow the diet prescribed by your doctor.

What happens after the treatment?

- A nurse will observe the person for signs of blood loss, lung complications, fever, a perforated esophagus, or other complications.
- The nurse will monitor the person's vital signs and maintain an intravenous line, as ordered by the doctor.
- The person will receive any pain medication prescribed by the doctor. (See *Recovering from sclerotherapy*.)

CATHETER ABLATION FOR AN IRREGULAR HEARTBEAT

This is a new procedure for treatment of symptomatic sustained irregular heartbeats. It involves placing a special large-tipped electrode catheter inside the heart through the arterial or venous system and using direct-current or radio-frequency energy to disrupt abnormally conducting pathways in the heart. Currently, radio-frequency energy is the preferred method of ablation because it can deliver a more localized and discrete focus of energy with fewer complications.

Catheter ablation is most effective for treatment of fast abnormal heartbeats that originate above the ventricle.

Why is this procedure done?

Catheter ablation is done to completely eliminate certain sustained irregular heartbeats and to control irregular heartbeats in people for whom previous drug therapy and other treatments have been unsuccessful.

When shouldn't this procedure be done?

Catheter ablation should not be performed when the origin of the irregular heartbeat cannot be precisely located or when multiple origins are present.

What happens during the procedure?

Catheter ablation is performed in the cardiac catheterization lab. A number of electrode catheters are placed through the skin into an appropriate vein or artery and are then guided by X-ray to the precise location in the heart. Electrocardiograms are recorded from surface leads and leads placed in the heart at various stages of the procedure. The irregular heartbeat is induced to identify the precise location of the problem. This area is then eradicated as follows.

Radio-frequency energy slowly heats the tissue and results in destruction of the origin of the abnormal heartbeat. Energy is delivered through the catheter for 20 to 30 seconds or up to 2 minutes if needed. This can be repeated several times. The procedure is done with the person awake or lightly sedated and causes only minimal chest wall discomfort.

Direct-current ablation, performed less commonly, uses a standard defibrillator. It produces a larger area of damage, destroying the origin of the abnormal heartbeat along with normal surrounding tissue. It also stimulates skeletal muscle and nerves, necessitating general anesthesia. Cryoablation, freezing with nitrous oxide, is performed primarily in the operating room, often with resection of the lining of the heart cavities. Laser ablation and microwave ablation are currently being evaluated.

What are the possible complications?

Complications include the risks associated with other forms of catheterization: venous or arterial damage, blood clots, compression of the heart by fluid or blood, perforation of the heart, and death. In some cases, the scar tissue created by catheter ablation becomes a new focus for an irregular heartbeat. Normal conduction tissue may be damaged by the procedure, resulting in heart block. The overall risk of this procedure is low; however, complications are more likely with direct-current ablation.

What happens after the procedure?

- During and after catheter ablation, the electrocardiogram is monitored for recurrence or worsening of the abnormal heartbeats. A temporary or permanent pacemaker may be required.
- A nurse will monitor the person's vital signs and watch for complications, such as low blood pressure, shortness of breath, and distended neck veins.
- Puncture sites are observed for bleeding or hematoma.
- Before discharge, a nurse will teach the person how to care for himself or herself at home.
- The person should adhere to the drug regimen or any other therapies as prescribed by the doctor.

REMOVAL OF PLAQUE FROM THE CORONARY ARTERIES

In this procedure (also known as *atherectomy*), atherosclerotic plaque (deposits containing cholesterol) is extracted from the coronary arteries using a disposable catheter with a cutting head that slices away or pulverizes the plaque. The excised plaque is suctioned out of the artery to prevent clot formation and its complications.

The decision to perform this procedure is based on the results of an electrocardiogram, a treadmill stress test, cardiac enzyme levels, and angiography (an X-ray study of the coronary arteries to determine the site and extent of the disease).

Why is this procedure done?

Plaque is removed from the coronary arteries to restore oxygenated blood flow to the heart, to relieve chest pain, and to prevent heart attack. This procedure is performed on people who have chest pain that is unresponsive to medical therapy and on those who are candidates for balloon angioplasty (widening of the coronary arteries using a balloon catheter) or coronary artery bypass grafting. If complications such as perforation occur during the procedure, one of the above procedures is done on an emergency basis.

For people who have had a coronary artery bypass graft, removal of plaque is an alternative if grafted veins have less than a 50% reocclusion rate. (Grafted veins are thicker than native coronary arteries, so perforation is less likely to occur than when plaque is removed in the actual coronary artery. Also, grafted veins may not open as well with the balloon technique, so plaque removal is a better option.)

When shouldn't this procedure be done?

Plaque should not be removed when it is located where blood vessels divide into two branches or when it may be angular in shape or located in an angle of a vessel. This procedure also shouldn't be performed in a person with vessels that have developed weakenings in the wall, with ulcerated lesions, with lesions severely hardened with calcium, or with blockages that resist passage of a guide wire.

Plaque is removed from the coronary arteries to restore oxygenated blood flow to the heart, to relieve chest pain, and to prevent heart attack.

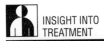

INSIGHT INTO
TREATMENT

How plaque is removed

A method of cutting away and removing plaque, directional coronary atherectomy uses a bullet-shaped probe that has an opening on one side of the casing. The benefits of this technique include less trauma to the blood vessel, less risk of emergency bypass surgery, fewer recurrences of the blockage, and increased safety and predictability.

Using a guide wire, the doctor inserts the catheter into the narrowed vessel.

A tiny, rotating cup shaves off the plaque that projects into the chamber.

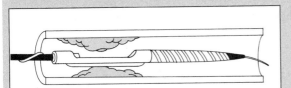
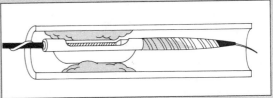

The doctor inflates the balloon to force the open side of the catheter against the opposite vessel wall. This squeezes the plaque into the casing chamber.

Then the doctor rotates the instrument and removes more plaque until serial X-rays of the coronary arteries show improved blood flow.

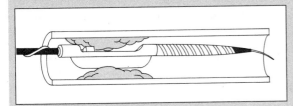
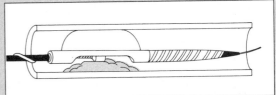

What happens before the procedure?

- The day before the procedure, the person takes medication to prevent his or her blood from clotting.
- The person may be asked to bathe and shampoo twice with an antiseptic skin cleaner on the day before the procedure.
- The nurse or doctor explains the procedure to the person and asks if he or she is allergic to X-ray dye, shellfish, or iodine.
- On the morning of the procedure, an intravenous catheter is inserted.
- A sedative is given as prescribed by the doctor.

What happens during the procedure?

Plaque removal is performed in the cardiac catheterization lab with the open-heart surgical team on standby in case emergency surgery

Recovering from plaque removal

After you've been discharged from the hospital, follow these important guidelines.

Take special precautions

- Make sure you know the dose, schedule, and side effects of drugs prescribed by your doctor. Take your medications exactly as prescribed.
- Notify your doctor promptly if you have chest pains.

Other instructions

- Follow your doctor's instructions about diet and lifestyle changes that will reduce the risk that your coronary artery disease will recur.
- Regular exercise is important for improving cholesterol levels. So follow your doctor's instructions regarding exercise carefully.
- Keep your follow-up appointments with your doctor as scheduled.

becomes necessary. The doctor performs the procedure; nurses and cardiovascular technicians assist and are involved in setting up for the procedure and monitoring the person.

At the start of the procedure, the person receives several medications to control blood pressure, dilate the coronary arteries, and prevent blood clots.

To place the plaque-removing device in the coronary artery, the doctor inserts a needle into an artery in the groin, then inserts a guide wire, advancing it through the plaque. When the guide wire is in place, the cutting head of the plaque-removing device is advanced over the guide wire and positioned against the plaque. The cutting head is then activated, and plaque and other debris and blood are immediately suctioned out.

Periodically, the procedure is evaluated by angiography. If the plaque is not reduced by 20% to 30%, or if plaque has not been suctioned out, larger blades can be inserted because the guide wire remains in place. (See *How plaque is removed,* page 67.)

What are the possible complications?

The most common complication of plaque removal is chest pain. Other common complications include injury to the lining of the blood vessel, recurring plaque formation, hematoma, and bleeding at the insertion site.

Less common but more serious complications include blood vessel perforation, reduced blood flow to the heart, and tearing of the blood vessel wall.

What happens after the procedure?

- A pressure dressing is applied to the insertion site and pressure is applied for at least 20 minutes.
- An electrocardiogram and a blood test to evaluate coagulation are obtained and vital signs are checked every 15 minutes for the first hour. The intravenous line will be maintained for administration of medication to keep the person pain-free.
- The puncture sites in the groin will be checked at least once an hour for hematoma and bleeding.
- The person will stay in bed for 24 hours after the procedure and then remain in a cardiac monitoring area for several days. (See *Recovering from plaque removal.*)

BALLOON ANGIOPLASTY

Balloon angioplasty (also known as *percutaneous transluminal coronary angioplasty*) is a method of improving blood flow that's an alternative to coronary artery bypass grafting. Balloon angioplasty was first performed in 1977 and has rapidly become the procedure of choice for improving coronary blood flow in many people with coronary artery disease. This procedure, which uses a tiny balloon catheter to widen a narrowed coronary artery, is favored over bypass surgery in certain people.

Perhaps more than 50% of the 300,000 balloon angioplasties performed annually in the United States are performed for blockages in more than one artery. The usual initial success rate is 90% to 95%. In people with only one blocked vessel or chest pain that does not respond to medical treatment, angioplasty has proved to relieve symptoms better than medical therapy. However, the procedure's effect on long-term survival and how it compares with coronary artery bypass grafting and other methods of improving blood flow are still unknown. Currently, fewer than 4% of people who have had balloon angioplasty require emergency coronary artery bypass surgery.

A recent advance—laser angioplasty—makes it likely that more people will undergo some form of angioplasty in the future (see *Laser angioplasty*, page 70).

A major disadvantage of balloon angioplasty is the 1% to 5% rate of acute complications, including tears in the coronary artery, closure of the blood vessel, heart attack, the need for emergency coronary artery bypass grafting, and a 30% to 50% rate of recurring blockage of the artery after the procedure.

Recently, balloon angioplasty has also emerged as an alternative to peripheral bypass surgery for many people with peripheral vascular disease of the legs.

Why is this procedure done?

Balloon angioplasty is performed to improve coronary blood flow by enlarging the diameter of diseased coronary arteries. The procedure is used to treat single and multivessel coronary artery disease, coronary artery disease in which there is more than one blockage in a single artery, and blockages in grafts placed to bypass coronary arteries. Balloon angioplasty is usually reserved for vessels with at least 60% narrowing.

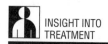

Laser angioplasty

Laser angioplasty shows great promise in vaporizing arterial blockages and may also be used to remove calcified plaque. With this procedure, which uses a pulsed beam, it's easier for doctors to remove the blockage without destroying the vessel wall.

What it's used for

Laser angioplasty allows cardiologists to treat complex artery blockages without the hazards of open-heart coronary artery bypass surgery. It is most effective for treating diffuse disease; long, calcified lesions or lesions at the beginning or end of an artery; totally blocked vessels; and diseased saphenous vein grafts. Laser angioplasty is not effective against lesions caused by blood clots.

How it's done

To perform the procedure, the doctor threads a laser-containing catheter into the diseased artery. When the catheter nears the blockage, the doctor rotates it, advancing it until the blockage is destroyed.

This procedure takes about 1 hour and requires only local anesthesia. For optimal results, most people (about 50% to 70%) also undergo balloon angioplasty both before and after laser angioplasty.

Complications

Complications of laser angioplasty include a higher rate of tearing of the coronary arteries and recurring blockage than occurs following balloon angioplasty.

Balloon angioplasty is also performed as an emergency treatment during the first 12 hours after the onset of a heart attack, especially when clot-dissolving therapy is not appropriate and when the person has acute episodes of severe chest pain.

When shouldn't this procedure be done?

Balloon angioplasty is rarely used in arteries that have been totally blocked for an extended period because such old lesions are tough and rigid and therefore difficult to dilate with the balloon. The procedure is also not recommended for long lesions involving a large segment of the artery or for blockages at the beginning or end of the artery.

What happens before the procedure?

- A doctor will explain the procedure to you and tell you to expect a hot, flushing sensation or transient nausea when the dye is injected.
- If you're not allergic to aspirin, you'll take it before the treatment to help prevent blood clot formation in the artery after angioplasty.
- You'll be told to expect chest discomfort or pain for 1 to 3 minutes while the balloon is inflated within the coronary artery.

- You'll be asked if you're allergic to shellfish, iodine, or the dye used in the procedure.
- Food and fluid are restricted for at least 6 hours before the procedure.
- Pulses in your leg are located and marked with indelible ink so that they can be checked later.

What happens during the procedure?

Balloon angioplasty is performed in the cardiac catheterization lab under local anesthesia. You're awake but sedated and must lie flat on a hard table during this time. You may be asked to take deep breaths to permit the balloon catheter to be clearly seen. The procedure takes 1 to 4 hours.

The cardiologist begins by cleaning and anesthetizing the catheter insertion site, then inserts a guide wire through the skin into an artery in the arm or groin. With X-ray guidance, the doctor threads the catheter into the coronary artery, confirms the presence of the blockage by angiography (X-ray examination of blood vessels after a dye is injected into an artery or vein), and then introduces a small, balloon-tipped catheter through the guide wire. After positioning the balloon tip in the blocked coronary artery, the doctor repeatedly inflates it with normal saline solution and the X-ray dye. The inflated balloon compresses the cholesterol-containing deposits against the arterial wall, thereby widening the diameter of the artery.

To confirm successful angioplasty, angiography is repeated. The catheter is left in the artery for up to 24 hours to provide emergency access in case coronary blockage develops. You'll receive intravenous blood thinners during this time.

What are the possible complications?

Balloon angioplasty avoids many of the risks of surgery, and its incidence of serious complications has steadily declined, but it is not without risk. The most dangerous complication is tearing of the artery during dilatation, which can lead to coronary artery rupture, compression of the heart caused by bleeding, reduced blood flow to the heart, heart attack, or death. Because of the procedure's potentially serious complications, the surgical team should be available in case coronary artery bypass surgery becomes necessary.

The most common complications of balloon angioplasty are acute closure of the blocked artery, which can occur soon after the procedure, or reblockage, which can occur up to 6 months later. Acute closure is the sudden narrowing of the vessel due to blood clot forma-

Recovering from balloon angioplasty

After you've been discharged from the hospital, follow these important guidelines.

Take special precautions
▪ Notify the doctor of any bleeding or bruising at the arterial puncture site.
▪ Make sure you know the dosage, schedule, and possible side effects of prescribed drugs. Take all medications exactly as prescribed by your doctor.

Other instructions
▪ Resume your normal activities. Most people experience increased exercise tolerance after the procedure.
▪ Keep follow-up appointments with your doctor, particularly if chest pain recurs.

tion within 24 to 48 hours after the procedure. Reblockage is the narrowing of the vessel because of increased thickness of the blood vessel wall that occurs within 3 to 6 months after angioplasty. Late reblockage affects up to 50% of people who undergo balloon angioplasty. However, if the procedure is repeated to treat reblockage, the long-term success rate is about 85%.

Other possible complications include coronary artery spasm, bleeding, allergic reactions to the X-ray dye, and abnormal heart rhythms during the procedure. Heart attack and local reactions where the needle was inserted may also occur. Infrequently, blood clot formation can lead to a stroke.

What happens after the procedure?

▪ You'll be sent to the intensive care unit or recovery area for monitoring.
▪ Every 15 minutes for the first hour, your blood pressure, heart rate and rhythm, and respirations will be checked. The pulses in your leg will also be checked. The doctor will be notified if pulses are absent.
▪ You'll receive intravenous fluids to promote elimination of the X-ray dye.
▪ The arterial catheter will be removed 6 to 24 hours after the procedure, and direct pressure will be applied to the insertion site for 30 minutes or until the bleeding stops. Then a pressure bandage will be applied to avoid bleeding or bruising.
▪ You'll receive blood tests to check for evidence of a heart attack. (See *Recovering from balloon angioplasty.*)

BALLOON ENLARGEMENT OF A NARROWED HEART VALVE

This procedure to enlarge the opening of a narrowed heart valve (also known as *balloon valvuloplasty*) was first performed in 1979 on children with congenital heart disease. Since then, it has been performed on thousands of adults and children in the United States. In most cases, this procedure results in improved valve function with relief of valvular obstruction. It provides curative results with less than 30% incidence of reblockage. Nevertheless, the treatment of choice for valvular heart disease is usually still surgery—either valve replacement or surgical opening of the narrowed valve—because balloon enlargement leaves residual narrowing, and reblockage rates are as high as 75% in adults with narrowed aortic valves.

Why is this procedure done?

Balloon enlargement of a narrowed heart valve is done to enlarge the valve opening and improve mobility of valve leaflets, thereby correcting valve tightening. It is the procedure of choice for many heart and blood vessel defects and offers a conservative alternative for people who are poor candidates for surgery.

What happens before the procedure?

- The treatment is explained to you and your family, along with its risks, alternatives, and expected outcome.
- An intravenous line is inserted for administration of medications.
- Your groin area is shaved and cleaned with an antiseptic.
- You'll be told that you'll feel a brief stinging sensation when the local anesthetic is injected.
- Food or fluids are restricted for at least 6 hours before the procedure.

What happens during the procedure?

Typically, you're awake during the procedure, which may take up to 4 hours. The doctor performs the balloon enlargement in a cardiac catheterization lab, using local anesthesia. After preparing and anesthetizing the catheter insertion site, the doctor inserts a catheter into the appropriate artery, then passes the balloon-tipped catheter through the catheter and, guided by X-ray, slowly threads it into the heart. After positioning the deflated balloon in the valve opening, the doctor repeatedly inflates it with normal saline solution and X-ray dye. The pressure of the inflated balloon causes the valve leaflets to split apart, allowing them to open and close freely and widening the valve's opening.

Throughout the procedure, the doctor asks you to take deep breaths (so that he or she can see the catheter clearly) and to answer questions about how you're feeling.

Once valve function is improved, the balloon-tipped catheter is removed. The other catheter is left in place for 6 to 12 hours in case the procedure must be repeated.

SELF-HELP

Caring for yourself after heart valve enlargement

After you've been discharged from the hospital, keep in mind the following:
• You can resume normal activities.
• Notify the doctor promptly of any bleeding or bruising at the puncture site or any recurring symptoms of valvular leakage, such as breathlessness or decreased exercise tolerance.
• Keep all scheduled follow-up visits with your doctor.

What are the possible complications?

Balloon enlargement of a narrowed heart valve can have serious complications. It can worsen valve leakage by misshaping the valve so that it doesn't close completely. Another serious complication is embolism (when pieces of the calcified valve break off and travel to the brain or lungs). The procedure can also severely damage the delicate valve leaflets, requiring immediate surgery to replace the valve.

Other complications include bleeding and hematoma at the arterial puncture site, abnormal heart rhythms, reduced blood flow to the heart, heart attack, puncture of the heart, and circulatory problems below the catheter entry site.

What happens after the procedure?

• Your electrocardiogram is continuously monitored.
• The leg in which the catheter was inserted will be immobilized and its pulses and skin condition will be monitored.
• A sandbag is placed over the insertion site to minimize bleeding until the catheter is removed.
• You'll receive intravenous fluids to aid elimination of the X-ray dye and possibly intravenous blood thinners or medications to widen the coronary arteries.
• Your vital signs are monitored every 15 minutes for the first hour, every 30 minutes for the next 2 hours, and then hourly for the next 5 hours.
• The catheter insertion site will be observed for bleeding. If bleeding occurs, the nurse will apply direct pressure to it and notify the doctor.
• Your heart sounds will be checked frequently to assess the function of the heart valve. (See *Caring for yourself after heart valve enlargement.*)
• After the doctor removes the catheter, direct pressure will be applied over the puncture site for at least 30 minutes. Then a pressure dressing will be applied.

DEFIBRILLATION

Defibrillation is delivery of a brief electric shock to the heart during a life-threatening abnormal heart rhythm. This burst of electric current allows the heart's natural pacemaker to regain control of the heart's rhythm.

Life-threatening heart rhythm disturbances cause cardiac output (the amount of blood pumped by the heart) to drop to zero. If zero output persists for more than 4 to 6 minutes, irreparable brain damage results from lack of oxygen in the blood. Once the emergency situation is identified, defibrillation must be performed immediately. Recent research has shown that when advanced cardiac life support (including defibrillation) is given to a person within 5 minutes, about 40% of victims are successfully resuscitated.

The person receiving defibrillation must have no pulse and be unresponsive. No matter what the electrocardiogram indicates, a person who is alert or has a pulse should never be defibrillated. Defibrillating an alert person could trigger lethal heart rhythm disturbances and cardiac arrest. The person who has an abnormal heart rhythm with a pulse may be a candidate for synchronized cardioversion instead. (See "Cardioversion," page 90.)

Why is this procedure done?

Defibrillation is performed to correct life-threatening abnormal heart rhythms when the person has no pulse. It is performed by a health professional specially skilled in advanced cardiac life support and is administered with other resuscitation measures, such as mechanical ventilation, CPR, and emergency medications.

What happens before the procedure?

- The person who discovers the emergency calls for help and begins CPR.
- CPR is continued while the defibrillator equipment is being prepared.
- The defibrillator is set up and electrocardiogram leads are attached to the person.
- Conductive gel or paste is applied to the defibrillator paddles, or two gel pads are placed on the person's bare chest.

SELF-HELP

Recovering from defibrillation

After you've been discharged from the hospital, follow these important guidelines:

- Take your pulse for a full minute before taking prescribed medication, and notify the doctor if you experience palpitations, dizziness, faintness, or any changes in your normal pulse rate and rhythm.
- Make regular medical follow-up appointments for routine electrocardiograms and evaluation of your response to medication.

- Lack of a pulse is verified by checking for a pulse in the neck, and the presence of a life-threatening abnormal heart rhythm—or no rhythm at all—is verified on the heart monitor.
- The charge is selected and the prepared paddles are placed on the person's chest. They should not be placed over a permanent pacemaker or on a woman's breast.
- All caregivers are told to stand clear before the defibrillator delivers the electric shock.

What happens during the procedure?

- The person's pulse and heart rhythm are continuously monitored.
- Medications are administered as necessary to treat possible causes of the life-threatening heart rhythm.
- Defibrillation and other resuscitation measures continue until the person's cardiac condition stabilizes or the doctor orders discontinuation.

What are the possible complications?

The most common complication of defibrillation is a skin burn from the defibrillator paddles. Other potential complications include injury to the heart muscle, abnormal heart rhythms, and blood clots. Safety precautions must be taken to avoid delivering electric shocks to the emergency health care team.

What happens after the procedure?

- The person's cardiac status, breathing, and vital signs are monitored until he or she is stabilized.
- An electrocardiogram and chest X-ray are taken.
- The person's skin and the defibrillator paddles are cleaned to remove conductive gel or paste.
- The person's skin is checked for burns and ointment is applied if necessary.
- The intravenous line is maintained in case additional medication is needed. (See *Recovering from defibrillation*.)

REMOVAL OF FLUID AROUND THE HEART

This procedure (also known as *pericardiocentesis*) is the removal of excess fluid from the pericardial sac (the sac that surrounds the heart).

Why is this procedure done?

Fluid around the heart is removed to relieve compression of the heart and increase the heart's ability to pump blood. It may also be done to provide a sample of fluid for laboratory evaluation. This procedure may be performed in acute or chronic inflammation of the pericardial sac.

What happens before the procedure?

- The procedure is explained to you.
- You'll receive tranquilizers or sedatives, if ordered by the doctor.
- An intravenous catheter will be inserted for administration of medications.
- The needle insertion site on your chest may be shaved and will be cleaned with an antiseptic solution.
- Electrocardiogram electrodes are put in position.

What happens during the procedure?

The doctor typically performs this procedure at the bedside in the critical care unit, with the nurse assisting. After the insertion site has been shaved and cleaned, the doctor administers a local anesthetic at the puncture site, then inserts the needle that will remove the excess fluid.

The doctor very slowly and cautiously removes the fluid, then removes the needle and places a bandage over the insertion site.

What are the possible complications?

This procedure carries some risk of potentially fatal complications, such as inadvertent puncture of internal organs (particularly the heart, lung, stomach, or liver), tearing of the myocardium or a coronary artery, or initiation of life-threatening irregular heart rhythms.

SELF-HELP

Recovering from fluid removal

After you've been discharged from the hospital, follow these important guidelines:
- Notify the doctor immediately if you experience chest pain, shortness of breath, or palpitations.
- Make sure you keep follow-up medical appointments. They're very important.

What happens after the procedure?
- Your vital signs are monitored every 15 minutes for 1 hour, every 30 minutes for the next 2 hours, and then every 4 hours for 16 hours or until you're stable.
- Your electrocardiogram is continuously monitored.
- A nurse will watch you closely for signs of fluid collecting around the heart. The doctor will be notified if such signs occur. (See *Recovering from fluid removal*.)

VALSALVA'S MANEUVER

Valsalva's maneuver is a procedure in which the person forces an expiration against closed vocal cords (as when trying to exhale while holding one's breath). This maneuver can correct certain abnormal heart rhythms and has been known to relieve angina by stimulating a nerve that leads to the heart.

Why is this treatment done?
Valsalva's maneuver is done to help correct certain abnormal heart rhythms and to assist with diagnosis of heart abnormalities during echocardiography (an ultrasound test that shows the size, shape, and motion of various structures within the heart).

Rarely, it can also be used for people with mild coronary disease who suffer from chest pain. Valsalva's maneuver should be initiated only by a doctor.

When shouldn't this treatment be done?
Valsalva's maneuver should not be performed in patients with severe coronary artery disease, recent heart attack, or a moderate to severe reduction in blood volume.

What happens before the treatment?
- A nurse will explain the treatment and what it's intended to accomplish. If you have chest pain, the maneuver will diminish your heart's workload and thereby relieve the pain. For someone with an abnormally fast heart rhythm originating in the atrium, the maneuver tem-

porarily raises the blood pressure, causing the heart to respond by beating more slowly.

- You'll be told you may feel faint or dizzy during the procedure.

What happens during the treatment?

Because Valsalva's maneuver can cause a slow heart rate, when it's first performed you'll be placed on a heart monitor with emergency equipment nearby; an intravenous line will usually be in place. To perform Valsalva's maneuver in the traditional manner, you'll lie on your back, inhale deeply, and bear down (as in defecation). If you don't faint or experience dizziness or irregular heart rhythms, you'll continue to hold your breath and bear down for 10 seconds. You'll then exhale and breathe quietly. If the maneuver is successful, your heart rate will begin to slow before you exhale.

What are the possible complications?

Valsalva's maneuver can cause mobilization of blood clots, bleeding, abnormal heart rhythms originating in the ventricle, or cardiac arrest.

What happens after the treatment?

- Your vital signs are checked when the procedure is completed, and your electrocardiogram is monitored continuously for at least 12 hours to ensure that abnormal heart rhythms don't return.
- If the treatment was unsuccessful, the doctor will probably prescribe some form of drug therapy. (See *Performing Valsalva's maneuver at home.*)

 SELF-HELP

Performing Valsalva's maneuver at home

If you've been taught how to perform Valsalva's maneuver on yourself, keep in mind the following points:

- Make sure you lie down during the maneuver to prevent fainting or dizziness.
- Make sure you perform the maneuver for 10 seconds.
- Call your doctor immediately if the maneuver doesn't relieve symptoms.

CAROTID SINUS MASSAGE

Carotid sinus massage is a method for evaluating and terminating certain abnormally fast heart rhythms. It involves manual stimulation of blood pressure sensors in the carotid artery in the neck, a procedure that slows the heart rate and electrical conduction in the heart.

The response to carotid sinus massage varies, depending on the type of abnormal heart rhythm involved. This difference can be used to help diagnose the specific abnormal heart rhythm, but it limits the treatment's usefulness.

Why is this treatment done?

Carotid sinus massage is performed to slow the heart rate and stop abnormal heart rhythms and to differentiate between certain abnormal heart rhythms.

When shouldn't this treatment be done?

Carotid sinus massage should not be performed on people who have cholesterol-containing deposits in the carotid artery, people with cerebrovascular disease, or those who've had previous surgery on the carotid artery. The treatment should be used cautiously in elderly people, those receiving the heart medication Lanoxin, and those with heart block (a type of abnormal heart rhythm), high blood pressure, coronary artery disease, diabetes, or high levels of potassium in the blood.

What happens before the treatment?

- A nurse will explain the procedure and tell you to report if you feel light-headed.
- An intravenous line may be inserted.
- You'll be given an electrocardiogram.
- The pulses in your carotid artery will be checked.

What happens during the treatment?

Carotid sinus massage may be performed by a doctor or a specially prepared nurse. While the heart is continually monitored, the appropriate area of the carotid artery is located manually and then is massaged firmly in a circular motion for 3 to 5 seconds. The artery is released as soon as the electrocardiogram shows slowing of the heart rate. If the procedure has no effect, it will be performed on the other side, with both sides massaged simultaneously.

What are the possible complications?

Carotid sinus massage may cause life-threatening irregular heart rhythms or brain damage from reduced blood flow. If the carotid artery is totally blocked during carotid sinus massage, decreased blood flow to the brain may cause a stroke. Also, carotid sinus massage may cause cholesterol-containing deposits to be released into the circulation, which can also cause stroke.

What happens after the treatment?

- A nurse will monitor your vital signs.
- You'll receive another electrocardiogram.
- Your heart will be monitored continually for at least 4 hours to assess the effects of the treatment and to watch for recurrence of the abnormal heart rhythm. (See *Caring for yourself after carotid sinus massage.*)
- You'll be watched closely for signs or symptoms of complications.

STOCKINGS THAT PREVENT BLOOD CLOTS

Also known as *antiembolism stockings,* these stockings help decrease the risk of blood clots forming in veins located deep below the surface of the skin. The stockings compress superficial leg veins, thereby forcing blood into the deep veins instead of allowing it to pool in the legs and form clots. They can provide equal pressure over the entire leg or a graded pressure that is highest at the ankle and decreases to the knee or thigh.

Why is this treatment done?

These stockings are used to decrease the risk of blood clots in the deep veins. They benefit people with a previous history of blood clots or blood disorders, heart and blood vessel or lung disease, cancer, diabetes, obesity, infection of the blood, inflammatory bowel disease, varicose veins, or a decreased ability to walk; those who have had surgery involving the thigh, calf, pelvis, or abdomen; those who have had total hip or knee replacement; those with hip fractures, multiple injuries, or pelvic and spinal injuries; and those who are underweight and over age 40.

For people with chronic problems with their veins, special compression cuffs may be ordered during and after surgery.

When shouldn't this treatment be used?

These stockings should not be used on people with certain skin diseases or open skin lesions, gangrene, conditions resulting in poor circulation, severe fluid retention in the lungs or body, recent vein ligation, or blood vessel or skin grafts.

 SELF-HELP

Caring for yourself after carotid sinus massage

After you've been discharged from the hospital, follow these important guidelines:
- Make sure you take your pulse as instructed for 1 full minute each morning before you get out of bed and whenever you feel chest pain, palpitations, dizziness, or faintness.
- Notify your doctor if any of the above symptoms occur or if you have a pulse rate less than 60 beats per minute or greater than 100 beats per minute.

SELF-HELP

Using stockings at home

After you've been discharged from the hospital, follow these important guidelines:
- Remember to wear the stockings at all times until your activity level returns to normal or the doctor says you no longer need them.
- Follow the instructions you received in the hospital about how to apply the stockings correctly. These instructions will include the care and inspection of the stockings and how to order additional pairs if needed.

What happens before the treatment?

- Your legs are measured so that the stockings fit properly. Your legs need to be clean and dry. Powder may be applied beforehand to ease application if you're not allergic to it.
- You're instructed about the application, care, and purpose of the stockings. You should wear the stockings in bed and while walking to provide continuous protection against blood clots.

What happens during the treatment?

The stockings may be applied by a nurse, you yourself, or a caregiver as medically appropriate. Many doctors order application of stockings before surgery. The stockings are worn continuously until the risk of developing blood clots has diminished. Studies have demonstrated that increased blood flow persists for 30 minutes after the stockings are removed, possibly because of the increased strength in the outside of the vein produced by the compression. (See *How to apply stockings.*)

While you're wearing the stockings, the following precautions will be taken:

- Your legs are evaluated daily—or every 4 hours if you feel faint pulses or swelling. If complications occur, the stockings are removed and the doctor notified immediately.
- The stockings are removed at least once a day to inspect and wash the legs.

What are the possible complications?

Reduced blood flow in the arteries (characterized by cold and bluish toes, dusky toenail beds, decreased or absent pulses in the feet, and leg pain or cramps) or increased congestion in the veins can occur if the stockings roll down, producing a tourniquet effect. These complications can be avoided by measuring, applying, and wearing the stockings properly. Less serious complications are allergic reactions or skin irritations. (See *Using stockings at home.*)

How to apply stockings

Stockings that prevent blood clots are usually applied in the morning before getting out of bed.

To apply stockings
- Lightly dust your ankle with talcum powder to ease stocking application.
- Insert your hand into the stocking from the top, and grab the heel pocket from the inside. Turn the stocking inside out so that the foot section is inside the stocking leg.
- Hook the index and middle fingers of both hands into the foot section. Ease the stocking over your toes, stretching it sideways as you move it up the foot. You may want to point your toes to help ease the stocking on.
- Center the heel in the heel pocket. Then gather the loose material at the ankle and slide the rest of the stocking up over the heel with short pulls, alternating front and back.

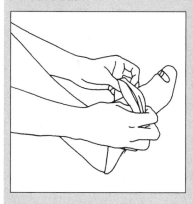

- Insert your index and middle fingers into the gathered stocking at the ankle, and ease the stocking up the leg to the knee.

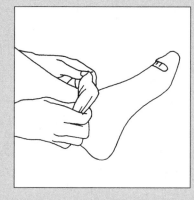

- Stretch the stocking toward the knee, front and back, to distribute the material evenly. The stocking should fit snugly and remain unwrinkled.

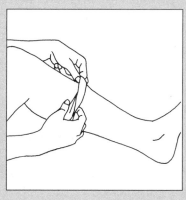

- Follow the appropriate directions at right for the length of stocking that you're applying.

For a knee-length stocking
- Make sure the top of each stocking is below the crease at the back of the knee. If the top of the stocking sits in the crease, it can put pressure on the vein and decrease circulation to the leg.
- Repeat the steps to apply the second stocking.

For a thigh-length stocking
- Keep the leg extended and stretch the rest of the stocking over the knee. Then flex your knee, and pull the stocking over the thigh until the top is 1 to 3 inches (3 to 8 centimeters) below the buttock.
- Stretch the stocking from the top, front, and back to distribute the fabric evenly over the thigh.
- Gently snap the fabric behind the knee to eliminate gaps that could reduce pressure.
- Repeat the steps to apply the second stocking.

For waist-length stockings
- Extend the stockings to the top of the thigh and then over the buttocks to the waist.
- Place the adjustable belt that accompanies the stockings around your waist to help hold them in place.

CARDIOPULMONARY RESUSCITATION (CPR)

CPR is performed to support and maintain breathing and circulation when heart rate and breathing are failing or have stopped.

An individual can have respiratory arrest without cardiac arrest. However, if respiratory arrest is not corrected, cardiac arrest will soon follow. Rescue breathing is initiated for respiratory arrest; rescue breathing and chest compressions are initiated for cardiac arrest.

Recent studies have indicated that a new method using alternating chest and abdominal compressions (double thrust resuscitation technique) significantly improves cardiac output (the amount of blood pumped by the heart) and blood flow to the brain and heart, compared with chest compressions alone. In one study, this new method improved survival by 18%. This method is currently under study and is not yet recommended for general use.

About two-thirds of sudden deaths due to coronary artery disease take place outside of the hospital and occur within 2 hours after the onset of chest pain. Many of these deaths can be prevented by prompt recognition, prompt notification of the emergency medical service system, initiation of CPR, early defibrillation (delivery of a brief electric shock to the heart to correct an abnormal heart rhythm), and early initiation of advanced cardiac life support measures.

How to remember the steps of CPR

You can remember the steps of CPR easily by thinking of the letters A, B, and C—for airway, breathing, and circulation. However, since the National Conference on Emergency Cardiac Care and Cardiopulmonary Resuscitation in February 1992, the new steps to follow for CPR are A, A, B, and C: The first A stands for access into the emergency medical service system. (For details, see *How to perform CPR*, pages 85 to 88.)

External chest compressions and rescue breathing may be ineffective in supporting life, even when properly performed, if they're not begun soon enough. Basic life support is usually successful if medical procedures such as defibrillation can be performed within 8 to 10 minutes. If CPR or definitive care is delayed, irreversible brain damage or death can result. There are exceptions—for example, a drowning victim who has been in cold water or someone who has suffered

(Text continues on page 88.)

How to perform CPR

You can perform CPR quickly in almost any situation without assistance or equipment. To follow the correct sequence for CPR, remember the letters A, A, B, and C: **A**ccess the emergency medical service system, open the **A**irway, restore **B**reathing, and restore **C**irculation.

One-person adult CPR

If you're the only rescuer, follow this procedure for CPR on an adult:

- Gently shake the person's shoulders and shout "Are you okay?" This simple action ensures that you don't start CPR on a conscious person.
- Quickly scan the person for major injuries, particularly to the head and neck.
- Access the emergency medical service system.
- Place the person in a supine position on a hard, flat surface, such as the floor. If you suspect a head or neck injury, move the person as little as possible to reduce the risk of paralysis.

Open the airway

- If you suspect a neck injury, use the head-tilt, chin-lift maneuver. Place one hand on the person's forehead and the fingers of the other hand on the bony portion of the lower jaw near the chin. Gently push the person's forehead back and pull upward on the chin, making sure the teeth are almost touching.

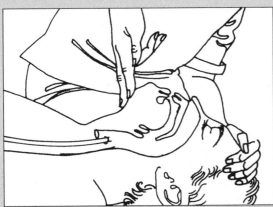

- If you suspect a neck injury, open the airway using the jaw-thrust maneuver. Curve your index fingers under the person's jaw by his or her ears. With a strong, steady motion, lift the jaw upward and out-

ward. This maneuver opens the airway without moving the neck.

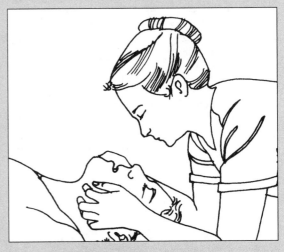

Restore breathing

- Keep the person's airway open as you place your ear over the person's mouth and nose and look toward the feet. Listen for the sound of air moving and watch for chest movement. You may also feel air on your cheek.

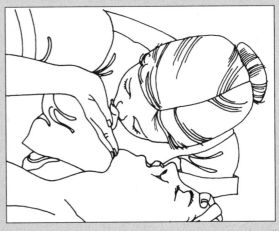

(continued)

How to perform CPR *(continued)*

- If you detect signs of breathing and neck trauma is not suspected, place the person in the recovery position by rolling him or her onto the side to help protect the airway.
- If you don't detect breathing once you've opened the airway, begin rescue breathing. Pinch the person's nostrils shut with the thumb and index finger of the hand you have on the forehead.
- Take a deep breath and cover the person's mouth with yours, creating a tight seal. Give two full breaths, taking a deep breath after each to allow enough time for the person's chest to relax and to prevent stomach distention. Each breath should last 1½ to 2 seconds.

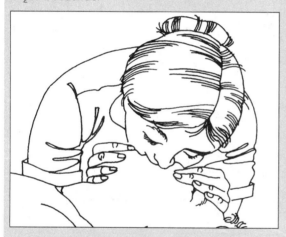

- If the first attempt to give the person a breath doesn't work, reposition the person's head and try again. If that doesn't work, suspect a foreign body (such as dentures) blocking the airway. If you see an object, follow the procedure for clearing a foreign-body airway obstruction.

Restore circulation

- Keep one hand on the person's forehead so the airway remains open. With your other hand, palpate the carotid artery closer to you by placing your index and middle fingers in the groove between the windpipe and the muscle next to it in the neck. Palpate the artery for 5 to 10 seconds.

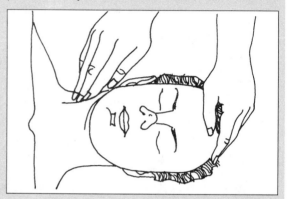

- If you detect a pulse, don't begin chest compressions. Instead, continue rescue breathing, giving 10 to 12 breaths per minute (or one every 5 seconds). Recheck the pulse every 2 to 3 minutes.
- If you don't detect a pulse and help hasn't arrived yet, start chest compressions. First, spread your knees apart for a wide base of support. Then, using the hand closer to the person's foot, locate the lower margin of the rib cage.

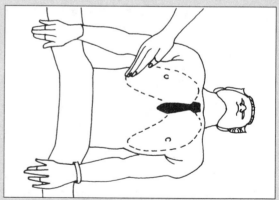

- Move your fingertips along the margin to the notch where the ribs meet the breastbone. Place your middle finger on that notch and your index finger next to it. Your index finger should be on the bottom half of the person's breastbone, just above the lowest point of the breastbone.

How to perform CPR *(continued)*

- Put the heel of your other hand on the person's breastbone, next to your index finger. The long axis of the heel of your hand should align with the long axis of the breastbone.

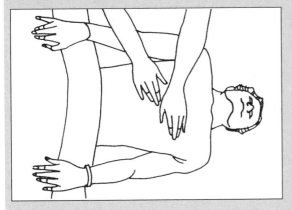

- Take your fingers off the notch, and put that hand directly on top of your other hand.

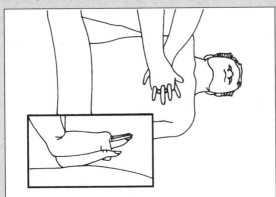

- Make sure your fingers don't rest on the person's chest. Proper hand position keeps the force of the compressions on the breastbone equal and reduces the risk of a rib fracture, lung puncture, or tearing the liver.
- With your elbows locked, arms straight, and shoulders directly over your hands, you're ready to start chest compressions. Using the weight of your upper body, compress the person's breastbone 1½ to 2 inches (4 to 5 centimeters), delivering the pressure through the heels of your hands.

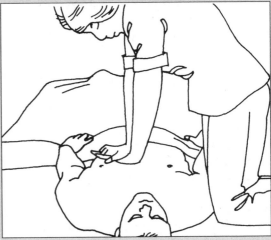

- After each compression, release the pressure and allow the chest to return to its normal position so that the heart can fill with blood. To prevent injuries, don't change your hand position during compressions.
- Give 15 compressions at a rate of 80 to 100 compressions per minute. Count "one and two and three and..." up to 15, compressing on the number and releasing on "and."
- After 15 compressions, give 2 breaths. Then find the proper hand position again and deliver 15 more compressions. Continue this pattern for four full cycles.
- Palpate the carotid artery again. If you still don't detect a pulse, continue CPR in cycles of 15 compressions and 2 breaths, beginning with breaths.
- Every few minutes, check for breathing and a pulse. If you detect a pulse but no breathing, give 10 to 12 breaths per minute and check the pulse. If you detect both a pulse and breathing, check the person's breathing and pulse closely. Don't stop CPR until breathing and a pulse return, you turn CPR over to someone else, or you become too exhausted to continue.

(continued)

How to perform CPR *(continued)*

Child and infant CPR

Perform CPR on a child or an infant as you would on an adult, with the following key variations:

- If you discover an unresponsive child or infant and you're alone, continue your assessment and perform CPR for 1 minute, if indicated, before you notify the emergency medical service system.
- Deliver rescue breaths at a rate of 20 breaths per minute for an infant or a child, with each breath taking 1½ to 2 seconds. Inflate a child's or an infant's lungs with smaller volumes of air at faster rates. You need two hands to maintain the airway for a child.
- When doing chest compressions, use the same landmarks as with an adult to find proper hand placement. (Because you need to give 100 compressions per minute, you don't have time to start at the notch and work upward; you need to visualize hand placement.) Give chest compressions with only one hand for a child and two or three fingers for an infant (as shown at left). Depress the breastbone only 1 to 1½ inches (2.5 to 3.8 centimeters) for a child and ½ to 1 inch (1.3 to 2.5 centimeters) for an infant.

- Hand (finger) placement for an infant can be maintained because the other hand alone will keep the airway open; once correct hand placement is achieved, your fingers need not leave the infant's chest. You need to give at least 100 chest compressions per minute for an infant.

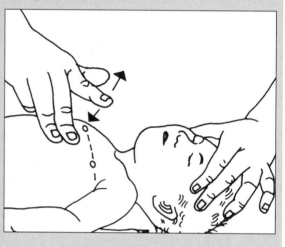

from exposure to low temperatures. However, CPR should be initiated regardless of how much time has elapsed since the arrest.

Why is this procedure done?

CPR is performed to restore and maintain breathing and circulation and to provide oxygen and blood flow to the heart, brain, and other vital organs until more advanced methods can be begun. It should be performed in situations in which either breathing or pulse is absent. Some common causes of respiratory and cardiac arrest are ineffective beating of the heart, electric shock, drowning, drug reactions or overdose, asphyxiation, allergic reactions, trauma, exposure to cold, blocked breathing passages, or severe shock.

What happens before the procedure?

- Although HIV infection has not been proved to be transmitted by saliva, the Centers for Disease Control and Prevention advises keeping mouthpieces, masks, or other ventilation devices available for immediate use in areas where the need for resuscitation is predictable. Because of this recommendation, mouth-to-mask rescue breathing is taught to all health care providers who are trained in two-rescuer CPR; furthermore, in health care facilities, masks are positioned at or near the bedside in case rescue breathing is necessary.

If a person collapses or suddenly becomes unconscious, the rescuer does the following:

- He or she calls out for help, determines if the person is responsive, and then notifies the emergency medical service system.
- The rescuer checks for breathing and a pulse and begins CPR only if the person is not breathing and does not have a pulse. If the person has a pulse but is not breathing, only rescue breathing is performed, not chest compressions; frequently, establishing an open breathing passage alone will resolve the situation.
- If the person was eating or could have had a foreign object in his or her mouth immediately before breathing stopped, the rescuer performs an abdominal thrust to clear the airway. Abdominal thrusts are performed only after the rescuer has been unsuccessful in delivering a breath and has tried repositioning the airway first. It's important to keep in mind that people can become unconscious or collapse and not require rescue breathing or chest compressions.

What happens during the procedure?

CPR can be performed by any trained person. CPR training can follow American Heart Association or American Red Cross guidelines and recommendations. Both organizations teach the same methods but use different terminology, and both recommend that family members or people who live with high-risk patients get training in CPR.

CPR includes rescue breathing, whereby the rescuer administers mouth-to-mouth breaths to the victim to provide oxygen to the lungs. Then the rescuer applies external chest compressions to help circulate the blood through the heart to the vital organs.

CPR may be administered to an adult by the one-rescuer or the two-rescuer technique; the principles are the same for both. Only one-rescuer CPR is taught to nonprofessional rescuers. Variations of the adult method are used for infants and children.

What are the possible complications?

Even properly performed CPR can cause complications. The most common problem associated with rescue breathing is stomach distention, which is caused by giving too much air during breathing. It can lead to vomiting, which then poses the risk of vomit going into the lungs. Stomach distention is common in children. If vomiting occurs, turn the victim on his or her side and wipe out the mouth; then return the victim to his or her back and continue resuscitation measures.

Improper hand placement or strong compressions performed on a person with frail bones may cause rib or sternal fractures. A fractured rib can puncture a lung and result in a collapsed lung by pressure from air that escapes from the puncture site. Bone fractures can also lead to fat or bone marrow particles traveling through the bloodstream and blocking circulation.

Too-deep compressions can result in bruising of the heart, abnormal heart rhythms, or excess fluid in the sac around the heart. Incorrect positioning of the hands during compressions may result in tearing of the liver.

CARDIOVERSION

Cardioversion is the delivery of a synchronized electric current to the heart muscle. It's used to convert a fast abnormal heart rhythm, which is either unstable or does not respond to medical treatment, to a normal heart rhythm.

In cardioversion, unlike defibrillation, the electric current must be discharged at a precise time during the heartbeat. Discharge at the wrong time could precipitate a life-threatening heart rhythm disturbance.

Why is this treatment done?

Cardioversion is done to restore a normal heart rhythm and rate in people with a fast abnormal heartbeat.

When shouldn't this treatment be done?

Cardioversion should not be done on people with atrial fibrillation (a type of heart rhythm disturbance) if they have not received blood thinners for at least 3 weeks, on those who have a toxic reaction to the heart medication Lanoxin, or on those with third-degree heart block (another type of heart rhythm disturbance).

What happens before the treatment?

- The procedure is explained to the person (if time permits).
- The person's electrocardiogram is monitored, and vital signs are checked frequently.
- Blood tests may be done to check the level of potassium in the blood and, if the person is taking Lanoxin, its levels in the blood may also be checked.
- Blood thinners are administered to reduce the risk of blood clots.
- An intravenous line is inserted for administration of emergency medications.
- The person signs a consent form.
- A sedative is administered because cardioversion may be extremely uncomfortable.
- Food and fluids are restricted 8 to 12 hours before the procedure, if possible, to reduce the risk of vomiting during cardioversion.

What happens during the treatment?

Cardioversion can be performed as a scheduled procedure or an emergency procedure. The person is sedated or given light anesthesia. In scheduled cardioversion, a nurse typically assists the doctor. In an emergency, many hospitals authorize specially skilled nurses to perform the procedure.

Cardioversion is performed with a defibrillator (a device that applies a brief electric shock to the heart); however, the synchronized button on the defibrillator must be activated. The person is connected to the defibrillator's electrocardiogram leads. It's important that the electric current be discharged at an exact point during the heartbeat, as monitored on the electrocardiogram.

Paddles are positioned as for defibrillation and then charged to the desired energy level. The discharge buttons are pressed and held until all the current is released while pressure is applied to each paddle. To ensure safety, the operator should state "all clear" and check that no one is touching the person or the bed before discharging the current. If the first cardioversion doesn't correct the abnormal heart rhythm, the procedure may be repeated at a higher energy level.

SELF-HELP

Caring for yourself after cardioversion

After you've been discharged from the hospital, follow these important guidelines:

- Before leaving the hospital, you will have been taught how to take your pulse. If, while taking your pulse at home, you detect an abnormally fast heart rate, notify the doctor immediately and call an ambulance if there is no one to drive you to the emergency department.

- If skin burns resulted from the cardioversion procedure, follow the doctor's or nurse's instructions about how to care for them and how to observe for signs of infection.

What are the possible complications?

Cardioversion may cause other abnormal heart rhythms and may release blood clots into the circulation. Skin burns may result from the placement of the paddles if the conductive gel pads are dry or improperly placed.

What happens after the treatment?

- Heart rhythm, vital signs, pulses in the arms and legs, and mental status are monitored.

- The person is observed for complications, including skin burns. (See *Caring for yourself after cardioversion*.)

2

TREATING RESPIRATORY DISORDERS

DRUG THERAPIES

BRONCHODILATORS

Bronchodilators relax the smooth muscles that line the respiratory passages. They help control certain respiratory conditions that are associated with reduced air flow through the respiratory passages. These conditions include bronchial asthma, chronic bronchitis, and emphysema.

The bronchodilator theophylline and its derivatives provide long-term control of asthma and other breathing problems. These drugs are available in varied oral, injectable, and suppository forms.

What are bronchodilators used for?
Bronchodilators are used to prevent and treat chronic obstructive pulmonary disease.

What are some commonly used bronchodilators?
- aminophylline, known by the brand names Aminophyllin, Phyllocontin, and Somophyllin-DF
- dyphylline, known by the brand names Dilor and Lufyllin
- oxtriphylline, known by the brand name Choledyl
- theophylline, known by the brand names Aerolate, Elixophyllin, Slo-Phyllin, Theo-Dur, and Uniphyl
- theophylline sodium glycinate, known by the brand name Synophylate

What are the possible side effects?
- Low blood pressure, palpitations
- Nausea, vomiting, diarrhea
- Headache, nervousness, twitching

What are the guidelines for taking bronchodilators?
- If you're sensitive to caffeine, chocolate, and theobromine, tell your doctor, who may place you on a different medication.
- If you have a viral infection or have had a recent viral immunization, tell your doctor because these conditions slow the rate of drug

metabolism. Metabolism is also slowed in people with heart disease and liver disease.

- Tell your doctor if you have peptic ulcer disease because these drugs can worsen this problem.
- Expect the doctor to take frequent blood samples, especially at the start of therapy.
- If you smoke, try to stop. Smoking worsens lung disease; it also causes the body to metabolize these drugs at a faster rate than normal, reducing their effectiveness.
- Call your doctor if you feel any unusual symptoms while taking your medication.
- Don't exceed the prescribed dosage. If you miss a dose, take it as soon as you remember, unless it's time for your next dose. Never double the dose.
- Take the drug with food and a full glass of water to reduce stomach upset.
- Don't dissolve, crush, or chew a sustained-release medication.
- Avoid large amounts of caffeine-containing beverages or foods because they can increase central nervous system stimulation. Don't take any other medications, including nonprescription ones, without first checking with your doctor.

ADRENERGICS

The sympathetic nervous system is responsible for the fight-or-flight reflex. When a person is aroused by a potentially life-threatening situation, blood pressure and heart rate increase, the cardiac output (volume of blood that the heart expels per minute) increases, air flow in and out of the lungs increases, blood flow to skeletal muscle increases, and the pupils of the eye dilate. All of these effects prepare the person to fight or run from a dangerous situation.

Adrenergic drugs can mimic this response. They're useful in treating low blood pressure, certain types of heart and lung disease, and certain eye diseases.

What are adrenergics used for?
- To improve air flow into the lungs
- To relieve nasal congestion

- To increase cardiac output
- To reverse the effects of severe allergic reactions

What are some commonly used adrenergics?
- albuterol, known by the brand names Proventil and Ventolin
- bitolterol, known by the brand name Tornalate
- epinephrine, known by the brand names Adrenalin, Bronkaid Mist, and Primatene Mist
- isoetharine, known by the brand name Bronkosol
- isoproterenol, known by the brand names Aerolone, Isuprel, and Vapo-Iso
- metaproterenol, known by the brand names Alupent and Metaprel
- phenylephrine, known by the brand name Neo-Synephrine
- pirbuterol, known by the brand name Maxair
- pseudoephedrine, known by the brand names Sinufed, Sudafed, and Sufedrin
- terbutaline, known by the brand names Brethaire and Brethine

What are the possible side effects?
- Reduced blood flow to vital organs, fingers, and toes
- Changes in heart rate (either slowed or increased), chest pain, irregular heartbeats
- Restlessness, anxiety, weakness, nervousness, dizziness, temor
- Insomnia, headache
- Severe breathing difficulty
- Blanching of the skin

What are the guidelines for taking adrenergics?
- Epinephrine can cause severe high blood pressure when combined with some antidepressants and certain antihistamines. Be sure to tell your doctor about all drugs that you're taking, including nonprescription ones.
- Tremors are an annoying but common side effect of adrenergics. However, if you develop a hand tremor that interferes with daily activities, call your doctor.
- If you're taking a nasal decongestant, headaches may occur. Reduce the dosage.
- Use nasal decongestants only for short periods. With repeated use, the nasal passages fail to respond and congestion may actually worsen.
- If you're taking an inhalant bronchodilator, check your pulse before taking the drug. Notify your doctor if your resting heart rate in-

Tremors are an annoying but common side effect of adrenergics. However, if you develop a hand tremor that interferes with daily activities, call your doctor.

creases more than 10 beats per minute after starting treatment. Don't take any over-the-counter inhalants without your doctor's approval because these products contain epinephrine.

- If you're using a nebulizer, learn how the machine works and follow instructions for disassembly and cleaning. The nebulizer can be a source of infection if it is not thoroughly rinsed and air-dried between treatments.

CORTICOSTEROIDS

Corticosteroids mimic the effects of natural hormones produced by the body. These hormones play an important role in maintaining good health. They're involved in blood sugar regulation, fluid and electrolyte balance, regulation of the immune system, and many other processes.

Most corticosteroids are excellent at fighting inflammation. They may be given alone or in combination, depending on the person's condition, and may be taken orally, topically, or by injection. Corticosteroids have many uses, such as the treatment of severe asthma, suppression of inflammation in serious food and drug allergies, and emergency treatment of shock.

What are corticosteroids used for?
- To reduce inflammation
- To suppress the immune system

What are some commonly used corticosteroids?
- beclomethasone, known by the brand names Beclovent and Vanceril
- betamethasone, known by the brand name Celestone
- cortisone, known by the brand name Cortone
- dexamethasone, known by the brand names Decadron and Hexadrol
- fludrocortisone, known by the brand name Florinef
- flunisolide, known by the brand name AeroBid
- hydrocortisone, known by the brand names Cortef and Hydrocortone

- methylprednisolone, known by the brand names Medrol and Meprolone
- paramethasone, known by the brand name Haldrone
- prednisolone, known by the brand names Delta-Cortef and Prelone
- prednisone, known by the brand names Deltasone, Meticorten, and Orasone
- triamcinolone, known by the brand names Aristocort and Kenalog

What are the possible side effects?

- Swelling of the ankles, legs, or feet
- Congestive heart failure, heart rate disturbances, blood pressure changes
- Muscle weakness, fractures of the long bones or spine
- Nausea, vomiting, peptic ulcers
- Menstrual irregularities, growth suppression in children, altered fat distribution
- Decreased ability to fight infection
- Acne, abnormal hair growth, impaired wound healing
- Emotional instability, visual disturbances

What are the guidelines for taking corticosteroids?

- Don't abruptly stop taking corticosteroids after long-term, high-dose therapy; you could die. Drug dosage should always be decreased gradually and the drug discontinued under a doctor's close supervision.
- Weigh yourself regularly during therapy to detect any increases caused by drug-induced appetite stimulation and fluid retention.
- Because corticosteroids may cause stomach upset when given orally, take the drug with milk or food.
- Call the doctor if you suffer insomnia or changes in behavior such as sudden mood swings.
- Corticosteroids may delay healing, so be especially careful if you have recently had surgery. Watch for signs of infection, such as abnormal breath sounds.
- Make sure your doctor knows all of the other drugs you are taking, including nonprescription ones. If you're taking corticosteroids by mouth, avoid taking aspirin and drinking alcohol because these substances irritate the stomach and may lead to an ulcer.

Because corticosteroids may cause gastrointestinal upset when given orally, take the drug with milk or food.

- If you're taking the drug once a day, take the dose in the morning to mimic the body's natural pattern of corticosteroid release. If you're taking a divided dose, take the larger dose in the morning.
- If you're taking the drug every other day and you miss a dose, take it as soon as you remember. Otherwise, take the dose the next morning and then omit the next day, resuming an alternate-day schedule. If you're taking the drug daily, take the missed dose as soon as you remember, unless it's almost time for the next dose; never double the dose. If you're taking the drug several times daily, take a missed dose as soon as you remember or double the dose if it's time for your next dose.
- Report minor stress or illness, such as a cold or a tooth extraction, so that the doctor can increase the dosage.
- Corticosteroids impair resistance to infection. As a result, you must avoid exposure to anyone with a known or suspected infection, and you must also avoid any vaccinations or immunizations during therapy and withdrawal.
- Carry an identification card specifying the name and dosage of the prescribed drug.
- If you're taking an inhaled drug for asthma, be sure to rinse your mouth after taking the drug to prevent fungal infections. If you experience tongue, lip, or inner cheek pain, call the doctor.

COUGH SUPPRESSANTS

These drugs relieve coughs caused by various conditions, including viral upper respiratory infections. They effectively suppress coughs that don't produce phlegm; these coughs can cause tiredness and interfere with sleep or daily activities. Prescription cough suppressants, such as codeine and hydrocodone, are derived from opium. Their use is limited because of the potential for abuse and the range of side effects, from stomach upset to nervous system depression. The nonopiate cough suppressants, dextromethorphan and diphenhydramine, are common ingredients in over-the-counter cough and cold remedies.

What are cough suppressants used for?

These drugs are used to relieve a cough that doesn't produce phlegm.

What are some commonly used cough suppressants?

Opiate cough suppressants

- codeine, found in many prescription products, such as Bromphen DC with Codeine, Cheracol, and Robitussin A-C
- hydrocodone, found in many prescription products, such as Chlorgest-HD, Hycodan, and Hycotuss
- hydromorphone, known by the brand name Dilaudid Cough

Nonopiate cough suppressants

- benzonatate, known by the brand name Tessalon
- dextromethorphan, found in many nonprescription remedies, such as Benylin DM, Hold, and Robitussin DM
- diphenhydramine, found in many nonprescription remedies, such as Nytol Maximum Strength and Tylenol Cold Night-Time

What are the possible side effects?

Opiate cough suppressants

- Nervous system depression, dizziness, seizures
- Constipation, nausea and vomiting
- Palpitations, low blood pressure
- Itching
- Allergic reactions

Nonopiate cough suppressants

- Sedation, dizziness
- Constipation
- Allergic reactions

What are the guidelines for taking cough suppressants?

- Tell your doctor if you have any side effects, including constipation, dizziness, rash, or itching.
- Drink plenty of fluids and eat high-fiber foods to prevent constipation.
- Be sure to tell your doctor about all of the other medicines you're taking, including nonprescription drugs.
- Take the drug with food or milk to help prevent an upset stomach. Take the syrup form undiluted, and do not drink liquids afterward. The syrup may provide some of the cough relief by coating an irritated throat.
- These drugs may cause drowsiness. Avoid driving and other hazardous activities that require alertness until your reactions are known.

Alternatives to cough suppressants

Not every person with a cough needs a cough suppressant. An expectorant, which liquefies secretions and promotes their expulsion, may be more useful for a person with pneumonia, bronchitis, cystic fibrosis, or tuberculosis. The following expectorants are commonly used.

Acetylcysteine

This drug is usually given through a face mask or mouthpiece. It helps treat acute and chronic bronchopulmonary diseases. Acetylcysteine should not be given to people with reactive airways because it may cause bronchospasm.

Guaifenesin

A common ingredient in over-the-counter cough remedies, guaifenesin liquefies secretions and promotes expulsion but can cause drowsiness and gastrointestinal upset.

Terpin hydrate

This elixir liquefies secretions and promotes expulsion. The recommended dosage shouldn't be exceeded because of terpin hydrate's high alcohol content.

- Use sugarless hard candy, ice chips, or sugarless gum to relieve dry mouth.
- Use a vaporizer at night to minimize the drying effects of room air. Hot tea with honey and lemon, other hot beverages, and hard candy or lozenges may also help relieve a cough.
- Avoid oversedation by not exceeding the recommended dosage. (See *Alternatives to cough suppressants*, page 101.)

SURGERIES

TRACHEOTOMY

A tracheotomy is the surgical creation of an opening through the neck into the trachea. An incision is made between the tracheal rings, and a tube is inserted through the opening to allow the passage of air and removal of secretions. A tracheotomy may be temporary or permanent, depending on the person's condition.

Why is this procedure done?
- To provide access to the lower airway, permitting breathing and removal of secretions (particularly if endotracheal intubation, the treatment of choice in an emergency, is impossible)
- To provide an airway for an intubated person who needs prolonged mechanical ventilation
- To bypass an upper airway obstruction caused by trauma, burns, epiglottitis, or a tumor

What happens before the procedure?
- A nurse will help you establish an alternative communication system — a letter board, a magic slate, or flash cards — so you can communicate comfortably while your speech is limited.
- You must get diagnostic studies performed.

What happens during the procedure?
In an emergency, a tracheotomy may be performed at the bedside. Elective, permanent tracheotomy is performed in the operating room using general anesthesia. The surgeon makes a vertical incision

in the midline of the neck from the lower border of the thyroid cartilage to slightly above the suprasternal notch. The trachea is exposed, and a second vertical incision is made between the third and fourth tracheal rings. Then a tracheostomy tube is inserted to permit access to the airway.

What are the possible complications?

- A tracheotomy can cause serious complications. Within 48 hours after surgery, a person may develop a hemorrhage at the site, bleeding or swelling within the tracheal tissue, aspiration of secretions, collapsed lung, pneumomediastinum, cardiac tamponade, or subcutaneous emphysema.
- After 48 hours, complications may include stomal or pulmonary infection, ischemia and hemorrhage, airway obstruction, hypoxia, and irregular heartbeats.

What happens after the procedure?

- The nurse provides chest physical therapy to help mobilize secretions.
- You receive oxygen.
- A nurse monitors your hydration and nutritional status and evaluates your ability to swallow. The nurse also arranges for a consultation with a dietitian to modify your diet as needed. (See *Recovering from a tracheotomy*.)

LUNG SURGERY

The surgical removal of part or all of a lung to spare healthy lung tissue from disease is known as a *thoracotomy*. Removal of an entire lung is called a *pneumonectomy*. This procedure is done only when a less radical approach cannot remove all the diseased tissue. After pneumonectomy, chest cavity pressures will stabilize. Over time, fluid will fill the cavity once filled by lung tissue. *Lobectomy* is the removal of one of the five lung lobes. After lobectomy, the remaining lobes expand to fill the entire pleural cavity.

Segmental resection, removal of one or more lung segments, preserves more functional tissue than lobectomy. *Wedge resection* removes a small portion of the lung without regard to segments. It preserves

Recovering from a tracheotomy

After you've been discharged from the hospital, follow these important guidelines.

Report any problems
If you experience any breathing problems, pain in the chest or stoma (the artificial opening created in your neck), or any change in the amount or color of secretions, promptly call your doctor.

Protect the stoma
- Make sure you and a family member learn how to care for your stoma and tracheostomy tube.
- It's important not to get water in the stoma, so avoid swimming, and wear a stoma shield or direct the water below the stoma when showering.
- Remember to place a foam filter over your stoma in winter, thereby warming the air you breathe, and to wear a bib over the filter.

Other instructions
- Bend at your waist when coughing to help expel secretions, and keep a tissue handy to catch them.
- Wear loosely buttoned collars or scarves to disguise the stoma.
- Consider joining a community support group, which you and your family may find helpful.

Four types of lung surgery

Lung excision may be total (pneumonectomy) or partial (lobectomy, segmental resection, or wedge resection). These illustrations show the extent of each of these surgeries for the right lung.

PNEUMONECTOMY

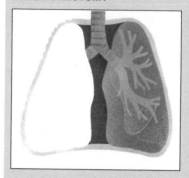

SEGMENTAL RESECTION

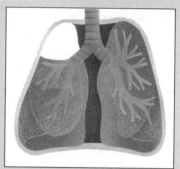

LOBECTOMY

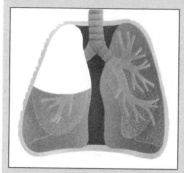

WEDGE RESECTION

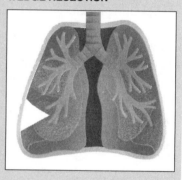

the most functional tissue but can treat only a small, well-circumscribed lesion. Remaining lung tissue needs to be reexpanded after both segmental and wedge resection. (See *Four types of lung surgery*.)

Why is this procedure done?

Lung surgery removes diseased or damaged lung tissue. Pneumonectomy is usually performed to treat lung cancer but may also be used to treat tuberculosis, bronchiectasis, or lung abscess. Lobectomy can treat lung cancer, tuberculosis, lung abscess, emphysematous blebs or bullae, benign tumors, or localized fungal infections. Segmental resection is commonly used to treat bronchiectasis. Wedge resection is reserved for small, well-circumscribed lesions. Any of these procedures also may be performed when an injury destroys part of the lung.

What happens before the procedure?

- Before surgery, the doctor will explain the procedure and answer any questions you may have. You will learn about mechanical ventilation and what to expect in the intensive care unit.
- You learn coughing and deep-breathing techniques that you will need to use after surgery to help reexpand your lung.
- Your doctor will order a number of diagnostic tests, such as pulmonary function tests, electrocardiogram, chest X-rays, arterial blood gas analysis, bronchoscopy and, possibly, cardiac catheterization.
- You or a member of your family must sign a consent form.

What happens during the procedure?

After you receive general anesthesia, the surgeon makes an incision through a space between the ribs and then spreads the ribs and exposes the lung area. In a pneumonectomy, the surgeon ties together and cuts the pulmonary arteries and veins, clamps the main stem bronchus leading to the affected lung, divides it, closes it with nonabsorbable sutures, and then removes the lung.

In a lobectomy, the surgeon removes the affected lobe and binds together and cuts the appropriate arteries, veins, and bronchial passages. In a segmental resection, the surgeon removes the affected segment and binds together and cuts the appropriate artery, vein, and bronchus. In a wedge resection, the surgeon clamps and excises the affected area and then sutures it. In both segmental and wedge resection, the surgeon inserts two chest tubes to drain fluid and aid lung reexpansion. After completing the excision, he or she closes the chest cavity and applies a dressing.

What are the possible complications?

Complications of lung surgery include severe bleeding, infection, collapsed lung, bronchopleural fistulas, and empyema.

What happens after the procedure?

- You may have chest tubes in place, and you may receive oxygen or be connected to a ventilator.
- If you had a pneumonectomy, lie only on your operative side or your back until your condition is stabilized.
- If you had a wedge or segmental resection, you will have chest tubes in place.
- A nurse will encourage you to do coughing and deep-breathing exercises as soon as you are stabilized.

- You will perform passive range-of-motion exercises the evening of surgery and two or three times daily thereafter. (See *Recovering from lung surgery*, page 105.)

INHALATION THERAPIES

MECHANICAL VENTILATION

Mechanical ventilation artificially controls or supports breathing. It can supply oxygen, reduce shortness of breath, and allow fatigued muscles to rest and become reconditioned. Because it also supports spontaneous breathing, mechanical ventilation allows healing to take place until normal breathing can resume. The ventilator delivers air to the lungs through an endotracheal or tracheostomy tube.

Ventilators are available in four types: negative-pressure, pressure-cycled, volume-cycled, and high-frequency. Each type is classified according to the mechanism that cycles the ventilator.

Why is this treatment done?
- To provide oxygen when you can't breathe on your own or when your breaths aren't sufficient to expand your chest and deliver enough oxygenated air to your lungs
- To support ventilation during general anesthesia
- To help control or support respiratory mechanics in certain disorders, such as respiratory infections, which fill the lungs with secretions and interfere with breathing; pulmonary emboli; adult respiratory distress syndrome; central nervous system disorders such as brain stem injury; neuromuscular diseases such as Guillain-Barré syndrome; and flail chest and other musculoskeletal disorders

What happens before the treatment?
- You typically need an endotracheal tube inserted before mechanical ventilation.
- A nurse places you in a semi-upright position, if possible, to promote lung expansion. Your position will be changed every 2 hours.

SELF-HELP

Using a ventilator at home

If you'll be using a ventilator at home, a nurse will teach you or a family member how to check the device and its settings, the nebulizer, and the oxygen equipment at least once a day. Make sure you follow these guidelines:

- Inform the fire department and electric and phone companies that you have a ventilator and oxygen in the home.
- Refill the humidifier as necessary.

Know when to call your doctor
- Call the doctor if you experience chest pain, fever, shortness of breath, or swollen arms or legs.
- Learn to measure your pulse rate, and report any changes in rate or rhythm.

- If you can be weighed at home, report a weight gain of 5 pounds (2.3 kilograms) or more within a week.

Perform daily tracheostomy care
- Be sure to perform daily tracheostomy care using the technique that the nurse or respiratory therapist taught you. If you're using nondisposable items, keep them clean.
- Try to bring your ventilator along if you need hospital treatment for an acute problem. It may be possible to stabilize you without hospital admission.
- Keep emergency numbers handy, and call your doctor or respiratory therapist if you have any questions or problems.

- A nurse will help you establish an alternative communication system because you'll be unable to speak after the endotracheal tube passes through your larynx.

What happens during the treatment?

Each of the four types of ventilators operate differently.
- Negative-pressure ventilators work by alternately removing and replacing air from a container that either encloses the entire body (except for the head) or just the front and sides of the chest and upper abdomen. Removing air creates a negative pressure in the chamber that forces the chest wall to expand, pulling air into the lungs. As the device's diaphragm returns to normal position, it allows the chest wall to fall, causing exhalation.
- Pressure-cycled ventilators stop inhalation when they reach a preset pressure and then allow passive exhalation.
- Volume-cycled ventilators, the most commonly used type, stop inhalation when they've delivered a preset volume of gas, regardless of the pressure needed to deliver it, and then allow passive exhalation.
- High-frequency ventilators use high respiratory rates (usually four times the normal rate) and small tidal volumes (less than or equal to your dead-space volume) to keep the lungs ventilated.

Managing ventilator problems at home

A person's home caregiver must know how to handle certain common ventilator problems and when to call for emergency help. It's important to remain calm when a ventilator problem develops.

Blocked tracheostomy tube
- Disconnect the person from the ventilator.
- Provide oxygen, using a handheld resuscitation bag.
- Suction the person.
- Irrigate the tube with normal saline solution if necessary.
- Reconnect the person to the ventilator, and check his breathing.
- If breathing difficulty persists, call for an ambulance.

Water in the tubing
- Disconnect the tubing from the ventilator.
- Empty the water from the tubing, and reconnect the tubing to the ventilator.

Incorrect cuff pressure
Inflate or deflate the cuff to the correct pressure.

- Additional treatments, such as continuous positive airway pressure and positive end-expiratory pressure, may be used during mechanical ventilation to help keep your lungs expanded and aid in oxygenation.
- A bite block may be used with an oral endotracheal tube to prevent you from biting the tube and obstructing gas flow.

What are the possible complications?

Mechanical ventilation can cause irregular heartbeats, asynchronous breathing, a collapsed lung, decreased cardiac output, infection, and oxygen toxicity. You also may experience psychological reactions, including anxiety, fear, and loss of control.

What happens after the treatment?

You may receive instructions for continuing the treatment at home. (See *Using a ventilator at home,* page 107, and *Managing ventilator problems at home.*)

CONTINUOUS POSITIVE AIRWAY PRESSURE

Continuous positive airway pressure (CPAP) is an adjunct to mechanical ventilation. Positive pressure is applied to the airways, forcing you to exhale against it. In nasal CPAP, used to treat obstructive sleep apnea (cessation of breathing), high-flow compressed air is directed into a mask that covers only your nose. The pressure supplied through the mask serves as a splint, preventing an unstable upper airway from collapsing during inhalation.

CPAP may be delivered through an artificial airway or a mask by means of a ventilator or a separate high-flow generating system. To receive CPAP, you must have the ability to breathe spontaneously.

Why is this treatment done?
- To improve oxygenation in acute respiratory disorders
- To prevent closure of upper airway passages in obstructive sleep apnea
- To prevent airway and alveolar collapse in newborns with respiratory distress syndrome
- To help wean a person from mechanical ventilation

- To treat pulmonary edema, bronchiolitis, pneumonitis, viral pneumonia, and postoperative atelectasis
- To provide an alternative to intubation and mechanical ventilation in mild to moderate respiratory disorders

When shouldn't this treatment be done?

- CPAP is not used in people with untreated hypovolemia caused by hemorrhage; dehydration; neurogenic, anaphylactic, or septic shock; or drug-induced decreased cardiac output or compromised circulation. In such people, the extra pressure generated by CPAP would aggravate circulatory problems.
- CPAP is not used in people with injury or disease affecting only one lung. The therapy would magnify the difference in blood distribution and ventilation between the two lungs.
- Because CPAP delivered by mask can cause nausea and vomiting, it shouldn't be used in people who are unconscious or at risk for vomiting.

What happens before the treatment?

- A nurse or doctor explains the treatment to you or your caregiver.
- A nurse records your vital signs and breath sounds.
- The doctor will probably order arterial blood gas levels and pulmonary function studies.
- If you will be receiving nasal CPAP for sleep apnea, your doctor may tell you to use a nasal decongestant spray before treatment.

What happens during the treatment?

- CPAP is usually performed by a respiratory therapist or a nurse, but policies vary among health care facilities. If you have a tracheostomy or endotracheal tube, the respiratory therapist connects the T-piece on the CPAP device to your airway.
- A nurse monitors your heart rate, blood pressure, and urine output.
- If you're wearing a mask and your condition permits, a nurse will remove it briefly every 2 to 4 hours to provide fluids and mouth and skin care. The length of time the mask is off increases as your ability to maintain oxygenation without CPAP improves.

What are the possible complications?

- The main risks of CPAP and other types of positive-pressure devices are a collapsed lung, pneumomediastinum, and pneumopericardium.

Using continuous positive airway pressure at home

If you're using continuous positive airway pressure (CPAP) for sleep apnea (cessation of breathing), a nurse will teach you and your caregiver how to perform the treatment at home.

Your sleeping partner will be told to monitor you for symptoms, and you'll be asked to demonstrate use of the system to make sure your can prevent excess leakage and maintain the prescribed pressures. You'll learn how to clean the mask and change the air filter.

Points to remember
- You must use CPAP every night even if you feel better after the initial treatments.
- Episodes of apnea will recur if you don't use CPAP as directed. If symptoms recur despite consistent use of CPAP, call the doctor.
- If you have a weight problem, losing weight may allow you to reduce the frequency of CPAP treatments.

- People with neurologic disorders are at risk because CPAP can increase intracranial pressure.
- Other complications of CPAP include gastric distress, particularly if you swallow air during the treatment. This is most common when CPAP is delivered without intubation. Rarely, CPAP causes barotrauma or lowers cardiac output.

What happens after the treatment?

You receive instructions for continuing the treatment at home. (See *Using continuous positive airway pressure at home*.)

OXYGEN THERAPY

Oxygen therapy, delivered by nasal tubes, mask, or transtracheal catheter, helps maintain oxygen levels in the bloodstream and reduces the work of breathing.

The type of equipment used depends on your condition and on the amount of oxygen you need. Inexpensive, disposable, and easy to use, nasal tubes permit talking, eating, and easy movement. However, they can cause nasal drying, can dislodge easily, and can't deliver high oxygen concentrations.

Some masks can deliver oxygen concentrations of nearly 100%, but only if the mask is tight-fitting. Other masks allow you to rebreathe the first one-third of exhaled air, which contains oxygen, not carbon dioxide. Masks may be confining, however, and may interfere with eating and talking. That can affect your willingness to use a mask, making it impractical for long-term oxygen therapy.

Transtracheal catheters permit highly efficient, continuous delivery of oxygen without hindering your mobility. They don't interfere with eating or talking and can be concealed by a shirt or scarf. They also avoid the complications of nasal delivery systems such as drying mucous membranes.

Why is this treatment done?

- Oxygen therapy maintains proper oxygen levels in the arteries, thus decreasing the heart's workload and making breathing easier. (Low oxygen levels in the arteries can be a result of heart, lung, or neuromuscular disorders.)

- Oxygen therapy may also be needed for conditions associated with high metabolic demands, such as massive injury or severe burns.

What happens before the treatment?
- A nurse tells you, your roommate, and visitors not to smoke.
- A nurse checks your heart and lungs.

What happens during the treatment?
The procedure varies according to the type of delivery device.
- *Nasal tubes:* A nurse inserts the curved prongs into your nose, following the nostrils' natural curvature. The tubing is hooked behind your ears and under your chin.
- *Simple mask:* Oxygen flows through an entry port at the bottom of the mask and exits through large holes on the sides of the mask. The nurse places the mask over your nose, mouth, and chin; presses the flexible metal edge to fit the bridge of your nose; and then adjusts the elastic band around your head to hold the mask firmly but comfortably over your cheeks, chin, and bridge of your nose. Gauze padding ensures comfort and a proper fit.
- *Partial rebreather mask:* This mask has an attached reservoir bag that conserves the first third of your exhalation and fills with oxygen before your next breath. The nurse applies it the same way as the simple mask.
- *Nonrebreather mask:* This mask has an attached reservoir bag and three one-way valves. These valves prevent entrance of room air and allow you to breathe only the source gas from the bag. The nurse applies this mask the same way as the simple mask.
- *Venturi mask:* This mask is connected to a Venturi device that mixes a specific volume of air and oxygen. It delivers the most precise oxygen concentrations.
- *Transtracheal catheter:* You receive oxygen through a catheter that the doctor inserts into your trachea.

What are the possible complications?
- High oxygen concentrations continued for 24 or more hours can lead to oxygen poisoning, which can cause lung damage and result in permanent disability.
- High oxygen concentrations in a person whose blood has too much carbon dioxide can eliminate the person's stimulus to breathe, worsening respiratory failure.

Using oxygen therapy at home

If you'll be receiving oxygen at home, you and your doctor will select the oxygen device that's best suited for you. The choice will depend on your needs and on the availability and cost of each system.

You'll be taught how to use the ordered oxygen equipment safely and effectively. You'll also learn how to clean and care for the catheter, if you have that type of device.

Points to remember

- Keep the skin surrounding the catheter insertion site clean and dry to prevent infection.
- Make sure you get regular follow-up care so your response to oxygen therapy can be evaluated.
- Never increase the flow rate without checking with the doctor first.

- Pressure applied by the oxygen delivery device can cause skin irritation and necrosis.
- Aspiration can occur if a person, especially one who is comatose, vomits within a mask.

What happens after the treatment?

- A nurse will monitor your condition.
- You'll learn how to use oxygen at home. (See *Using oxygen therapy at home.*)

*I*NCENTIVE SPIROMETRY

Normally, a person sighs every 6 to 10 minutes. But when deep breaths cause pain, a natural tendency to override the process leads to a pattern of taking shallow breaths that do little to open the airways. Incentive spirometry enhances natural sighing, inducing the person to take a deep breath and hold it. The spirometer also measures the amount of air inhaled to provide feedback on performance.

Why is this treatment done?

Incentive spirometry is used to encourage you to take deep breaths, especially after surgery (to prevent pulmonary complications such as pneumonia). It's also used in people with rib fractures (who are reluctant to breathe deeply because of pain) and in people with neuromuscular disease (who have weak respiratory muscles).

What happens before the treatment?

- A nurse or respiratory therapist will explain the procedure to you and tell you that you must sit to enhance lung expansion.

What happens during the treatment?

You perform the procedure yourself but initially you get direction from the nurse or respiratory therapist.

What are the possible complications?

Hyperventilation may occur if your perform breathing exercises too quickly.

What happens after the treatment?

- If you had surgery, a nurse will help you splint your incision before you cough.
- If additional treatments are needed at home, a nurse will explain how to use a disposable unit. (See *Performing incentive spirometry at home.*)

LIFE SUPPORT FOR NEWBORNS

This life support system for newborns, called *extracorporeal membrane oxygenation,* is an adaptation of cardiopulmonary bypass methods used during open-heart surgery. It diverts blood from the lungs and decreases the potentially damaging side effects associated with mechanical ventilation. In this way, it gives severely compromised lungs a chance to rest and heal. During this therapy, a machine removes a baby's venous blood, passes it through a membrane oxygenator, and then returns it to the circulation. Babies can usually remain on this life support system for several days (up to 17 days have been reported), perhaps long enough for their lungs to heal.

This type of life support has not been very successful in adults.

Why is this treatment done?

- To provide oxygen while allowing the lungs to recover and heal (only after ventilatory support has failed to improve oxygenation)
- To "buy time" in life-threatening respiratory failure that is potentially reversible within 2 weeks

When shouldn't this treatment be done?

- This treatment shouldn't be used for babies with central nervous system damage, irreversible shock, pulmonary fibrosis, multiple organ failure, intracranial bleeding, congenital anomalies incompatible with life, heart anomalies, or blood clotting disorders, or in babies who have been receiving mechanical ventilation for more than 10 days.
- Premature infants of less than 35 weeks' gestation and those weighing less than 4.5 pounds (2 kilograms) aren't candidates for this procedure because they have the greatest risk of intracranial bleeding.

 SELF-HELP

Performing incentive spirometry at home

If you'll be performing incentive spirometry at home, make sure you follow these important guidelines.

Inhale slowly and deeply
First, exhale normally. Then place your lips tightly around the mouthpiece of the incentive spirometer and inhale slowly and deeply. Try to reach the goal, which you can see. Depending on the type of spirometer used, you may be forcing the ball to the top of the chamber, compressing the bellows, or lighting up the different color panels. If you have difficulty achieving your goal, suck in as if you were sipping through a straw. Breathing in slowly ensures an even distribution of air to the lungs.

Hold your breath
- After breathing in, hold your breath for 3 seconds and then remove the mouthpiece, exhaling normally. A 60-second rest between consecutive deep breaths helps prevent fatigue and dizziness. Repeat this exercise 5 to 10 times per hour.
- If you have a neuromuscular disease, continue therapy as directed by your doctor. Notify him if your capacity to breathe in declines.

SELF-HELP

Care after life support is removed

After you've been discharged from the hospital, follow the important guidelines below.

Know when to call your doctor
Promptly notify the doctor of fever, bleeding, bruising, changes in mental status, shortness of breath, or chest pain. Signs of respiratory distress include bluish discoloration of the skin, increased respiratory rate, and congestion.

Other points to remember
▪ Activity levels should follow the doctor's instructions or the assigned rehabilitation program.
▪ Depending on the underlying reason for the life support, you may get additional home care instructions from the doctor.

What happens before the treatment?
▪ A doctor or nurse explains the procedure to the infant's parents.
▪ The doctor orders an ultrasound test of the head to rule out intracranial bleeding.
▪ The parents must sign a consent form.

What happens during the treatment?
▪ Insertion is a surgical procedure that is usually performed at the patient's bedside in the intensive care unit by an operating room team.
▪ There are two approaches: venoarterial and venovenous. The venoarterial approach is more common. In this technique, a doctor inserts a catheter into the right atrium by way of the right internal jugular vein. The blood is drained into a membrane oxygenator. While blood travels this extracorporeal circuit, oxygen is infused and carbon dioxide is removed. After passing through the circuit, the blood is returned to the body.
▪ In the venovenous approach, blood is drained by gravity into the extracorporeal circuit. After blood is oxygenated and carbon dioxide is removed, the blood is reinfused into the venous system rather than the arterial system.
▪ A nurse monitors the infant's vital signs closely.
▪ The nurse suctions the infant thoroughly.

What are the possible complications?
▪ This treatment can cause mechanical and physiologic complications, including internal and external bleeding and blood poisoning.
▪ Mechanical difficulties, although uncommon, can be life-threatening.

What happens after the treatment?
The operating room team goes to the intensive care unit, where they remove the catheter. (See *Care after life support is removed.*)

OXYGEN CHAMBER THERAPY

A person placed in an oxygen chamber (also known as a *hyperbaric chamber*) is exposed to oxygen that's at a much higher pressure than normal atmospheric pressure. The person breathes 100% oxygen while the pressure within the chamber is increased to up to three times the normal atmospheric pressure.

Why is this treatment done?

Oxygen chamber therapy is performed to improve oxygen delivery to body tissues in people with decompression sickness, severe carbon monoxide poisoning, or gas gangrene.

When shouldn't this treatment be done?

A person with an untreated collapsed lung shouldn't be placed in an oxygen chamber. Other conditions that require specific precautions include upper respiratory infections, chronic sinusitis, seizure disorders, emphysema with carbon dioxide retention, and uncontrolled high fever as well as a history of spontaneous lung collapse, thoracic surgery, reconstructive ear or eye surgery, pulmonary lesions on a routine X-ray or computed tomography scan (commonly called a CAT scan), viral infections, congenital spherocytosis, or optic neuritis.

What happens before the treatment?

- You may be given a mild sedative.
- A nurse will demonstrate techniques of ear clearing, such as yawning, swallowing, or chewing motions, and evaluate your ability to ventilate the middle ear.
- An ear, nose, and throat specialist examines you if ear problems are anticipated.
- If you smoke, stop. Smoking narrows the blood vessels and makes treatment less effective.

What happens during the treatment?

You're placed in a chamber that can accommodate one person or one that can accommodate up to 10 persons. In a single-person chamber, you lie on a cart that slides inside the chamber; its hull, made of clear acrylic plastic, allows you to see outside of the chamber. The chamber is filled with compressed oxygen, and you breathe from the surrounding environment.

In multiplace chambers, oxygen is supplied from the wall by a mask, a hood, or an endotracheal tube.

Caring for yourself after oxygen chamber therapy

After you've been discharged from the hospital, follow the important guidelines below.

▪ Notify the doctor if you experience any side effects, especially apprehension, sweating, confusion, visual changes, ringing in the ears, nausea, vomiting, or twitching.

▪ If you had ear surgery, avoid getting water in your ears.

▪ Keep in mind that a small amount of bleeding from the ears is normal.

What are the possible complications?

Oxygen chamber therapy may be associated with barotrauma (rupture of the eardrum membrane, sinus barotrauma, lung barotrauma, and air embolism), oxygen poisoning (chronic lung fibrosis or seizures), visual acuity changes (worsening nearsightedness and hastened growth of cataracts), and numbness and tingling in the extremities.

What happens after the treatment?

The nurse will provide instructions on how to care for yourself at home. (See *Caring for yourself after oxygen chamber therapy.*)

OTHER TREATMENTS

REMOVING FLUID OR AIR FROM THE LUNGS

Removing fluid or air from the lungs with a needle or catheter inserted through the chest wall is called *thoracentesis*. The underlying cause of such fluid accumulation must be identified and corrected to prevent the fluid or air from reaccumulating.

Why is this procedure done?

▪ To identify diseases of the lungs' lining
▪ To relieve pressure on the lungs and respiratory distress, which may occur in emphysema, tuberculosis, or cancer
▪ To medicate the lungs

What happens before the procedure?

▪ The doctor may prescribe sedation.
▪ You may feel a stinging sensation during injection of the local anesthetic and some pressure during needle insertion and fluid withdrawal. It is important to remain still during the procedure to reduce the risk of lung injury.
▪ The doctor orders a chest X-ray or ultrasound to identify the exact location of the fluid.

What happens during the procedure?

▪ Fluid drainage is typically performed at the bedside by a doctor with a nurse's assistance.

▪ After you're properly positioned and your skin prepared, the doctor administers a local anesthetic at the puncture site. Next, using sterile technique, he or she inserts the needle through the chest wall and into the pleural space. The doctor may introduce a Teflon catheter into the needle, remove the needle, and attach a stopcock and syringe or drainage tubing to the catheter. He or she then slowly and carefully aspirates the pleural fluid and, after the needle or catheter is removed, applies pressure to the puncture site before applying a sterile dressing. (See *Positions for fluid removal.*)

What are the possible complications?

Complications include pneumothorax, reaccumulation of fluid, mediastinal shift, and hypovolemic shock. Air embolism, a rare complication, may occur if air enters a superficial pulmonary vessel because of injury to the visceral pleura. Infection may result if contamination occurs during the procedure. There's a risk of hemorrhage in people with a bleeding disorder.

What happens after the procedure?

▪ The nurse helps you into a comfortable position.
▪ The nurse monitors your vital signs and respiratory status.
▪ The nurse tells you and your family to notify the doctor if fever, shortness of breath, or rapid heartbeat occurs.

CHEST DRAINAGE THERAPY

Chest drainage therapy is used to relieve the accumulation of air, fluid, or pus in the lungs. A chest tube is inserted and connected to a suction or a water-seal drainage system. This drainage system permits air and fluid to leave the chest and not be drawn back in during inspiration. When all of the air and fluid have been removed and the lung fully reexpands, the chest tube is removed.

Positions for fluid removal

Fluid can be removed from the lungs with a person in several positions, which are illustrated below.

LEANING ON A TABLE

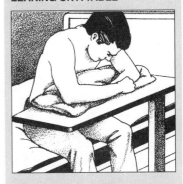

STRADDLING A CHAIR

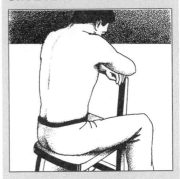

SEMI-UPRIGHT POSITION IN BED

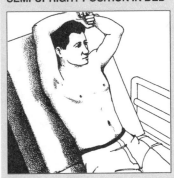

Why is this procedure done?

- Chest drainage therapy is done to remove air, blood, or pus from the pleural space, permitting the lung to reinflate. After heart surgery, chest drainage therapy is used to remove blood from the chest cavity.
- Chest drainage therapy is performed for people with a collapsed lung, blood in the pleural cavity, chylothorax, empyema, or pleural effusion. All people who undergo major lung surgery, except those having a pneumonectomy, will require chest drainage.

When shouldn't this procedure be done?

The procedure should not be done when a collapsed lung is not life-threatening or when blood clotting time is prolonged. With a life-threatening collapsed lung, chest drainage typically must be performed as an emergency procedure.

What happens before the procedure?

- If time permits, a nurse will explain the procedure to you.
- A nurse will take your vital signs and give you a sedative.
- You'll be asked to sign a consent form.

What happens during the procedure?

- In most cases, you're awake when the chest tubes are inserted and receive a local anesthetic. The doctor inserts the chest tube by connecting one end of the tube to the chest drainage system and stabilizing the other end by suturing the tube into place. The doctor then applies petroleum gauze and a dry sterile dressing and, to prevent dislodgment, tapes the chest tube to your chest wall. All tube connections are taped, and suction is regulated.
- The doctor most commonly uses a disposable water-seal drainage system. This compact, one-piece unit is composed of three compartments. The first compartment collects the fluid drained from the chest; the second compartment — the water-seal chamber — allows pleural air to escape but prevents the return of atmospheric air. The third compartment controls suction; the amount of water in this chamber determines the degree of suction.
- Disposable waterless systems are also available. In these systems, no water is added to the suction-control chamber; instead, a screw-type valve or spring is used to regulate suction.
- You'll receive a chest X-ray to verify tube placement and to assess the outcome of treatment. You may get daily X-rays to monitor your progress.

- A nurse will monitor you for signs and symptoms of complications.
- A nurse will check your dressing to make sure that it's airtight, clean, dry, and intact.
- A nurse will check the collection chamber, assessing the drainage for amount, color, consistency, and rate of flow.

What are the possible complications?

Tension pneumothorax, a life-threatening complication, can result from a blocked or dislodged chest tube or from a malfunctioning chest drainage system. Other complications may include lung puncture when the chest tube is inserted, bleeding, and infection.

What happens after the procedure?

- The nurse applies an airtight, sterile petroleum gauze dressing to the site after the chest tube is removed.
- A nurse will monitor you for signs of respiratory distress.
- Before you leave the hospital, a nurse will teach you how to clean the wound site and change dressings.
- Make sure you report any signs of infection.
- Be sure to keep all follow-up appointments with your doctor.

CHEST PHYSICAL THERAPY

Chest physical therapy is a collective term that includes coughing and deep-breathing exercises, postural drainage, and chest percussion and vibration. Together, these techniques aid elimination of secretions and reexpansion of lung tissue and promote efficient use of respiratory muscles. Chest physical therapy is often combined with other treatments, such as suctioning, incentive spirometry, nebulizer treatments, and administration of expectorants and other drugs.

Successful treatment with chest physical therapy produces improved breath sounds, improved partial pressure of arterial oxygen, and increased sputum production and air flow.

Why is this treatment done?

- To mobilize pulmonary secretions (especially from peripheral lung areas) in immobile people and in people with bronchitis, cystic fibrosis, bronchiectasis, or pneumonia; neuromuscular diseases (Guillain-Barré syndrome, myasthenia gravis, tetanus); chronic obstructive pulmonary disease; diseases associated with aspiration (cerebral palsy or muscular dystrophy); or postoperative pain associated with impaired breathing

▪ To increase clearance of tracheobronchial mucus and promote maximum ventilation

Successful treatment with chest physical therapy produces improved breath sounds, improved partial pressure of arterial oxygen, and increased sputum production and air flow.

When shouldn't this treatment be done?

Chest physical therapy is not performed when a person has pulmonary bleeding and is spitting up blood or after a hemorrhage. Other reasons for not doing chest physical therapy include fractured ribs, an unstable chest wall, lung contusions, tuberculosis, untreated pneumothorax, acute asthma or bronchospasm, pulmonary embolism, lung abscess or tumor, head injury, and recent heart attack.

What happens before the treatment?

A nurse will give you pain medication to minimize discomfort. If you've had surgery, a nurse will splint your incision during therapy.

What happens during the treatment?

▪ For hospitalized patients, chest physical therapy is typically performed by a respiratory therapist or a nurse. If such therapy is required after discharge, it can be performed by a family member. (See *How to perform chest physical therapy at home.*)

▪ You will be told to cough while performing deep-breathing exercises. This helps prevent obstruction by keeping your airways clear and open. Coughing dislodges and removes secretions from the respiratory system; deep breathing after coughing increases the amount of air in the lungs' air sacs and makes the cough more effective.

▪ After listening to your chest and reviewing chest X-rays, your doctor will instruct you to lie in a position that will result in the most effective drainage.

▪ The nurse performs percussion by hitting the chest with cupped hands, a percussion cup, or a mechanical percussion and vibration device. This procedure mechanically dislodges thick, stubborn secretions from the bronchial wall so that they can be spit out or suctioned.

▪ The nurse or therapist uses vibration during postural drainage, either with percussion or as an alternative to it for a patient who's frail, in pain, or recovering from thoracic surgery or injury. Vibration in-

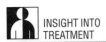

INSIGHT INTO
TREATMENT

How to perform chest physical therapy at home

As you review this guide, keep in mind that coughing and deep-breathing exercises are performed together and that they are followed by postural drainage (body positioning to drain fluid), which is performed in conjunction with percussion (tapping) and vibration.

Coughing
- Assume a comfortable, upright position.
- Inhale deeply through your nose and exhale in three short huffs.
- Inhale deeply and cough three times with your mouth slightly open.
- Repeat this exercise two or three times.

Deep breathing
- Assume a seated position or lie down with the head of the bed elevated. Put one hand on the middle of your chest and the other on your abdomen just below the ribs. This permits you to feel your diaphragm rise and fall.
- Inhale slowly and deeply, pushing your abdomen out against your hand to provide optimal distribution of air to the lungs' air sacs. Then purse your lips and exhale. Contract your abdomen at the same time.
- Breathe this way for 1 minute and then rest for 2 minutes. Gradually progress to a 10-minute exercise period four times a day.

Postural drainage
- Assume the position that most effectively loosens and drains the area.
- Remain in this position for 10 to 15 minutes while another person performs percussion and vibration, as discussed below. If necessary, assume another position for further drainage.

Percussion
- Have the person who will be percussed breathe slowly and deeply, using his or her diaphragm to promote relaxation.
- Cup your hands with your finger flexed and your thumb tight against your index finger. Percuss each lung segment for 1 to 2 minutes, rhythmically alternating your hands. Listen for a hollow sound to gauge the effectiveness of your technique.

Vibration
- Have the person who requires vibration inhale deeply and exhale slowly through pursed lips. While the individual exhales firmly, place your hands flat against the chest wall on the lung segment being drained. Position your hands side by side with your fingers extended.
- Vibrate the chest wall by quickly contracting and relaxing the muscles of your arms and shoulders to generate fine vibrations. Stop vibrating while the person inhales. Vibrate over each lung segment while the person exhales five times.

creases the speed and turbulence of exhaled air, loosens secretions, and propels them into the larger bronchi so that they can be spit out or suctioned.

What are the possible complications?
Complications of chest physical therapy are few. The head-down position used in postural drainage can result in an oxygen deficiency or

a decrease in blood pressure. Vigorous percussion or vibration may cause rib fracture.

What happens after the treatment?

- If your gag reflex is diminished or if you have difficulty spitting out secretions, the nurse may use suction.
- You'll receive oral hygiene after therapy because secretions may taste foul or have an unpleasant odor.

BRONCHOSCOPY

This surgical procedure allows the doctor to see the trachea and tracheobronchial tree through a bronchoscope, a slender, flexible tube with mirrors and a light at its end. Bronchoscopy can be performed on anyone, even if an endotracheal or tracheostomy tube is in place.

Why is this procedure done?

- To remove an obstruction in the breathing passages
- To remove foreign bodies, tumors, mucus plugs, or excessive secretions from the tracheobronchial tree
- To inspect the tracheobronchial tree for asymptomatic cancer before chest surgery

What happens before the procedure?

- A doctor or nurse will explain that, although you won't be able to speak during the procedure, you'll be able to breathe. Oxygen will be administered through a nasal cannula, a face mask, or an endotracheal tube.
- You won't be allowed to eat or drink for 6 to 12 hours before the procedure. In some cases, food, fluids, and oral drugs also will be withheld for about 2 hours after the procedure, until the gag reflex returns.
- Just before the procedure, a nurse will administer a preoperative sedative, an I.V. infusion, and the prescribed medication. If you wear dentures, you'll be instructed to remove them.

How a flexible bronchoscope works

Inserted through the person's nostril and into the bronchi, the flexible fiber-optic bronchoscope has four channels (see enlargement). Two light channels (A) provide a light source; one visualizing channel (B) allows direct examination; and one open channel (C) can accommodate biopsy forceps, a cytology brush, an anesthetic, or oxygen, as well as suctioning or lavage.

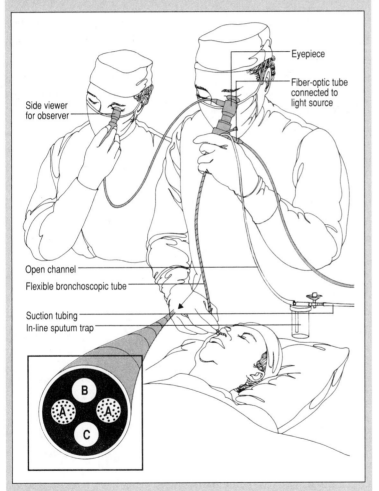

Side viewer for observer

Eyepiece

Fiber-optic tube connected to light source

Open channel
Flexible bronchoscopic tube

Suction tubing
In-line sputum trap

Recovering from a bronchoscopy

After you've been discharged from the hospital, follow these important guidelines:
- If the bronchoscopy was performed on an outpatient basis or in the emergency room, promptly report any shortness of breath, pain, or prolonged bleeding to your doctor.
- Avoid straining your voice, but understand that your sore throat and hoarseness are temporary.
- Report signs of infection, such as a fever or thick yellow sputum.

What happens during the procedure?

- When bronchoscopy is performed for diagnostic purposes, biopsy forceps, a brush, or a catheter may be passed through the bronchoscope to obtain specimens for lab analysis.
- In most cases, the doctor performs bronchoscopy with a flexible fiber-optic bronchoscope. (See *How a flexible bronchoscope works,* page 123.) However, a metal bronchoscope is used to remove a foreign body, excise endobronchial lesions, and control excessive spitting up of blood.
- During the procedure, you're in a sitting position or lying flat. You're asked to place your arms at your sides and breathe through your nose.
- A local anesthetic is sprayed into your nose and mouth to suppress the gag reflex. (General anesthesia may be used for children or extremely apprehensive people.)
- After the anesthetic takes effect, the doctor introduces a lubricated bronchoscope into the upper airway. When he or she can see the vocal cords, the doctor instills Xylocaine to continue suppressing the gag reflex and to anesthetize the vocal cords. The doctor then advances the bronchoscope through the larynx and into the windpipe and bronchi, and removes mucus, secretions, or a foreign body or withdraws a specimen for lab analysis. After removing the foreign body, mucus, or specimen, the doctor withdraws the bronchoscope.

What are the possible complications?

A transbronchial biopsy may result in a collapsed lung. Some rare complications of bronchoscopy include hypoxemia, hemorrhage (most likely to occur with biopsy), laryngeal swelling or laryngospasm, bronchospasm, infection, and tracheal or bronchial perforation.

What happens after the procedure?

- The nurse will place you on your side, with the head of the bed slightly elevated.
- A nurse will check your vital signs until you are stable.
- The nurse will give you a basin and instruct you to spit out saliva rather than swallow it.
- You must rest quietly and refrain from talking. The nurse may give you medicated lozenges for hoarseness or a sore throat. (See *Recovering from a bronchoscopy.*)

HEIMLICH MANEUVER

Also called an *abdominal thrust,* the Heimlich maneuver relieves the sudden airway obstruction that occurs when a foreign body lodges in the throat or bronchus or when a person aspirates (chokes on) blood, mucus, or vomit. In this procedure, pressure applied below the diaphragm elevates the diaphragm and forces sufficient air from the lungs to create a forceful cough, which expels the obstruction. A variation of the abdominal thrust, the chest thrust, is used on pregnant women or markedly obese people.

Obstruction of an airway by a foreign body usually occurs when the person is eating. In adults, the most common cause is an accidentally aspirated piece of meat, although various other foods and foreign bodies can block the airway.

Foreign bodies can cause complete or partial airway blockage. The Heimlich maneuver and its variations shouldn't be performed on a person with a partial airway obstruction who has sufficient air exchange to maintain adequate ventilation; such a person can cough forcefully enough to dislodge the foreign body. However, a partial airway obstruction can progress to poor air exchange and complete obstruction; therefore, if the partial obstruction with good air exchange persists, call the emergency medical service system, a coordinated, community-wide system for responding to emergency situations that is usually activated with a phone call.

The Heimlich maneuver becomes necessary when an individual develops a weak, ineffective cough and a high-pitched noise when inhaling and has increased difficulty breathing. In complete airway obstruction, the person can't speak, breathe, or cough and often clutches the neck with his or her thumbs and fingers — the universal distress signal.

An obstructed airway can lead to brain damage and death in minutes without successful intervention. For this reason, it's necessary to call for emergency help as soon as airway obstruction is identified.

Why is this procedure done?

The Heimlich maneuver is performed to relieve airway obstruction in conscious or unconscious adults who have suddenly developed a foreign body airway obstruction.

What happens before the procedure?

- A rescuer should call the emergency medical service system.
- Foreign body airway obstruction should be confirmed before a Heimlich maneuver is performed.

What happens during the procedure?

The Heimlich maneuver can be performed by anyone who has been taught the technique. Before performing it, however, a rescuer has to make sure the person has a completely obstructed airway or a partially obstructed airway with poor air exchange. The person who has a complete obstruction won't be able to answer when asked if choking; if the person has poor air exchange, he or she will have a weak cough and may not be able to speak easily. If the person is unconscious and the airway is obstructed, he or she won't be breathing, and the air that the rescuer attempts to blow into the lungs will meet with resistance.

When the rescuer has established that the person requires the Heimlich maneuver, he or she performs forceful inward and upward maneuvers below the diaphragm (or, if appropriate, chest thrusts) until the foreign body is dislodged. Once dislodged, the foreign body is usually visible in the person's mouth and can be removed by the rescuer with a finger-sweep if the person's unable to remove it alone.

For an unconscious victim, adult CPR is performed. If the airway is obstructed, the rescuer will meet resistance when attempting to ventilate the person. Because the tongue is the most common cause of airway obstruction, the airway may not have been properly opened, so the rescuer repositions the airway and again attempts ventilation. If the rescuer still meets resistance, he or she may attempt to clear the obstructed airway by performing five abdominal maneuvers (or chest thrusts, if indicated), then a blind finger-sweep, and trying ventilation again. This sequence — thrusts, finger-sweep, and ventilation — is repeated until ventilation succeeds or the obstruction is relieved. For a child or an infant, the sequence and procedures are different. (See *How to clear a blocked airway.*)

Points to remember

- When the Heimlich maneuver is performed on a conscious victim, each thrust should be a separate and distinct movement that's forceful enough to create an artificial cough that will dislodge the obstruction.

(Text continues on page 129.)

How to clear a blocked airway

If you determine that a person's airway is totally blocked, follow these guidelines for performing the Heimlich maneuver.

For a conscious adult

- Tell the person you're going to try to dislodge the foreign body.
- Standing behind the person, wrap your arms around his or her waist. Make a fist with one hand and place the thumb side against the person's abdomen, slightly above the navel and well below the bottom of the breastbone. Then grasp your fist with the other hand, and squeeze the person's abdomen with a quick inward and upward thrust (see below).

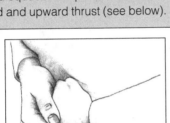

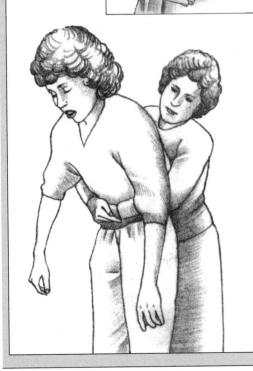

- Repeat this maneuver until the object is dislodged or the person becomes unconscious. If the person becomes unconscious, lower him or her carefully to the floor and continue trying to dislodge the obstruction using the technique for an unconscious person, beginning with a finger-sweep.

For an unconscious adult

- If you come upon an unconscious person, ask any witnesses what happened. Begin CPR and try to ventilate the person. If you can't ventilate him or her, reposition the head and try again.
- If you still can't ventilate the person, kneel astride his or her thighs.
- Place the heel of one hand on top of the other. Then place your hands between the person's navel and the bottom of the breastbone at the midline. Push inward and upward with five quick abdominal thrusts.

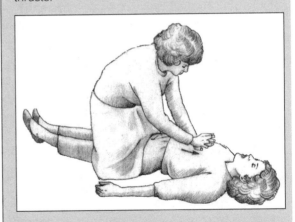

- After delivering the abdominal thrusts, open the person's airway by grasping the tongue and lower jaw with your thumb and fingers. Lift the jaw to draw

(continued)

How to clear a blocked airway *(continued)*

the tongue away from the back of the throat and perform a finger-sweep (see below).

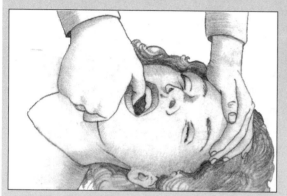

- If you can see the foreign body, remove it by inserting your index finger deep into the person's throat at the base of the tongue. Using a hooking motion, remove the object. Keep in mind that some clinicians object to a blind finger-sweep—using your finger when you can't see the obstruction—because the finger acts as a second obstruction. They believe that in most cases, the jaw lift described above should be enough to dislodge the obstruction (see below).

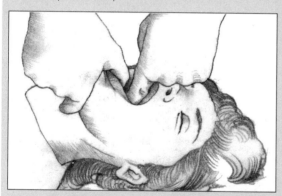

- If you can't remove the object, try to ventilate the person. If you can't, repeat the abdominal thrust maneuver described above in sequence until you clear the airway.

- If you are able to remove the obstruction, determine if the person is breathing; if not, proceed with CPR.

For an obese person or a woman in advanced stages of pregnancy
- If the person is conscious, stand behind him or her and place your arms under the armpits and around the chest (see below).

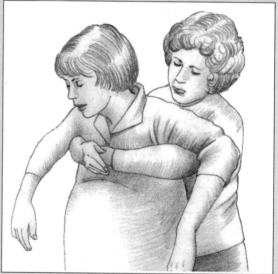

- Place the thumb side of your clenched fist against the middle of the breastbone, avoiding the margins of the ribs and the bottom of the breastbone. Grasp your fist with your other hand, and perform a chest thrust with enough force to expel the foreign body. Continue until the person expels the obstruction or loses consciousness.
- If the person loses consciousness, carefully lower him or her to the floor.
- Kneel close to the person's side and place the heel of one hand just above the bottom of the breastbone. The long axis of the heel of your hand should align with the long axis of the person's breastbone. Place the heel of your other hand

How to clear a blocked airway *(continued)*

on top of that, making sure your fingers don't touch the person's chest (see below). Deliver each thrust forcefully enough to remove the obstruction.

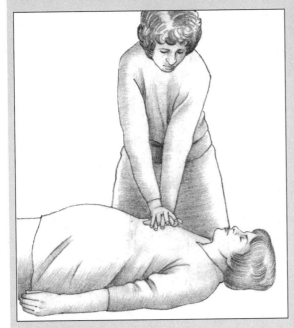

For a child
- If the child is conscious and can stand, perform abdominal thrusts using the same technique as you would with an adult, but with less force.

- If the child's unconscious or lying down, kneel at his or her feet; if the child is large, kneel astride his or her thighs. If the child's lying on a treatment table, stand by his or her side. Deliver abdominal thrusts as you would for an adult, but use less force. (Never perform a blind finger-sweep on a child because you risk pushing the foreign body farther back into the airway.)

For an infant
- Whether or not the infant is conscious, place him or her face down and straddling your arm, with the head lower than the trunk. Rest your forearm on your thigh and deliver five back blows between the infant's shoulder blades with the heel of your hand.
- If this action doesn't remove the obstruction, place your free hand on the infant's back. Supporting the neck, jaw, and chest with your other hand, turn the infant over onto your thigh, keeping the head lower than the trunk.
- Position your fingers. To do so, imagine a line between the infant's nipples; place the index finger of your free hand on his or her breastbone, just below this imaginary line. Then place your middle and ring fingers next to your index finger, and lift the index finger off the infant's chest. Deliver five chest thrusts, but at a slower rate than for a child or adult. (As with a child, never perform a blind finger-sweep.)

- Hold a conscious victim securely because he or she may lose consciousness and need to be lowered to the floor.
- If the person vomits, turn him or her to one side, quickly do a finger-sweep, and then return the person to a supine position. Repeat the maneuver as necessary.
- Even if efforts to clear the airway don't seem effective, you should keep trying. As oxygen deprivation increases, smooth muscles and skeletal muscles relax, which makes the maneuver more likely to succeed.
- For a child, perform a finger-sweep only if you can see the object.
- For an unconscious infant in whom partial or complete obstruction is established, perform five back blows and five chest thrusts

SELF-HELP

How to avoid a blocked airway

To help prevent a blocked airway, keep in mind the following.

Eating tips

- Cut food into small pieces and chew it thoroughly before swallowing.
- Don't laugh or talk when chewing or swallowing.
- Avoid drinking excessive amounts of alcohol before or during meals.

Advice for parents

- Don't allow your children to walk, run, or play when they have food or anything else in their mouths. Also try to keep small objects away from infants and small children.
- Parents should also learn how to perform the Heimlich maneuver correctly and how to recognize the universal sign of foreign body airway obstruction.

identical to the chest compressions recommended for infant CPR. Next, check the mouth and do a finger-sweep if you see the obstructing object; then attempt ventilation. Repeat this sequence until you've successfully ventilated the infant or removed the obstruction.

- For a conscious infant, perform only back blows and chest thrusts.

What are the possible complications?

A major complication associated with abdominal or chest thrusts is laceration or rupture of the underlying organs, such as the liver or lungs. Vomiting may also result.

What happens after the procedure?

- If the person was unconscious, observe him or her closely. Nausea and vomiting may develop after the person regains consciousness and can breathe independently. He or she should also be evaluated for injuries that may have occurred.
- Afterwards, the emergency medical service team will transport the person to the hospital for further evaluation.
- The person may feel achiness, which often follows this procedure. (See *How to avoid a blocked airway*.)

$\boxed{3}$

TREATING DIGESTIVE TRACT DISORDERS

DRUG THERAPIES

ANTACIDS

Antacids act within the digestive tract to reduce acidity. Because they're usually safe for self-medication, antacids are available without prescription. However, problems can occur if they're used improperly.

Antacids come in powder, tablet, and liquid forms. After ingestion, antacids begin to act almost immediately and their effects last for 1 to 3 hours, depending on whether they were taken with food or another medication.

What are antacids used for?
- To relieve heartburn
- To help heal peptic ulcers
- To strengthen the protective lining of the digestive tract
- To help treat diseases associated with excess stomach acid production such as Zollinger-Ellison syndrome

What are some commonly used antacids?
- aluminum hydroxide, known by the brand names AlternaGEL, Alu-Cap, Basaljel, Dialume, and Nephrox
- aluminum hydroxide with magnesium hydroxide, known by the brand names Gelusil and Maalox
- calcium carbonate, known by the brand names Alka-Mints, Chooz, Rolaids Calcium Rich, Titralac, and Tums
- dihydroxyaluminum sodium carbonate, known by the brand name Rolaids
- magaldrate, known by the brand name Riopan
- magnesium oxide, known by the brand names Mag-Ox 400 and Maox
- sodium bicarbonate

What are the possible side effects?
- Magnesium-containing antacids, which have a laxative effect, may cause diarrhea.

- Aluminum-containing antacids can cause constipation, which may lead to intestinal blockage. They may also cause serious electrolyte imbalances.
- Calcium carbonate, magaldrate, magnesium oxide, and sodium bicarbonate may actually enhance stomach acid output.
- Sodium bicarbonate commonly causes stomach distention and gas. Serious electrolyte imbalances may occur when it's given in large doses.

What are the guidelines for taking antacids?

- Don't use an antacid if you have any symptoms of gastrointestinal or rectal bleeding, an intestinal blockage, or appendicitis.
- Calcium-containing antacids should not be used if you have hypercalcemia, constipation, hemorrhoids, hypoparathyroidism, or sarcoidosis.
- Aluminum-containing antacids should not be used if you have constipation, chronic diarrhea, a stomach outlet obstruction, or hemorrhoids.
- Magaldrate should not be used if you have severe kidney disease, ulcerative colitis, a colostomy or ileostomy, diverticulitis, chronic diarrhea, or a stomach outlet obstruction.
- Magnesium-containing antacids should not be used if you have severe kidney disease, ulcerative colitis, a colostomy or ileostomy, diverticulitis, or chronic diarrhea.
- Sodium bicarbonate-containing antacids should not be used if you have kidney or liver disease, congestive heart failure, swelling, or toxemia of pregnancy.
- Pay attention to your bowel movements and report any changes in your normal pattern. If you develop constipation or diarrhea, call your doctor, who may then change the drug or reduce the dosage.
- Don't take antacids indiscriminately. You should know that many drugs that are taken orally interact with antacids. Because they change the acidity of the stomach, drugs with protective, enteric coatings may release their contents prematurely if taken with an antacid. This premature release may cause stomach irritation or reduce the effectiveness of the enteric-coated medication because it may bind to the antacid and not be absorbed. This interaction may be especially dangerous if you're taking antibiotics, anticonvulsants, or certain cardiovascular drugs such as Lanoxin or Coumadin. Check with your doctor or pharmacist before taking antacids with other drugs.
- If you're taking a liquid antacid, shake the suspension thoroughly before pouring. If you're taking antacid tablets, chew each tablet well before swallowing and follow the dose with a full glass of water.

> *Don't use an antacid if you have any symptoms of gastrointestinal or rectal bleeding, an intestinal obstruction, or appendicitis.*

- If a particular antacid is recommended by your doctor, don't switch brands without his or her advice.
- If you experience headache, confusion, weakness, malaise, or loss of appetite, discontinue the drug and call your doctor.

HISTAMINE$_2$-RECEPTOR ANTAGONISTS

Most of us are familiar with histamine. The itching, swelling, and "flare-up" reaction that occurs after a bee sting is caused by the body releasing histamine in the area of the injury. But histamine has many other functions as well. One important action is the regulation of acid production by the stomach.

How can one substance function so differently? Histamine attaches to receptors within the area that it's released, and the response that occurs is a function of the type of receptor present. The allergic reaction is mediated by histamine$_1$ receptors, and drugs used to treat the reaction are called *antihistamines* or *histamine$_1$ blocking agents*. The release of stomach acid is mediated by another set of histamine receptors called *histamine$_2$ receptors*. Scientists have developed drugs that can effectively block these receptors and dramatically reduce the stomach's ability to secrete acid.

What are histamine$_2$-receptor antagonists used for?

- To reduce stomach acid secretion
- To treat ulcers
- To treat certain hypersecretory conditions such as Zollinger-Ellison syndrome
- To prevent gastrointestinal bleeding in critically ill patients
- To treat gastroesophageal reflux disease

What are some commonly used histamine$_2$-receptor antagonists?

- cimetidine, known by the brand name Tagamet
- famotidine, known by the brand name Pepcid
- nizatidine, known by the brand name Axid
- ranitidine, known by the brand name Zantac

What are the possible side effects?

- Headache, dizziness; confusion or agitation, although rare, may occur in elderly or critically ill patients
- Muscle pain
- Nausea, diarrhea or constipation
- Skin rashes, itching
- Breast tenderness

What are the guidelines for taking histamine$_2$-receptor antagonists?

- Make sure your doctor knows about all of the other drugs you are taking, including nonprescription drugs. Some of these histamine$_2$-receptor antagonists can interfere with the way your body metabolizes certain drugs. Your doctor may need to adjust the dosage of these other drugs while you're taking the histamine$_2$-receptor antagonist.
- If your doctor tells you to take antacids, be sure to separate doses of the two drugs by at least 1 hour. Antacids can interfere with the absorption of other drugs.
- Be aware that for maximum effectiveness, you need to complete the full course of therapy.
- Take a missed dose as soon as you remember. However, if it's almost time for your next dose, omit the missed dose and resume the regular schedule with the next dose. Don't take a double dose.
- Watch for and immediately report any signs of bleeding disorders: easy bruising, bloody stools, or bloody vomit. Also report any other side effects.
- During the initial part of therapy, avoid driving or other potentially hazardous activities that require good coordination and alertness until the side effects of the drug on your central nervous system are known.
- Avoid smoking. Smoking causes the stomach to increase acid production, thereby worsening the disease.
- Avoid other substances that irritate the gastrointestinal tract, including alcohol, hot drinks, caffeine-containing products, and aspirin.

CHOLINERGIC BLOCKERS

Also known as *anticholinergics*, cholinergic blockers are among the most widely used drugs. These agents block the effects of the neurotransmitter acetylcholine on many organ systems, including the heart, digestive tract, and brain.

What are cholinergic blockers used for?
- To reduce stomach acid secretion and intestinal motility
- To prevent motion sickness

What are some commonly used cholinergic blockers?
- anisotropine, known by the brand name Valpin 50
- atropine (generic)
- belladonna elixir (generic)
- clidinium bromide, known by the brand name Quarzan
- dicyclomine, known by the brand name Antispas, Bentyl, Spasmoject
- glycopyrrolate, known by the brand name Robinul
- isopropamide, known by the brand name Darbid
- methantheline, known by the brand name Banthine
- propantheline, known by the brand name Pro-Banthine
- scopolamine (generic)

What are the possible side effects?
- Headache, restlessness, dizziness, disorientation, hallucinations, confusion, insomnia
- Increased heart rate, palpitations, chest pain
- Dry mouth, thirst, constipation, nausea, vomiting
- Urinary hesitancy, urine retention
- Hot, flushed skin
- Widened pupils, blurred vision, sensitivity to light

What are the guidelines for taking cholinergic blockers?
- Watch for side effects and report them to your doctor, who may want to reduce the dosage.
- During therapy with a cholinergic blocker, be alert for palpitations and rapid heart rate. If the drug makes it difficult for you to urinate,

During therapy with a cholinergic blocker, be alert for palpitations and rapid heart rate. If the drug makes it difficult for you to urinate, call your doctor who may recommend that you urinate before taking a dose.

call your doctor who may recommend that you urinate before taking a dose.

- Make sure your doctor knows about all other medications you're taking, including nonprescription medicines. Don't take any other drugs without checking with him or her first.
- Don't take anticholinergics with antacids and absorbent antidiarrheals such as Kaopectate because they may decrease the absorption and reduce the therapeutic effects of anticholinergics.
- Avoid overexertion in hot or humid weather. These drugs decrease sweating and may cause your body temperature to rise, possibly leading to heatstroke. Watch for and report early signs of heatstroke, such as fever, confusion, and dry skin and mucous membranes.
- Immediately report any abdominal pain, distention, or constipation.
- These drugs may cause dizziness, confusion, and visual problems. Avoid potentially hazardous activities that require alertness and coordination until your response to the drug has been determined. Elderly patients should take special care to remove objects that could cause falls, such as footstools and throw rugs.
- Avoid alcohol and depressant drugs (such as tranquilizers), which increase these drugs' sedative effects.
- Treat dry mouth with frequent sips of water, ice chips, sugarless gum, or hard candy.
- Take the drug as prescribed, generally 30 minutes to 1 hour before meals.

LAXATIVES

When used correctly, laxatives are safe and effective. Most are available for use without a prescription.

Laxatives may be bulk-forming agents, saline laxatives, stool softeners, hyperosmolar agents, lubricants, or stimulants.

- *Bulk-forming laxatives* (psyllium and methylcellulose) absorb water and expand, increasing the bulk and fluid content of stools. The increased bulk stimulates a bowel movement.
- *Stool softeners* (docusate salts) act like soaps and reduce the surface tension of bowel contents. This detergent activity increases the water content of the stools, forming a softer mass.

- *Hyperosmolar laxatives* (glycerin and lactulose) draw water into the colon, increasing bulk and promoting a bowel movement. They act rapidly, usually within 30 minutes to 12 hours.
- *Saline laxatives* (magnesium salts and sodium phosphates) also draw water into the intestine, producing distention and stimuating a bowel movement. Because they are ingested in large quantities, they actually clean out the bowels by producing large amounts of watery stools. Typically, the onset of action occurs soon after ingestion, usually within 30 minutes to 12 hours.
- *Lubricant laxatives* (mineral oils) create a barrier between the colon wall and the fecal mass, allowing the colon to transport stools more easily.
- *Stimulant laxatives* (bisacodyl, cascara sagrada, castor oil, senna, and phenolphthalein) stimulate the colon's smooth muscle directly. This results in increased propulsion of stools through the colon.

What are laxatives used for?

- Bulk-forming laxatives are generally considered mild laxatives that are use to treat chronic constipation.
- Stool softeners are also mild laxatives that are used to prevent constipation and straining during defecation. Many doctors prescribe these drugs when the patient may be at risk for developing constipation; risk factors include sudden immobility or the accompanying use of certain drugs such as narcotics.
- Hyperosmolar agents, such as glycerin and magnesium salts, treat constipation.
- Saline laxatives are used to prepare the bowel for diagnostic or surgical procedures.
- Lubricants, such as mineral oil, and stimulants, such as castor oil or senna, are also used to treat constipation.

What are some commonly used laxatives?

Bulk-forming agents

- calcium polycarbophil, known by the brand names Equalactin, Fiberall, FiberCon, FiberLax, and Mitrolan
- methylcellulose, known by the brand names Citrucel and Cologel

Saline laxatives

- magnesium citrate, known by the brand names Citroma and Citro-Nesia
- magnesium hydroxide, known by the brand names Milk of Magnesia and M.O.M.

- magnesium sulfate, known as epsom salts (generic)
- polyethylene glycol-electrolyte solution, known by the brand names CoLyte and GoLYTELY
- sodium phosphates, known by the brand name Fleet Phospho-Soda

Stool softeners
- docusate calcium, known by the brand names Pro-Cal-Sof and Surfak
- docusate potassium, known by the brand names Dialose, Diocto-K, and Kasof
- docusate sodium, known by the brand names Colace, Diocto, Dio-Sul, Doss 300, D-S-S

Hyperosmolar agents
- glycerin, known by the brand names Fleet Babylax and Sani-Supp
- lactulose, known by the brand names Cephulac, Duphalac, and (in Canada) Lactulax

Lubricants
- castor oil, known by the brand names Alphamul, Neoloid, and Purge
- mineral oil, known by the brand names Agoral Plain and Kondremul Plain

Stimulants
- bisacodyl, known by the brand names Bisco-Lax, Dulcolax, Theralax, and (in Canada) Laxit
- phenolphthalein, white, known by the brand names Alophen Pills and Modane
- phenolphthalein, yellow, known by the brand names Evac-U-Gen, Evac-U-Lax, Ex-Lax, and Feen-A-Mint Gum
- psyllium, known by the brands name Metamucil, Naturacil, and Perdiem Plain
- senna, known by the brand names Black Draught, Senokot, and X-Prep Liquid

What are the possible side effects?
- Most laxatives can cause nausea, vomiting, abdominal cramps, and diarrhea; overuse can cause fluid or electrolyte depletion.
- Excessive or long-term use may cause laxative dependence, a condition where you can't produce a bowel movement without using laxatives.

- Bulk-forming laxatives may cause gas; they can also cause intestinal obstruction or fecal impaction.
- Stimulant laxatives may cause intestinal cramps or increased mucus secretion.
- Saline laxatives can cause nausea and vomiting.

What are the guidelines for taking laxatives?

- Children and elderly people should use laxatives cautiously. If you ever question whether or not you can safely use a laxative, call your doctor.
- If you experience fever, rapid heart rate, dizziness or weakness, decreased urine output, or extreme thirst, stop taking the laxative and call your doctor.
- If you're taking other prescription medicines, check with your doctor before taking a laxative. If your prescription medicine causes constipation, he or she may switch you to another drug.
- Lubricant laxatives should not be taken with or immediately after meals because they delay passage of food from the stomach. Take lubricant laxatives on an empty stomach.
- Don't take oral drugs within 2 hours of taking a hyperosmolar laxative.
- Don't take a laxative if you are experiencing abdominal pain, nausea, or vomiting. These symptoms may indicate the presence of a serious condition that laxatives may worsen.
- Drink 6 to 8 glasses of water a day while taking these drugs.
- Tell the doctor if you don't have a bowel movement after taking the laxative as prescribed.
- You should understand that a daily bowel movement isn't essential to good health; it's more important to maintain a consistent pattern of elimination. Don't overuse laxatives — this may lead to dependence.
- Use alternative ways to prevent constipation, such as regular exercise and adequate fluid and fiber intake. Good dietary sources of fiber include bran and other cereals, fresh fruits, and vegetables.
- If your doctor prescribes polyethylene glycol-electrolyte solution to prepare you for a diagnostic test, understand that you'll need to drink approximately 1 gallon (4 liters) of fluid over about 3 hours. This drug will induce watery diarrhea within 30 to 60 minutes after ingestion that will clean the bowel and allow the doctor to visualize abnormalities in the intestine clearly.

If you experience fever, rapid heart rate, dizziness or weakness, decreased urine output, or extreme thirst, stop taking the laxative and call your doctor.

ANTIEMETICS

Antiemetics help control nausea and vomiting. The doctor will choose the right antiemetic for you based on what's causing your vomiting.

Vomiting may be a normal response. For example, drugs, poisons, or toxins produced by viruses and bacteria may act within the digestive tract to trigger the vomiting reflex. Other toxins may actually act within areas of the brain that control this response. Vomitng may also be caused by nontoxic stimuli. For example, motion sickness arises from excessive stimulation of certain sensory nerve endings within the inner ear.

There are several different types of antiemetics, and the correct drug choice will largely depend on the suspected cause of vomiting. For example, drugs used to treat motion sickness interfere with the transmission of signals from the inner ear to the vomiting center of the brain. Other potent antiemetics block the vomiting center in the brain. And some of the newer drugs used to prevent nausea and vomiting associated with cancer therapy act both in the gastrointestinal tract and the brain.

What are antiemetics used for?
These medications prevent or control nausea and vomiting.

What are some commonly used antiemetics?
Phenothiazines
- prochlorperazine, known by the brand names Compazine and Stemetil
- promethazine hydrochloride, known by the brand name Phenergan
- thiethylperazine maleate, known by the brand names Norzine and Torecan
- trimethobenzamide hydrochloride, known by the brand names Tebamide, Ticon, and Tigan

Cannabinoids
- dronabinol, known by the brand name Marinol

Serotonin antagonists
- ondansetron hydrochloride, known by the brand name Zofran

Miscellaneous agents
- benzquinamide, known by the brand name Emete-Con

- buclizine, known by the brand name Bucladin-S
- cyclizine, known by the brand name Marezine
- dimenhydrinate, known by the brand names Dommanate, Dramamine, Apo-Dimenhydrinate, and Nauseatol
- diphenidol, known by the brand name Vontrol
- meclizine, known by the brand names Antivert and Bonine
- metoclopramide, known by the brand names Reglan and Maxeran
- scopolamine, known by the brand name Tranderm-Scop

What are the possible side effects?

Phenothiazines
- Sedation, dizziness
- Low blood pressure
- Movement disorders
- Dry mouth
- Blurred vision
- Constipation
- Urine retention

Cannabinoids
- Rapid heart rate
- Dizziness
- Euphoria, muddled thinking, or psychotic episodes
- High abuse potential

Serotinin antagonists
- Headache

Miscellaneous agents
- Sedation, dizziness
- Dry mouth
- Urine retention

What are the guidelines for taking antiemetics?

- Don't take other drugs without first checking with your doctor. Because antacids interfere with phenothiazine absorption, the two shouldn't be given within 2 hours of each other. Avoid alcohol and over-the-counter preparations, such as cough and cold remedies or sleeping pills, which cause central nervous system depression.
- Promptly report chest pain, palpitations, or persistent headache.

Some antiemetics cause drowsiness and dizziness. Don't drive or perform any task requiring alertness until your response to the drug has been determined.

- Some antiemetics cause drowsiness and dizziness. Don't drive or perform any task requiring alertness until your response to the drug has been determined.
- Minimize dizziness by rising slowly from a sitting or lying position and by avoiding sudden bending or reaching. Be careful if you take hot showers.
- Chew sugarless gum, suck hard candy, or rinse with a mouthwash that doesn't contain alcohol if you experience problems with dry mouth.
- If you're taking a phenothiazine, use a sunscreen and wear protective clothing when outdoors. These drugs may increase your susceptibility to severe sunburn.

ANTIDIARRHEALS

Many people suffer from occasional bouts of diarrhea. There are a number of causes, including changes in diet, drug therapy, or infection.

In many cases, diarrhea is self-limiting and temporary, and it's often a symptom of some underlying illness. When poisons accumulate in the digestive tract, diarrhea may be an effective way for the body to rapidly eliminate them. Doctors often consider this when deciding whether or not to treat diarrhea.

What are antidiarrheals used for?
These medications treat acute, mild, or chronic stages of nonspecific diarrhea.

What are some commonly used antidiarrheals?
- difenoxin with atropine sulfate, known by the brand name Motofen
- diphenoxylate with atropine sulfate, known by the brand names Diphenatol, Lomotil, and Nor-Mil
- loperamide, known by the brand names Imodium and Imodium A-D
- paregoric (also known as camphorated tincture of opium)

What are the possible side effects?
- Dryness of the skin, lips, mouth, and throat
- Flushing

- Fever
- Rapid heart rate
- Urine retention
- Nausea, vomiting, dry mouth
- Dizziness, drowsiness
- Allergic reactions
- Constipation
- Intestinal blockage in patients with colon disease

What are the guidelines for taking antidiarrheals?

- You should avoid using antidiarrheals if you have a colon disease such as ulcerative colitis.
- If your diarrhea is the result of food, drug, or other poisoning, you should seek medical attention immediately. Don't take antidiarrheal drugs because they inhibit elimination of toxins from the gastrointestinal tract.
- Because they are opium derivatives, persons with a history of opioid dependence shouldn't use these drugs.
- Call your doctor if you suffer from fever, abdominal pain, bloody stools, dizziness, or other central nervous system effects. Certain side effects are especially severe in children, elderly patients, and patients with impaired kidney or liver function.
- Never exceed the prescribed dosage; doing so could produce drowsiness or other central nervous system side effects.
- Keep an accurate record of the amount and consistency of all stools and notify your doctor if no improvement occurs within 48 hours of starting drug therapy or if you have a fever.
- Maintain adequate fluid intake during treatment. Drinking fluids will not worsen your diarrhea. Rather, it helps replace the large amount of fluid lost in diarrhea.

SURGERIES

ESOPHAGEAL SURGERY

Esophageal surgery is rarely performed on adults and has major potential for serious complications. It may be performed to manage an emergency or to relieve serious symptoms associated with disease of the esophagus. Typically, esophageal surgery is attempted only after conservative measures or attempts to dilate the esophagus fail to produce results. Cancer of the esophagus is usually far advanced when it's diagnosed. Therefore, therapy usually consists of laser and radiation treatment and aims to relieve symptoms rather than to cure the disease. Radical surgery, while uncommon, is the only hope for a cure.

Esophageal surgery is done to remove an esophageal obstruction, repair traumatic damage to the esophagus, correct a problem in which food or digestive juices reverse from the stomach to the esophagus, or relieve a severe tightening of the esophagus.

Why is this surgery done?

Esophageal surgery is done to remove an esophageal obstruction, repair traumatic damage to the esophagus, correct a problem in which food or digestive juices reverse from the stomach to the esophagus, or relieve a severe tightening of the esophagus.

In an adult, esophageal surgery may be performed to treat a tear in the wall of the esophagus, usually from a traumatic injury. This is a surgical emergency. Esophageal surgery may also be warranted when food is unable to move from the esophagus to the stomach, when severe symptoms occur from weakening in the wall of the esophagus and caustic injuries such as those caused by ingestion of lye. Radical surgery to attempt a cure for esophageal cancer may be performed on certain people.

What happens before the surgery?

- The doctor or nurse will explain the surgery and what will happen before and afterward to you.
- If you are malnourished because of difficulty eating, you'll receive a high-protein, high-calorie, soft diet. If you can't tolerate oral feedings, you'll be fed through a tube in the stomach or a vein.
- You'll receive intravenous fluids and electrolytes, if necessary.
- You or a responsible family member will sign a consent form.

What happens during the surgery?

Surgery to increase the ability of food to move from the esophagus to the stomach requires an incision into the muscle that separates the esophagus from the stomach. This incision may be in the chest or stomach. Surgery to improve the ability of food to move from the throat to the esophagus requires an incision in the muscle at the top of the esophagus. Surgery to prevent food or digestive juices from reversing from the stomach up to the esophagus requires an incision on the lower end of the esophagus and stomach.

Esophagectomy, which removes the diseased or damaged part of the esophagus and then connects the remaining portions of the esophagus, may be necessary to remove esophageal cancer or fix tightening of the esophagus or a weakening in its wall. Radical esophageal surgery is most often attempted to remove tumors in the lower and middle esophagus. If insufficient esophageal tissue remains after removal of a large section of the esophagus, several procedures may be used to restore its function. In the most common procedure, the diseased portion of the esophagus is removed and the remaining segment is connected to the stomach. This procedure requires an incision into both the chest and abdomen.

What are the possible complications?

Esophageal surgery has the potential for causing serious complications. For example, radical surgery may result in leakage at the place where the end of the remaining esophagus was connected. The area between the lungs may become inflamed from food or stomach juices leaking into it. Severe inflammation can produce obstruction of large veins, the windpipe, and the esophagus. Hemorrhage, respiratory infection, and wound infection may also occur. If food and stomach contents continue to reverse up the esophagus after surgery, they can go into the breathing tube and cause pneumonia.

What happens after the surgery?

- You'll lie with your head elevated to reduce the likelihood of food and stomach contents reversing up your esophagus and going into your lungs.
- Your nurse will encourage you to turn, cough, and perform deep-breathing exercises.
- You'll receive pain medication as prescribed by your doctor.
- The nurse will monitor you closely for signs of complications, including fever, shortness of breath, signs of shock, and complaints of chest pain. Such symptoms will be reported to the doctor immediately.
- Your blood count will be checked regularly.
- You won't be able to eat or drink by mouth for several days after surgery but will be fed intravenously or through a tube in your stomach. After several days, you'll begin oral feedings with small amounts of water and gradually resume your diet as you're able to tolerate it.
- The nurse may refer you to community or home health care agencies as needed, especially after extensive surgery. When appropriate,

SELF-HELP

Recovering from esophageal surgery

After you've been discharged from the hospital, keep in mind the following.

Protect the esophagus
- Follow the instructions you received in the hospital about how to care for your incision and watch for signs of infection.
- If you smoke, you should try to stop. Nicotine has a detrimental effect on the muscle that prevents food from reversing from the stomach up to the esophagus.
- Avoid alcohol, aspirin, and effervescent over-the-counter products (such as Alka-Seltzer) because they may damage your tender esophagus.

- Avoid heavy lifting, straining, and coughing, which could rupture the weakened lining of your esophagus.

Other instructions
- Try to sleep with your head elevated to prevent stomach contents from reversing to the esophagus. You can use a wedge under your mattress or raise the head of the bed on blocks.
- Be alert for signs of breathing problems, such as wheezing, coughing, or shortness of breath at night. If they occur, report these symptoms to your doctor.
- Eat a high-protein, high-calorie, soft diet in frequent, small feedings if you had extensive surgery.

you and your family may also be informed about supportive organizations such as the American Cancer Society. (See *Recovering from esophageal surgery.*)

HERNIA REPAIR

A hernia repair corrects the protrusion of an organ through a weak area of muscle by herniorrhaphy or hernioplasty. *Herniorrhaphy,* the preferred surgery for inguinal and other abdominal hernias, returns the protruding intestine to the abdominal cavity and repairs the defect in the abdominal wall. *Hernioplasty,* which is used to correct more extensive hernias, reinforces the weakened area around the repair with plastic, steel, or tantalum mesh or wire.

Hernias of the abdominal wall may be inguinal, femoral, epigastric, umbilical, or incisional. *Inguinal hernia,* protrusion of part of the intestines through the inguinal canal (where the testicles descend to the scrotum), occurs in about 2% of adult males. *Femoral hernia* is protrusion of part of the intestine through the area where the femoral artery and vein pass from the abdomen to the thigh. *Epigastric hernia* results from a weakness in the upper abdominal muscles that allows the intestine to protrude through an area between the navel (umbilicus) and the breastbone. An *umbilical hernia* causes the intestine to protrude through the abdominal wall near the navel. *Incisional hernias* may appear after surgery involving the abdominal wall.

The protruding intestine may become trapped and twisted within the hernia and its blood supply may be diminished or cut off. This condition is known as a *strangulated* or *incarcerated hernia* and can lead to gangrene if not corrected surgically.

Hernia repairs may be performed on an outpatient basis with local anesthesia. Performed as an inpatient procedure, hernia repair usually requires a 3- to 5-day hospitalization.

Why is this surgery done?

Hernia repair returns the herniated organ to its original position and corrects the underlying defect in the muscle wall. Surgical repair is necessary when the herniated organ is painful and cannot be pushed back into place. If the intestine becomes strangulated or incarcerated, emergency surgery is required.

What happens before the surgery?

- Your doctor or nurse will explain the procedure to you.
- You or a responsible family member will sign a consent form.
- Your nurse will shave the surgical site and give you an enema to clean out your bowels.
- You'll receive a sedative.

What happens during the surgery?

Herniorrhaphy is performed under local, spinal, or general anesthesia, depending on your general state of health. After making an abdominal incision, the surgeon pushes the herniated organ back into the abdomen and repairs and strengthens the weakened area of the abdominal wall with sutures. A large hernia may require a hernioplasty. In this procedure, the abdominal wall is reinforced with plastic, steel, or tantalum mesh or wire. After the repair, the surgeon closes the incision and applies a bandage.

What are the possible complications?

Hernia repair is typically done quickly and produces few complications and minimal pain and bleeding after the surgery. The hernia recurs in 10% to 20% of people who've had hernia surgery.

SELF-HELP

Caring for yourself after a hernia repair

After you've been discharged from the hospital, keep in mind the following:

- Follow your surgeon's instructions to avoid lifting, bending, and pushing or pulling movement.
- Typically, you can resume your previous activities within 4 to 6 weeks.
- Watch for and notify your doctor of signs of infection, including fever, chills, sweating, and sleepiness as well as pain, inflammation, swelling, and drainage at the site of the incision.
- Keep follow-up appointments with your doctor.

What happens after the surgery?

- The nurse will monitor your vital signs until you're stable.
- You'll be taught how to get up from a lying or sitting position without straining your abdomen and how to protect the incision when you cough or sneeze.
- You'll be encouraged to walk soon after the procedure but warned against bending, lifting, or other strenuous activities. (See *Caring for yourself after a hernia repair*.)
- The nurse will check your incision for excessive bleeding, swelling, and inflammation and will report to the surgeon if these symptoms occur.
- You'll receive pain medication as ordered by your doctor.
- The nurse will administer a stool softener, if prescribed by your doctor, to prevent straining during defecation.

Stomach Resection

Stomach resection (removal of part of the stomach) can take various forms, depending on the location and extent of the disease. Names of stomach surgeries (except vagotomy) usually refer to the stomach portion removed. A partial gastrectomy (stomach removal) may be performed to reduce the amount of acid secreted by the stomach. A vagotomy may be performed to relieve ulcer symptoms by eliminating stimulation of stomach acid by the vagus nerve. A pyloroplasty may be performed to improve passage of food and stomach juices into the duodenum (the first part of the intestine) and prevent blockage.

Stomach resection for cancer depends on the extent of tumor involvement. Extensive tumors may be treated with total removal of the stomach and spleen because the splenic lymph nodes are a major site of cancer spread. The overall 5-year survival rate after stomach resection for cancer is about 12%.

Why is this surgery done?

Stomach resection is performed to control bleeding in the upper gastrointestinal tract by repairing a broken blood vessel or removing a bleeding area, to remove ulcerous or cancerous areas of the stomach, to reduce stomach acid production by removing those portions

Dumping syndrome

After stomach resection, rapid emptying of stomach contents into the small intestine produces dumping syndrome.

Early dumping syndrome

Early dumping syndrome, which may be mild or severe, occurs a few minutes after eating and lasts up to 45 minutes. Onset is sudden, with nausea, weakness, sweating, palpitations, dizziness, flushing, a rumbling noise from movement of gas through the intestines, explosive diarrhea, and increased blood pressure and heart rate.

Late dumping syndrome

Less serious than early dumping syndrome, late dumping syndrome occurs 2 to 3 hours after eating. Symptoms include profuse sweating, anxiety, tremor of the hands and legs accompanied by a sensation of spinning, exhaustion, palpitations, a throbbing headache, urine glucose, and a marked decrease in blood pressure and blood sugar.

These symptoms may persist for one year after surgery or for the rest of the person's life.

of the stomach that produce acid, or to relieve a blockage of the stomach.

Stomach resection may be necessary to remove diseased areas and prevent recurrence of ulcers if the disease doesn't respond to drug and dietary therapy and rest. In an emergency, it may be performed to control severe gastrointestinal bleeding resulting from a perforated ulcer. Additionally, stomach resection may be performed to remove foreign objects or stomach polyps (if they can't be removed by non-surgical techniques).

What happens before the surgery?

- The nurse will prepare you for surgery, depending on the nature of operation.
- If you have a stomach blockage, you may require several days' preparation to correct dehydration and fluid and electrolyte imbalance. A tube that goes through your nose to the stomach will be used to clean out your stomach.
- The nurse will insert an intravenous catheter to provide fluids and nourishment.
- On the night before surgery, your nurse may give you a laxative or an enema to clean out your bowels.
- As time permits, your doctor or nurse will explain the procedure and what will happen afterward to you.
- You or a responsible family member will sign a consent form.

Caring for yourself after a stomach resection

After you've been discharged from the hospital, follow the important guidelines below.

Know when to call your doctor
- Call your doctor immediately if you experience nausea, vomiting, or pain because these may indicate possible life-threatening complications, such as hemorrhaging, blockage, or tearing of the stomach.
- Promptly report to your doctor any fatigue, numbness, or tingling of the extremities; these symptoms may indicate a vitamin B$_{12}$ deficiency.

Other instructions
- To avoid dumping syndrome, eat small, frequent meals at regular intervals throughout the day; chew food thoroughly and drink fluids between meals — not with them; decrease intake of carbohydrates and salt while increasing fat and protein; and lie down for 20 to 30 minutes after a meal.
- Make sure you know the dose, schedule, and effects of drugs prescribed by your doctor and take them as ordered.

What happens during the surgery?

After you receive a general anesthetic, the surgeon will make an abdominal incision to expose the stomach and part of the intestine. Removal of the entire stomach requires a more extensive incision.

The rest of the procedure varies depending on the type of surgery. To complete the operation, the surgeon inserts abdominal tubes that permit drainage of fluids that accumulate after surgery, closes the incision, and applies a bandage.

What are the possible complications?

Stomach surgery carries a risk of serious complications, including hemorrhage, blockage, reduced bowel movement, anemia, incomplete filling of the lungs with air, chronic gastroparesis (delayed emptying of the stomach contents), and dumping syndrome. (See *Dumping syndrome*, page 151).

What happens after the surgery?

- After you've recovered from anesthesia, you'll lie with your head elevated to ease breathing and, if vomiting occurs, to prevent it from entering the lungs.
- The nurse will check your vital signs every 2 hours until your condition stabilizes.
- You'll be watched for signs of hemorrhage and shock. The incision tube that goes from your nose to your stomach and the abdominal drainage tubes will be checked for bleeding.
- You'll receive fluid and nourishment intravenously.
- The nurse will weigh you regularly and measure your intake of fluids and output of urine and other drainage.
- As you begin to recover, you'll begin taking nourishment by mouth and the tube going from your nose to your stomach will be removed.
- Throughout recovery the nurse will encourage you to cough, breathe deeply, and change position frequently. (See *Caring for yourself after a stomach resection*.)

BOWEL SURGERY WITH OSTOMY

An ostomy involves the resection of diseased sections of the colon and rectum and the creation of a stoma (intestinal opening) on the abdominal surface. Feces that would normally pass through the bowel are excreted through the stoma and safely collected in a specially designed surgical appliance.

Several surgical approaches may be used to create an ostomy, which is also known as a *colostomy* if it involves the large intestine or an *enterostomy* (ileostomy or jejunostomy) if it involves the small intestine.

An ostomy may be temporary or permanent. A temporary ostomy interrupts the intestinal flow to allow healing of inflamed or injured bowel segments. After healing occurs, usually within 10 weeks, the divided segments are reconnected to restore bowel integrity and function.

Permanent colostomies typically accompany a procedure that involves both an abdominal operation and a second incision and operation in the rectal area for removal of the remaining colon, rectum, and anus.

Severe, widespread obstruction of the colon or intractable inflammatory bowel disease may require total or near-total removal of the colon and rectum and creation of an ileostomy. A permanent ileostomy requires you to wear a drainage pouch over the stoma to collect the constant fecal drainage. In contrast, a Kock's (or continent) ileostomy doesn't require an external pouch. Connection of the ileum to the anus eliminates the need for a permanent ileostomy, establishes an ileal reservoir, and maintains elimination through the anal sphincter.

Why is this surgery done?

Bowel surgery with ostomy is performed to remove diseased sections of the colon and rectum and to create a stoma through the abdominal wall for the elimination of feces. This surgery is commonly performed for a variety of conditions, including inflammatory bowel disease, diverticulitis, and penetrating trauma. It is performed for advanced colorectal cancer if conservative surgery and other treatments fail or if the person develops acute complications, such as an obstruction or abscess.

What happens before the surgery?

- Your doctor or nurse will explain the procedure, including the type of ostomy you'll have and how feces will drain through it.
- You'll be reassured that after becoming comfortable with ostomy management, you should be able to resume normal activity with few restrictions.
- Your nutritional status will be carefully monitored. Typically, you'll receive intravenous nutrition to prepare for the stress of surgery. Your fluid intake and urine output will be measured and you'll be weighed daily. Your blood count will be checked frequently and transfusions given if necessary.
- If possible, arrangements will be made for you to meet with other people who have ostomies (from groups such as the United Ostomy Association) before surgery; these people can share their personal insights into the realities of living with and caring for a stoma.
- If you've been receiving cortisone therapy, it'll be continued before surgery but will be withdrawn gradually after the procedure. You may also receive antibiotics before surgery.

What happens during the surgery?

This surgery is performed in an operating room. You'll be given general anesthesia. The type of ostomy involved depends on the nature and location of the problem. (See *Reviewing types of ostomies* and *Types of ostomy surgery*, page 156.)

What are the possible complications?

Common complications of ostomy procedures include hemorrhage, infection of the bloodstream, obstruction of the intestines, and fluid and electrolyte imbalance from excessive drainage through the stoma. Inflammation of the membrane lining of the abdomen can also complicate recovery. Rarely, the bowel may push out of the abdominal cavity through the stoma and require surgery to replace it. Skin abrasion may occur around the stoma from contact with digestive enzymes in the drainage; irritation may result from the pressure of the ostomy drainage bag or pouch. Abrasion occurs more commonly with an ileostomy because of the higher concentration of digestive juices in ileal drainage.

What happens after the surgery?

- The nurse will measure your fluid intake and urine output, weigh you daily, and watch for signs of dehydration.

Reviewing types of ostomies

The type of ostomy depends on the person's condition. Temporary ones, such as a double-barrel or loop colostomy, help treat perforated diverticulitis, penetrating injury, and other conditions in which intestinal healing is expected. Temporary ostomies are also used to bypass an inoperable intestinal tumor. Permanent colostomy or ileostomy typically accompanies extensive abdominal surgery, often for removal of a malignant tumor.

PERMANENT COLOSTOMY

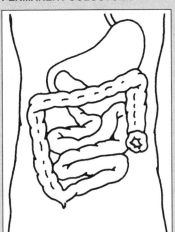

LOOP COLOSTOMY

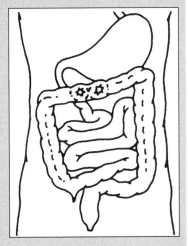

DOUBLE-BARREL COLOSTOMY

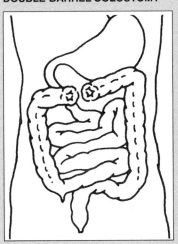

ILEOSTOMY

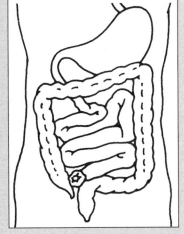

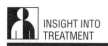

Types of ostomy surgery

Four types of ostomy surgery are described below.

Abdominoperineal resection

The surgeon makes a lower abdominal incision, divides the colon, and then brings the upper end of the colon out through another, smaller abdominal incision to create a permanent colostomy. Next, the surgeon makes a wide incision near the anus and resects the anus, rectum, and lower portion of the colon. After placing one or more drainage tubes in the abdomen and closing the abdominal wound, the anal wound is either left open and packed with gauze or is closed and several drainage tubes are placed in the closed wound.

Temporary loop colostomy

The surgeon brings a portion of intestine out through an abdominal incision, slips an ostomy bridge (a short plastic or glass rod) under the intestinal loop to support it on the outer abdominal wall, cuts into the intestine to create a temporary stoma (opening), and

then closes the wound around the exposed intestinal loop.

Temporary double-barrel colostomy

The surgeon divides the colon and brings both ends through an abdominal incision to create a proximal stoma for fecal drainage and a distal stoma leading to the inactive bowel. After inserting abdominal sump drains, the surgeon closes the incision around the stomas. Later, when the intestinal injury has healed or the inflammation has subsided, the loop or double-barrel temporary colostomy is discontinued, and the divided ends of the colon are reconnected to restore bowel integrity.

Ileostomy

The surgeon resects all or part of the colon and rectum and creates a permanent ileostomy by bringing a loop of the ileum out through a small abdominal incision. Typically, the incision is located in the right lower abdomen.

- The nurse will give you pain medication as ordered by your doctor.
- The nurse will carefully note the color, consistency, and odor of fecal drainage from the stoma. Excessive blood or mucus content, which could indicate hemorrhage or infection, are reported to the doctor.
- You'll be watched closely for signs of infection.
- Your incision will be kept clean and the bandage will be changed frequently.
- The nurse will check the stoma and the surrounding skin regularly for irritation and abrasion, which may result from contact with fecal drainage or from pressure caused by an overfilled or improperly fitted drainage pouch. (See *Recovering from ostomy surgery.*) Such problems will be corrected.
- You may feel anxious or depressed. These reactions should fade with adjustment to the ostomy. A counselor who's specially trained to work with people with ostomies will visit you if possible.

SELF-HELP

Recovering from ostomy surgery

When you've been discharged from the hospital after bowel surgery with an ostomy, keep in mind the following guidelines.

Avoid fluid loss

- Maintain a high fluid intake to help ensure fluid and electrolyte balance. This is especially important in times of increased fluid loss; for example, during periods of hot weather or bouts of diarrhea.
- Avoid alcohol, laxatives, and diuretics, which will increase fluid loss and may contribute to a fluid imbalance.
- If you experience persistent diarrhea through the stoma, notify your doctor.

Other points to remember

- Make sure you follow the instructions you received at the hospital regarding care of the stoma and surrounding area, application and removal of drainage bags, and recommended dietary modifications to prevent stoma blockage, diarrhea, gas, and offensive odor.
- If you have an incision in the rectal area, soaking in a tub of warm or hot water will help relieve the discomfort. You should avoid intercourse until the incision heals.
- Depression is common after ostomy surgery. Speak with a counselor if the feeling is severe or persists.

- You'll receive extensive instructions about care of the stoma and dietary recommendations. The nurse will show you how to apply, remove, and empty the drainage bag and, when appropriate, how to flush a colostomy with warm tap water to gain some control over elimination.

BOWEL RESECTION

This surgical procedure removes diseased portions of an intestine and then anastomoses (reconnects) the remaining edges of the intestine. If part of the large intestine is removed, the procedure is termed a *colectomy;* if part of the small intestine is removed, it's termed an *enterectomy.* Whenever possible, the surgeon will perform resection (removal) with reconnection to preserve bowel continuity. In some cases, particularly when there is not enough healthy intestine to reconnect, a temporary or permanent colostomy or ileostomy may be necessary.

Unlike people who undergo total colectomy or more extensive surgery, the person who has a simple resection and reconnection of the bowel usually retains normal bowel function.

Why is this surgery performed?

Bowel resection is done to remove diseased portions of the bowel and join the remaining segments to restore bowel integrity and function. Bowel resection and reconnection helps treat localized conditions that result in blockage of the bowel, including diverticulosis (with an area of acute diverticulitis, constriction, or abscess formation), intestinal polyps, and malignant or benign intestinal tumors.

This procedure is preferred for localized bowel cancer but not for widespread cancer, which usually requires creation of a temporary or permanent colostomy or an ileostomy. Bowel resection may also be used to remove the diseased segment of the bowel in inflammatory disorders of the bowel, such as Crohn's disease or colitis, when medical intervention fails to control the problem.

What happens before surgery?

▪ Your doctor or nurse will explain the procedure to you along with its potential risks and complications.

▪ You'll be informed that you'll wake up with a tube in your nose to drain air and fluid from the intestinal tract. The tube is usually removed within 2 to 3 days.

▪ The nurse will tell you that you'll begin walking the first day after surgery to help regain normal function of the intestines.

▪ You'll also be told to expect to have a tube coming out of the incision to drain fluids that accumulate after surgery, a urinary catheter, and an intravenous line, which will provide fluid replacement.

▪ To reduce the risk of lung complications after surgery, the nurse will teach you how to cough and deep-breathe properly. You'll be shown how to protect your stitches and reduce discomfort during coughing.

▪ Just before surgery, the nurse will administer antibiotics to reduce intestinal bacteria and laxatives or enemas to remove feces.

What happens during the surgery?

The surgeon performs the procedure after you're given a general anesthetic. The abdominal incision site varies depending on the site of the disease. Once the incision is made, the surgeon will remove the diseased portion of the colon and then connect the remaining healthy bowel segments to restore continuity.

If surgery is performed for removal of a malignant tumor, the surgeon removes the associated blood vessels and lymphatic channels as well as the cancerous structures as a unit in order to prevent spread of cancer cells into other nearby organs. The surgeon may wash out the area with an anticancer agent as a further precaution and may also take samples of the liver (the primary site for spread of the cancer) and abdominal lymph nodes in order to assess the severity of the cancer and guide continuing treatment.

What are the possible complications?

Complications of bowel resection and reconnection include bleeding, which can progress to hemorrhage and shock if severe; blockage of the intestine after surgery most often caused by the development of scar tissue; leakage of bowel contents where the stitches connect the bowel segments; and other problems common to abdominal surgery, such as wound infection and incomplete filling of the lung.

What happens after surgery?

- For the first few days after surgery, the nurse will measure your fluid intake and urine and drainage output and weigh you daily.
- The nurse will check your vital signs frequently and observe you closely for signs of complications.
- Your incision will be kept clean and the bandages changed often.
- You'll be observed for signs of infection, including sudden fever, especially when accompanied by abdominal pain and tenderness.
- The nurse will note the frequency and amount of all bowel movements as well as characteristics of stools. (See *Caring for yourself after a bowel resection*.)
- The nurse will encourage you to cough and breathe deeply to prevent lung complications. You'll be reminded to protect the incision during coughing.

*H*EMORRHOIDECTOMY

Hemorrhoidectomy is the surgical removal of hemorrhoidal varicose veins. Hemorrhoids are swollen or enlarged veins in the anorectal region that can be internal or external. *Internal hemorrhoids* aren't visible on inspection of the anal region unless they prolapse (enlarge and fall through the anal sphincter); typically, they lie above the sphincter. External hemorrhoids, which lie below the sphincter, are

 SELF-HELP

Caring for yourself after a bowel resection

After you've been discharged from the hospital, keep in mind the following guidelines.

Modify your diet
- Follow the diet prescribed by your doctor. You should avoid carbonated beverages and gas-forming foods.
- Because extensive bowel resection may interfere with absorption of nutrients from food, you should take vitamin supplements as prescribed by your doctor.

Other instructions
- Record the frequency and character of bowel movements and notify the doctor of any changes from your normal pattern. You should not use laxatives without the doctor's approval.
- Avoid abdominal straining and heavy lifting until the stitches are completely healed and the doctor allows unrestricted activity.

visible at inspection. People can have either internal or external hemorrhoids or both types.

Hemorrhoids can be extremely painful. They require surgical removal if they cause severe symptoms and conservative treatment is ineffective. Hemorrhoidectomy is performed in approximately 10% of people with problematic hemorrhoids.

Although you're usually discharged after hemorrhoidectomy on the day of surgery, healing of delicate anal and rectal tissues can be slow and painful. For this reason, treatment after surgery focuses on measures to increase your comfort and speed healing: pain control, sitz baths (immersion of the area into lukewarm or hot water), frequent changing of the bandage, and maintenance of a regular elimination schedule. (See *Ligating hemorrhoidal tissue.*)

Why is this surgery done?

Hemorrhoidectomy is done to remove hemorrhoids from the anus and rectum. This procedure is performed for internal hemorrhoids that are large, that prolapse but cannot be reduced, or are associated with external hemorrhoids that cause symptoms. Hemorrhoidectomy is also recommended for hemorrhoids that have ulcers, lack blood supply, or contain clotted blood.

When shouldn't this surgery be performed?

Hemorrhoidectomy shouldn't be performed on people who have a blood disease or certain stomach or intestinal cancers or during the first three months of pregnancy because of the risk of hemorrhage.

What happens before the surgery?

- Your doctor or nurse will explain the procedure to you.
- You'll be told that the bandages will be changed frequently after the surgery and that your anal area will be cleaned frequently.
- The nurse will give you an enema 2 to 4 hours before surgery and your anal area will be cleaned and shaved.
- You or a responsible family member will sign a consent form.

What happens during surgery?

Hemorrhoidectomy is performed in the operating room under local, spinal, or general anesthesia. After administration of the anesthetic, the surgeon opens up the anal opening, removes the hemorrhoid, and ties off the connecting blood vessels. He or she may place a small,

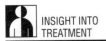

INSIGHT INTO
TREATMENT

Ligating hemorrhoidal tissue

Large internal hemorrhoids can sometimes be removed in the doctor's office by rubber-band ligation. The doctor inserts an anoscope to dilate the sphincter (anal muscle) and then uses grasping forceps to pull the hemorrhoid into position. Next the doctor inserts a ligator through the anoscope and slips a small rubber band over the stalk of the hemorrhoid to bind it and cut off its blood flow. Lack of blood within the hemorrhoid causes it to slough off naturally, usually within 5 to 7 days. People who undergo this therapy often experience bowel pressure or the urge to void for 24 to 48 hours after the ligation.

GRASPING THE HEMORRHOID

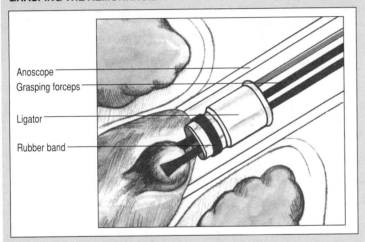

Anoscope

Grasping forceps

Ligator

Rubber band

LIGATING THE HEMORRHOID

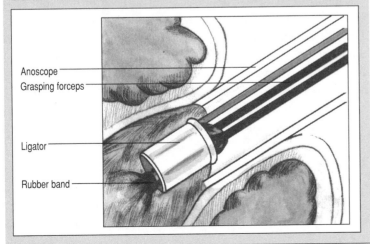

Anoscope

Grasping forceps

Ligator

Rubber band

SELF-HELP

Caring for yourself after a hemorrhoidectomy

After you've been discharged from the hospital, follow the important guidelines below.

Know when to call your doctor
- Check the bandage regularly and report any increased bleeding or drainage to your doctor.
- If you have trouble urinating after surgery, try sitting in a tub of warm water. If you still cannot urinate, you should notify your doctor.
- If you experience drainage of pus, fever, constipation, or rectal spasm, notify your doctor.

Reduce swelling and discomfort
- Soak your anal area in lukewarm or hot water three to four times daily and after each bowel movement to reduce swelling and discomfort and to help keep the area clean.
- To clean the anus: wipe gently with soft, white toilet paper (the dyes used in colored paper may cause irritation), clean the area with mild soap and warm water, and apply a sanitary pad.

Other instructions
- Avoid constipation with regular exercise and adequate intake of dietary fiber and fluids (8 to 10 glasses of water a day, 8 ounces each).
- Follow your doctor's instructions regarding the use of stool softeners. Don't overuse stool-softening laxatives because firm stools are necessary to widen the anal canal and prevent tightening of the opening.
- Take pain medication as prescribed by your doctor.
- Keep follow-up appointments with your doctor to check the operative area for infection and abscess formation.

lubricated tube in your anus to drain air, fluid, blood, and gas or may pack the area with petroleum gauze.

What are the possible complications?
Complications of hemorrhoidectomy include hemorrhage, difficulty urinating, anal constriction, and infection that can lead to abscess. The risk of hemorrhage, the most serious complication, is greatest during the first 24 hours after surgery and then again 7 to 10 days after surgery when the stitches are gone. Anal itch can result from mucus discharge or aggressive cleaning of the anus. In older people, hemorrhoidectomy sometimes requires stretching of the muscle at the anal opening to allow self-control of elimination.

What happens after surgery?
- You'll lie comfortably in bed; lying on your side is usually the most comfortable position.
- The nurse will administer pain medication as ordered by your doctor.

- The nurse will check your bandage frequently and report any excessive bleeding or drainage to your doctor. (See *Caring for yourself after a hemorrhoidectomy.*)
- Your vital signs will be checked frequently.

Appendectomy

Appendectomy is the surgical removal of an inflamed appendix. Commonly performed as an emergency procedure, this surgery aims to prevent imminent rupture or perforation of the inflamed appendix. When completed before the onset of such complications, an appendectomy is generally effective and uneventful. After an uncomplicated appendectomy, the person can be discharged from the hospital on the day of surgery.

However, if perforation or rupture occurs before the appendectomy, an abscess or peritonitis (inflammation of the lining of the abdomen and pelvis) can occur. If an abscess occurs, the appendectomy is postponed for 6 to 12 weeks, during which antibiotics are administered to control the infection. If inflammation of the lining the abdomen and pelvis occurs, an appendectomy is performed to remove the source of the infection.

Why is this surgery done?
An appendectomy is performed to remove an inflamed appendix.

What happens before the surgery?
- Your doctor or nurse will explain the procedure to you.
- The nurse will administer antibiotics as ordered by your doctor to prevent infection.
- You'll have an intravenous catheter for administration of fluids.
- You'll probably want to sit up in bed because this position tends to reduce the pain.
- You may have a tube in your nose that goes to your stomach to remove gas and fluid and reduce nausea and vomiting.

What happens during the surgery?
An appendectomy is usually performed under general anesthesia but may be done under spinal or local anesthesia. To remove the appen-

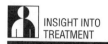

Laparoscopic appendectomy

Laparoscopic appendectomy is a new technique for removal of the appendix.

How is it done?
In this procedure, a trocar (a sharp pointed instrument) and a laparoscope (an instrument that permits the surgeon to see inside the abdomen) are inserted through a small incision under the navel to confirm appendicitis. With the help of a light source inserted through the laparoscope, the surgeon makes another small abdominal incision to allow insertion of a second trocar.

The surgeon then detaches the appendix, using instruments inserted through the trocars, and removes it from the abdominal cavity through a trocar without contaminating the incisions.

What are the advantages?
This technique is believed to be relatively safe, simple, and quick. If the surgeon is skilled in laparoscopic procedures, laparoscopic appendectomy can be performed in about 10 minutes.

Other advantages of this procedure include the absence of a large scar, reduced risk of injury to surrounding organs, and easy control of bleeding.

dix, an incision is made over the point of tenderness in the right lower abdomen, and the appendix is exposed and removed. After removal, the surgeon ties off the base of the appendix, removes excess fluid from the abdomen, and closes the incision. (For an alternative approach to this procedure, see *Laparoscopic appendectomy*.)

The incision usually heals without drainage. However, tubes are used to drain fluids that accumulate in the area if an abscess is discovered, or if rupture occurred or is imminent.

What are the possible complications?

Potential complications of appendectomy include inflammation of the lining of the abdomen and pelvis, which has a 10% mortality rate; abscess; obstruction of the intestines; and wound infection. (See *Recovering from an appendectomy*.)

What happens after surgery?

▪ You'll sit up in bed after recovery from anesthesia to decrease the risk of infecting the upper abdomen by exposure to contaminated fluid in the lower abdomen.
▪ You'll be encouraged to walk within 12 hours of surgery.
▪ Your nurse will encourage you to cough, breathe deeply, and change position frequently to prevent lung complications.

- If the appendix did not rupture or perforate, you will gradually resume oral foods beginning on the day of surgery.
- You'll be watched closely for signs of inflammation of the lining of the abdomen and pelvis including continuing pain and fever, excessive drainage from the incision, low blood pressure, rapid heart rate, paleness, and weakness. If this complication develops, emergency treatment may include insertion of a tube through the nose to the intestine, administration of intravenous fluids, and antibiotic therapy.

GALLBLADDER SURGERY

Gallbladder surgery is the removal of the gallbladder or gallstones in people with gallbladder or bile duct disease who fail to respond to drug therapy, dietary changes, and supportive treatments. Surgery is necessary to restore bile flow from the liver to the small intestine.

Cholecystectomy is surgical removal of the gallbladder. It's typically performed along with exploration of the tube that carries bile to treat cholecystitis (inflammation of the gallbladder) and cholelithiasis (gallstones).

Laparoscopic cholecystectomy (removal of the gallbladder through an instrument inserted into a small incision in the abdomen) is rapidly gaining favor in this country. Some experts estimate that by the end of the 1990s, laparoscopic procedures will replace about 80% of traditional abdominal surgeries. Laparoscopic cholecystectomy may not be performed in people with severe inflammation of the pancreas or the gallbladder, previous stomach surgery with resultant scar tissue, or extreme obesity (because available instruments aren't long enough). Laparoscopic cholecystectomy is never done in people who have severe cholecystitis with pus formation, yellow appearance of the skin due to obstruction in the flow of bile, increased pressure in the portal vein (vein that carries blood through the liver), or pregnancy.

Extracorporeal shock-wave lithotripsy is an alternative procedure that utilizes a computer and an ultrasound monitor along with a lithotriptor (shock-wave generator), which breaks up the gallstones so they are small enough to pass through the bile duct.

 SELF-HELP

Recovering from an appendectomy

When you've been discharged from the hospital, keep in mind the following:
- Watch for and immediately report to your doctor the following symptoms: fever, chills, sweating, nausea, vomiting, or abdominal pain and tenderness.
- If you are discharged on the day of surgery, you must return to have the stitches removed from the incision on the 5th or 7th day after surgery. Be sure to call the doctor's office to schedule an appointment to have this done.
- Keep follow-up appointments with your doctor.

Why is this surgery done?

Gallbladder surgery is done to correct obstruction of the flow of bile. Gallbladder surgery is performed most frequently on people with cholecystitis and cholelithiasis and less frequently for people with cancer of the gallbladder. It is also performed for inflammation of the pancreas caused by a gallstone, bleeding polyps in the gallbladder, a nonfunctioning gallbladder, gallstones in people with sickle cell anemia, gallstones that are larger than 3 centimeters even if they are not causing symptoms, and a gallbladder that is hardened by calcium deposits.

What happens before the surgery?

- Your doctor or nurse will explain the procedure and inform you about the tubes that will be in place after surgery (including a tube from your nose to your stomach).
- The nurse will teach you to perform coughing and deep-breathing exercises.
- You or a responsible family member will sign a consent form.
- You'll receive nutritional supplements, if necessary.

What happens during the surgery?

After you receive a general anesthetic (local anesthetic for a cholecystostomy), the surgeon will make an abdominal incision and remove the gallbladder in one of several ways. (See *Understanding gallbladder surgeries.*) After completion of the surgery and, if necessary, insertion of a drainage tube, the surgeon removes blood and debris from the abdomen, closes the incision, and applies a bandage.

What are the possible complications?

Although complications of gallbladder surgery are relatively rare, they can be serious. Peritonitis (inflammation of the membrane lining of the abdomen), for instance, may occur from blocked drainage of bile and resultant leakage of bile into the peritoneum. Also, a condition known as *postcholecystectomy syndrome,* which is marked by fever, yellow coloring of the skin, and pain, may occur. And, as in all abdominal surgeries, incomplete expansion of the lungs may be caused from shallow breathing because of pain from the incision.

Complications associated with laparoscopic cholecystectomy include injury to adjacent structures (such as the bowel or urinary bladder, blood vessels, or the bile duct) as well as hemorrhage, infection in the bloodstream, and peritonitis.

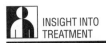

INSIGHT INTO
TREATMENT

Understanding gallbladder surgeries

Gallbladder surgeries include cholecystectomy and several less commonly performed procedures.

Cholecystectomy and common bile duct exploration

Through an incision in the upper abdomen, the surgeon isolates the gallbladder from the surrounding organs and inserts a balloon-tipped catheter to remove the gallstones in the biliary tract. The surgeon then removes the entire gallbladder and typically inserts a T tube into the common bile duct to compress the biliary tree and prevent bile peritonitis during healing. A second drain is sometimes inserted to drain the area under the liver.

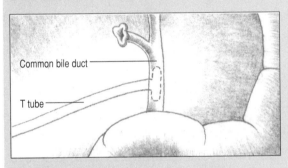

Common bile duct

T tube

Cholecystoduodenostomy or cholecystojejunostomy

In these procedures, the surgeon makes an incision under the right lower rib and connects the gallbladder to the duodenum or jejunum, preventing further yellow discoloration of the skin from a blockage in the common bile duct.

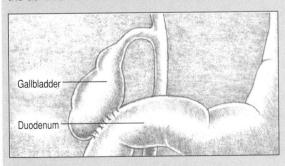

Gallbladder

Duodenum

Cholecystostomy

After administering a local anesthetic, the surgeon inserts a sharp pointed instrument with suction through a small incision in the gallbladder to decompress and aspirate the gallbladder and, using forceps, removes any retained gallstones or inflammatory debris. A large tube drain is inserted into the gallbladder and secured with stitches. Usually an emergency procedure, cholecystostomy is performed when bile flow is completely obstructed, pus formation or rupture is suspected, or the person is a poor surgical risk. This procedure typically controls pain and fever sufficiently so that the gallbladder can be removed later.

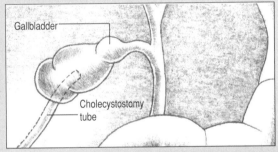

Gallbladder

Cholecystostomy tube

Choledochotomy

This procedure includes an incision into the common bile duct for exploration and removal of gallstones or other obstructions.

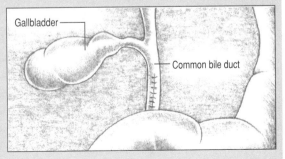

Gallbladder

Common bile duct

SELF-HELP

Caring for yourself after gallbladder surgery

After you've been discharged from the hospital, follow the important guidelines below.

Modify your diet
Eat a diet low in fats and high in carbohydrates and protein. As bile flow to the intestine increases, so will your ability to digest fats; when this happens, typically within 6 weeks, fats may gradually be added to your diet.

Other instructions
- If you have drainage tubes in place when you're discharged, follow your doctor's or nurse's instructions about how to take care of them.
- Be alert for signs of blockage of the flow of bile: fever, chills, tremors, yellow appearance to the skin, itchiness, pain, dark urine, and clay-colored stools.
- Keep follow-up appointments with your doctor.

What happens after the surgery?

- You'll lie with your head slightly elevated in the bed.
- The nurse will check frequently the amount and characteristics of drainage from the tube in your nose and drainage tubes in the incision. Your bandage will also be checked often and changed as necessary.
- After a few days, the tube in your nose will be removed and you'll begin to take food by mouth — first liquids and then soft solid food.
- You'll be watched closely for signs of complications.
- For several days after surgery, the nurse will check your vital signs and measure your fluid intake and urine and drainage output every 8 hours.
- You'll be encouraged to walk on the first day after surgery and to cough, breathe deeply, and perform breathing exercises every 4 hours.
- The nurse will administer pain medication as prescribed by your doctor.
- If you had a laparoscopic cholecystectomy, you'll be discharged the next day if there are no complications. (See *Caring for yourself after gallbladder surgery*.)

LIVER TRANSPLANT

Liver transplantation replaces a diseased liver with a healthy liver removed from a donor. This surgery is an accepted treatment for terminal liver disease. Since introduction of the surgery in 1963, rates of successful liver transplantations have improved remarkably. Before 1980 and the use of cyclosporine (a drug that suppresses the immune system, thereby helping to prevent rejection), only 38% of people with liver transplants survived for 1 year. Today, many transplant programs are reporting survival rates of 80% or more.

Types of transplants
There are three notable types of liver transplantation. In *orthotopic transplantation,* the surgeon removes the person's own liver and replaces it with a healthy donor's liver (from a recently brain-dead individual); in the second type, *heterotopic transplantation,* a donor liver is inserted at another site while the person's own liver remains in place; in the third type, *reduced-sized liver transplantation,* the surgeon

transplants a portion of a liver. This type of surgery is relatively new and is reserved for children.

Liver transplantations are typically reserved for terminally ill people who have a realistic chance of surviving the surgery and complications that arise afterward.

The most limiting factor in transplantation is the availability of donor organs, particularly for children. Many people who need livers are awaiting suitable donor organs. Often the wait proves fatal. And even if a compatible healthy liver is located and transplantation is performed, the person faces many obstacles to recovery.

Why is this surgery done?

Liver transplantation is performed to replace a terminally diseased liver with a healthy donor organ. It's performed for children and adults with severe, irreversible liver disease who can't be successfully treated by alternative medical and surgical methods.

When shouldn't this surgery be done?

A liver transplant should not be performed on people who test positive for HIV, those with advanced heart and lung disease or disease of the blood vessels in the brain, and those who actively abuse drugs or alcohol. In addition, people who have any potentially dangerous complications of liver disease, such as high blood pressure, brain disease, blood clotting disorders, or severe kidney disease, may not be suitable candidates for liver transplantation.

What happens before the surgery?

▪ You'll have a thorough physical exam, X-rays of your upper and lower gastrointestinal system, X-rays of the arteries of your liver, and an ultrasound test of your liver to determine if you're suitable for a liver transplant. In addition, you'll undergo an extensive battery of tests designed to match you with a donor.

▪ Your health care team will prepare you for surgery and will take steps to improve your nutritional and fluid status so you're as healthy as possible to withstand the extreme demands of transplantation.

▪ Your doctor or nurse will explain the procedure and what will happen afterward to you or, if the procedure is being performed on a child, to his or her parents.

▪ Your health care team will discuss the prospects of success and of complications after surgery with you. A successful transplantation doesn't guarantee a life free from medical problems. There is a need for lifelong follow-up care to minimize these problems.

- If possible, you and your family will visit the intensive care unit and meet staff members before the surgery.
- Your nurse will restrict your food and fluids for 8 to 12 hours before surgery.
- The nurse will administer drugs, such as cyclosporine and cortisone, to decrease your risk of rejection. The need for these drugs throughout your life will be explained to you.
- You'll be assured that the health care team will provide support through difficult times. You may be referred to a psychologist or psychiatric nurse specialist for further support both before and after the surgery.
- You or a responsible family member will sign a consent form.

What happens during the surgery?

In an orthotopic transplantation, the liver is removed from the donor and then flushed by injecting an electrolyte solution through a vein; then the organ is placed on ice. The combination of cold storage and electrolyte solution preserves the liver for up to 10 hours. Then the organ is transported in an ice-slush solution to the transplant center. Newer flush solutions containing high-molecular-weight sugars have extended the preservation time to approximately 36 hours.

To prepare the recipient for transplantation, the surgeon opens the abdomen, excises the diseased liver, and then quickly positions the donor organ in place and connects the blood vessels to restore circulation. After controlling all bleeding, the surgeon reconstructs the tube that carries bile. Finally, abdominal drainage tubes are inserted, the incision is closed, and a bandage is applied.

After surgery, you'll return to an intensive care unit with a breathing tube in place that will be connected to a ventilator. You'll also have a tube going from your nose to your stomach, a heart monitor, intravenous lines, and abdominal drainage tubes.

What are the possible complications?

Organ rejection and infection are the two major complications of a liver transplant. A successful transplant requires overcoming rejection, which results from differences between the donor and recipient. Kidney problems are common in transplant recipients and are usually caused by toxic reactions to the drug cyclosporine, which is given to help prevent rejection. Other complications include blood clots

SELF-HELP

Caring for yourself after a liver transplant

After you've been discharged from the hospital, keep in mind the important guidelines below.

Report any problems
- Be alert for early signs of organ rejection: pain and tenderness in the upper right side of the abdomen, right side of the body, or center of the back; fever; rapid heart rate; yellow discoloration of the skin; and changes in the color of urine or stools. Call your doctor immediately if any of these signs or symptoms develops.
- Watch for signs of liver failure, such as swelling of the abdomen, bloody stools or vomit, decreased urination, abdominal pain and tenderness, lack of appetite, or a change in mental function. If any of these symptoms develops, report it to your doctor.
- Watch for signs of infection, including a fever, weakness, sleepiness, and rapid heart rate. If any of these symptoms develops, report it to your doctor.

Take your medication
Be certain to take all medication prescribed by your doctor. Failure to take prescribed medication can trigger rejection, even of a liver that has been functioning well for years. You should be aware that the medication to prevent rejection can have side effects, such as infection, fluid retention, acne, glaucoma, diabetes, or cancer.

Other points to remember
- To reduce your risk of rejection, avoid contact with any person who has or may have a contagious illness.
- See your doctor regularly for follow-up examinations.
- You or your family may want to seek psychological counseling to help cope with the effects on your lives of your long-term and difficult recovery.

and leakage of bile. Psychological complications may arise as you change from a condition of severe illness to wellness.

What happens after the surgery?
- You'll continue to receive drug therapy to prevent rejection and you'll be monitored for signs of rejection and other complications. (See *Caring for yourself after a liver transplant.*)
- Although hospitalization after liver transplantation typically lasts 4 to 6 weeks, it can vary from 11 days to 5 months.

LIVER RESECTION

Resection or repair of the diseased or damaged liver may be performed for various liver problems, including cysts, abscesses, tumors (malignant and benign), tears, or crush injuries from blunt or penetrating trauma. Such surgery is usually performed only after conservative measures prove ineffective.

Resection of the liver is the removal of a significant portion of the organ. *Partial* or *subtotal resection* of the liver is removal of a portion of the liver. *Lobectomy* is the removal of an entire lobe of the liver.

Because liver cancer is often advanced at diagnosis, few such tumors are removable. Before the decision is made to resect the liver, thorough assessment must ensure that at least 15% of healthy liver tissue will remain after surgery and that the blood and bile systems will work properly. Resection for a metastatic tumor (a cancerous tumor that has spread from another location) requires that the primary tumor has been resected, that there are no other sites to which it has spread, and that the metastatic tumor does not involve the large veins of the liver. The probability of a successful resection increases if the tumor is solitary and is confined to one section of the liver.

Why is this surgery done?

Liver resection is performed to remove diseased areas or to repair injury to the liver. Resection or repair of the diseased or damaged liver may be performed for various liver problems, including cysts, abscesses, tumors (malignant and benign), tears, or crush injuries from blunt or penetrating trauma. Such surgery is usually performed only after conservative measures prove ineffective.

What happens before the surgery?

- Your doctor or nurse will explain the procedure to you.
- If surgery is not an emergency, the preparation may take up to 6 weeks. During this time, you will have a number of tests, including evaluation of blood clotting, blood chemistry tests, measurement of oxygen and carbon dioxide in the arterial blood, and blood typing and crossmatching.
- Preparation for surgery is based on the results of the above tests. For example, you may be transfused with blood or blood components or be given fluid and electrolyte replacements or protein supplements, as ordered by your doctor.
- You'll have additional diagnostic tests that help locate and identify disease, such as a liver scan, an ultrasound, a needle biopsy (removal and analysis of liver tissue), X-rays of the blood vessels in the liver, and X-rays of the gallbladder and bile ducts.

Types of liver resection

The illustration below indicates the various types of liver resection.

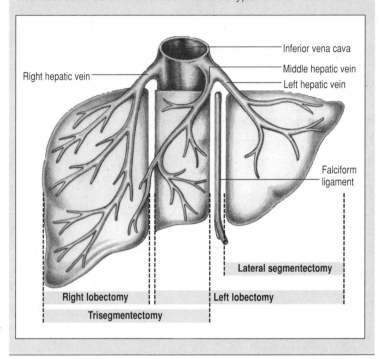

- The nurse will adminster vitamin supplements, as ordered by your doctor, to help improve liver function.
- Your nurse or doctor will explain that you'll have a tube going from your nose to your stomach, tubes in your chest, and catheters in arteries and veins for monitoring blood pressure, oxygen and carbon dioxide levels, and heart function.
- Because your liver is close to your right lung, liver surgery often interferes with normal breathing, increasing the risk of lung complications after surgery. To reduce this risk, the nurse will encourage you to practice coughing and deep-breathing exercises that you'll perform after surgery.
- You or a responsible family member will sign a consent form.

What happens during the procedure?
You'll receive a general anesthetic. The surgeon usually makes a vertical incision in your right upper abdomen and can quickly extend the incision if more damage is found than suspected. For emergency sur-

Caring for yourself after a liver resection

After you've been discharged from the hospital, keep in mind the following:

- See your doctor regularly for follow-up exams.
- Get adequate rest and follow your doctor's instructions regarding diet to conserve energy and reduce metabolic demands on the liver, thereby speeding healing.

gery when a tear in the liver or a crush injury is suspected, the extent of removal is determined during the surgery. The surgeon removes damaged areas of the liver, stitches any tears, and then carefully explores the surrounding area for additional injury. When all damage is repaired and bleeding controlled, the surgeon inserts a tube in the chest or drainage tubes in the abdomen to remove fluid, blood, and air; closes the incision; and applies a bandage.

In elective surgery, the technique depends on the location and extent of liver disease. (See *Types of liver resection,* page 173.)

What are the possible complications?

Liver resection frequently results in complications that occur with increasing frequency as the amount of liver removed increases. Because of the liver's anatomic location, surgery is typically performed through an incision that involves both the chest and abdomen. It therefore carries many risks associated with both chest and abdominal surgery: incomplete filling of the lungs, accumulation of fluid in the abdomen, kidney failure, and infection. In addition, impaired liver function due to surgery can result in such diverse complications as low blood sugar and brain disease. Because of the liver's fragility, acute hemorrhage remains a threat during and after surgery.

What happens after the surgery?

- The nurse will check your vital signs frequently.
- You'll be observed closely for signs of bleeding. An intravenous line will be maintained for possible emergency fluid replacement or blood transfusion.
- The nurse will administer pain medication as ordered by your doctor.
- You'll have blood tests taken and the results will be monitored for signs of complications.
- The nurse will check your bandage and drainage tubes frequently for excessive bleeding or drainage and change your bandage as necessary.
- You'll be encouraged to cough, breathe deeply, and change position frequently to prevent lung complications. (See *Caring for yourself after a liver resection.*)

PORTAL VEIN BYPASS

The portal vein is a short vein that carries blood from the stomach and intestinal organs to the liver. When pressure inside the portal vein becomes too high, it can cause swelling and bleeding of blood vessels in the esophagus. This surgery creates a bypass for blood in the portal vein, reducing pressure there. This, in turn, prevents or controls bleeding from swollen blood vessels in the esophagus. Typically, this surgery is done when the person does not respond to conservative treatments such as diet and drug therapy. If possible, it's performed after bleeding from the esophagus is under control and the person's condition has stabilized. However, emergency surgery may be necessary if compression of the esophagus or drugs that constrict blood vessels can't control bleeding from ruptured swollen veins in the neck.

Why is this surgery done?
Creation of a bypass for the blood in the portal vein is performed to reduce portal pressure and control bleeding from swollen veins in the esophagus by shunting blood away from the portal veins in people who have liver disease.

What happens before the surgery?
- The doctor or nurse will explain the procedure to you, as time permits.
- You'll be told that you'll return from surgery with a tube going from your nose to your stomach and tubes in your chest. You'll also be told that you'll be connected to a heart monitor and have catheters in your arteries and veins that will monitor your heart and circulation.

What happens during the surgery?
After you receive a general anesthetic, the surgeon makes an incision in the abdomen and performs one of three possible shunting (bypass) procedures. In *portacaval shunting,* the most commonly performed procedure, the portal vein is joined to the inferior vena cava.

In *splenorenal shunting,* the surgeon joins the splenic vein and the left renal vein.

Recovering from a portal vein bypass

After you've been discharged from the hospital, follow these important guidelines:

- Make sure you follow the diet and drug regimens prescribed by your doctor, including strict abstention from alcohol. It's also important that you get adequate rest to reduce the risk of bleeding and infection.
- Watch for and immediately report to your doctor the following symptoms of brain disease: disorientation, sleepiness, amnesia, slurred speech, tremors, or the inability to perform purposeful movements.
- Keep follow-up appointments with your doctor.

In *mesocaval shunting,* the surgeon joins the superior mesenteric vein to the inferior vena cava. However, this procedure is not as effective as the other shunts and carries the risk of blood clot formation.

A fourth type of shunt uses a device called a *transjugular intrahepatic portosystemic shunt,* by which an expandable balloon diverts blood from the portal vein to the hepatic vein.

What are the possible complications?
A delicate and complicated surgery, creation of a bypass for blood in the portal vein poses grave risks. For example, diversion of large amounts of blood into the inferior vena cava may cause heart failure. And diverting blood away from the liver inhibits the conversion of ammonia to urea, possibly causing brain disease, which can progress rapidly to coma and death. Other possible complications include hemorrhage, which can cause inflammation of the lining of the abdomen, and lung complications.

Due to complications, these bypass procedures have a mortality rate of approximately 25% to 50%. Research suggests that this surgery does little to prolong survival, with people dying from liver complications more commonly than from uncontrolled bleeding from the esophagus.

What happens after the surgery?
- The nurse will check your vital signs and measure your fluid intake and urine output hourly.
- You'll be watched closely for signs of complications. (See *Recovering from a portal vein bypass.*)
- You'll have liver function tests and electrolyte studies to assess your condition.
- The nurse will encourage you to cough, breathe deeply, and change position at least once every hour.
- The nurse will administer pain medication as ordered by your doctor.

*P*AROTIDECTOMY

This surgery removes the parotid gland, the largest of the salivary glands, located near the ear. A parotidectomy may be total or superficial, depending on the extent of parotid disease. *Total parotidectomy* is performed when infection or tumor involves the deep lobe of the parotid gland; *superficial parotidectomy* is done when only the superficial lobe is involved.

Why is this surgery done?
- To eliminate recurrent infection of the parotid gland
- To prevent the formation of abscesses in chronic inflammation of the parotid gland
- To remove tumors involving the parotid gland
- To remove a parotid duct stone

What happens before the surgery?
- Your doctor or nurse will explain the procedure to you.
- If you have chronic inflammation of the parotid gland, you'll receive antibiotics.
- You'll sign a consent form.

What happens during the surgery?
The surgeon makes an incision on the appropriate side of your neck. The area is carefully dissected and the facial nerve is identified. The affected parotid gland is removed. The facial nerve and its branches are examined to make sure they are intact and function normally. A drainage tube is inserted during surgery to remove excess fluid and a pressure bandage is applied.

What are the possible complications?
The major complications of parotidectomy include facial nerve paralysis, hematoma, and infection. A potentially serious complication is the complete loss of function of all the branches of the facial nerve.

The most common long-term complication is the appearance of a red area and sweating on the cheek in connection with eating, known as *Frey's syndrome.*

SELF-HELP

Caring for yourself after a parotidectomy

When you've been discharged from the hospital after a parotidectomy, keep in mind the following.

Protect the incision site
- Clean the incision with hydrogen peroxide and cotton-tipped applicators twice a day.
- Don't wash your hair until after the stitches are removed and your doctor gives permission.
- You may notice some numbness in the cheek and ear on the surgical side. The numbness may last for 3 to 6 months. Be sure to cover your face and ear in frigid weather to prevent frostbite because you may not feel the cold.

Other points to remember
- Take antibiotics as prescribed by your doctor.
- You may be instructed to remove the bandage at home (usually 24 hours after the drainage tube is removed).
- Make a follow-up appointment with your doctor for removal of stitches 5 to 7 days after surgery.

What happens after the surgery?
- You'll be hospitalized for 1 to 3 days.
- The nurse will monitor your vital signs and observe you for signs of hemorrhage or infection. (See *Caring for yourself after a parotidectomy*.)
- You'll be watched for signs of facial nerve damage, including the inability to smile, wink, or drink fluids.
- The nurse will check your bandage for drainage and change it as necessary. Excessive drainage or bleeding will be reported to your doctor.
- You'll receive pain medication as ordered by the doctor.

OTHER TREATMENTS

BOWEL TRAINING

Bowel training attempts to establish a regular pattern of elimination through changes in diet and lifestyle, supplemented as necessary by limited use of laxatives, enemas, or suppositories.

The success of a bowel-training program depends on the person's ability and willingness to follow the procedure and the presence of a

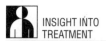

INSIGHT INTO
TREATMENT

Techniques to aid bowel training

If a person needs additional help defecating, the bowel-training program may also include mechanical stimulation, digital stimulation, or operant conditioning.

Mechanical stimulation
This technique uses stool softeners, enemas, laxatives, or glycerin suppositories and may be necessary early in the training program. However, after a routine is well established, these aids are gradually withdrawn so that the person can defecate consistently without them.

Digital stimulation
This technique involves using a lubricated finger to promote elimination. For a person with a spinal cord injury or other neurologic damage, it may be a necessary part of the training program. This procedure is performed by inserting a lubricated finger of a gloved hand about ½ to 1 inch (1 to 2 centimeters) into the person's rectum. Then the finger is gently rotated for 30 to 60 seconds.

Operant conditioning
This technique may be necessary to improve muscle tone in people who can't control their bowels. To accomplish this, a specially skilled nurse or technician inserts a balloon attached to a monitor into the rectum and inflates it. The person is instructed to contract the sphincter (anal muscle) against the balloon pressure and to check progress on the monitor. Another method of operant conditioning requires the insertion of measured amounts of water into the rectum. The person then holds the water as long as possible in an effort to control the sphincter. The water is held for longer periods as greater control of the sphincter is attained.

strong support system of family or friends. This program requires considerable time and patience to be effective. It requires sensitivity to the person's feelings of discomfort and embarrassment as well.

Why is this treatment done?
Bowel training helps the person establish a normal pattern of elimination. It can correct constipation and, in some cases, lack of control over one's bowels.

What happens before the treatment?
The medical team will evaluate your overall condition before establishing an elimination schedule to ensure your ability to withstand a prolonged and occasionally frustrating bowel-training program. They will take a complete history of your bowel habits, including your defecation patterns, use of laxatives, and regular dietary habits. After establishing your cooperation and stamina, your doctor will discuss the overall goal of the program, which is the establishment of

SELF-HELP

Caring for yourself after bowel training

After you've undergone bowel training, keep in mind the following:
- It's important never to ignore the urge to defecate.
- Follow the dietary instructions you've received.
- Although eating an adequate amount of fiber is important, excessive ingestion of bran can impair iron absorption.

a regular pattern of elimination based on your individual needs and abilities.

The requirements of the program will be explained to you, including your defecation schedule and need for adequate fluid intake, increased dietary fiber intake, and increased activity. (See *Caring for yourself after bowel training.*)

What happens during the treatment?

Bowel training requires a regular schedule for defecation. Toileting should follow each meal so that your attempts at defecation are made at about the same time every day. You should assume the normal position for defecation, so gravity can assist elimination, and you should remain in this position for at least 10 minutes but no longer than 30 minutes. You can help stimulate a scheduled bowel movement by leaning forward to increase abdominal pressure or by applying direct pressure to the abdominal wall and massaging the abdomen from right to left.

In addition to a regular schedule for defecation, essential components of a bowel-training program include an adequate fluid intake to promote softer stools and help stimulate normal movement of the intestines, increased intake of dietary fiber to add bulk to the stools and also to stimulate normal movement of the intestines, and an increased level of activity to stimulate and maintain intestinal activity. (See *Techniques to aid bowel training,* page 179.)

What are the possible complications?

No complications are associated with bowel training.

ENEMAS

Enemas involve instillation of a solution into the rectum and the colon, usually to stimulate intestinal movement by mechanically distending (enlarging) the colon and stimulating nerves in the rectal wall. There are several types of enemas. A *nonretention cleansing enema* instills a large volume of liquid to remove gas and feces from the rectum; it's usually expelled within 15 minutes. Another type, the *retention enema,* is introduced into the bowel and retained for approximately 30 minutes to 1 hour. For example, the oil retention enema is given to lubricate the rectum and anal canal and to soften hardened stools. The retention enema is also used to introduce medications that are absorbed through the rectum. A *return flow enema,* also called a *Harris flush,* is given to relieve gas.

Why is this treatment done?

Enemas are given to clean the lower bowel before tests or surgery, to relieve constipation, to relieve abdominal bloating and promote expulsion of gas, to deliver medications by the rectal route, and to lubricate the rectum and lower bowel. They're given when diet, exercise, and laxatives fail to relieve constipation. They're also sometimes used after barium X-rays to prevent retained barium from being impacted and before tests and surgery that require cleaning the bowel.

Certain enemas, such as the Harris flush, relieve gas or distention from obstruction of the bowel. The retention enema acts as a softener, soothing irritated tissues of the colon. It also facilitates medication administration by the rectal route.

When shouldn't this treatment be done?

Enemas shouldn't be given to individuals after recent colon or rectal surgery, to those with an acute abdominal condition for which the cause is unknown, or to those who've had a recent heart attack. Enemas should be administered cautiously to people with irregular heartbeats.

What happens before the treatment?

- The nurse will explain the procedure to you, including why it has been prescribed.
- If you have difficulty retaining enemas, a catheter with an inflatable balloon may be used.
- The solution will be warmed to reduce discomfort.

What happens during the treatment?

An enema is administered by a nurse or nursing assistant, or may be administered at home by you or a family member.

For a therapeutic enema, you lie on your left side with the right knee flexed. This will enhance the flow of enema solution into the intestine. If you have poor control of your sphincter (anal muscle), you may sit on a bedpan while lying in bed. To allow for easier insertion into the rectum, the tip of the enema tube is lubricated with a

SELF-HELP

Caring for yourself after an enema

When you're discharged from the hospital, keep in mind the following:
- Follow the nurse's instructions if you'll be receiving enemas at home.
- Don't give yourself an enema in a sitting or standing position because this may cause abrasions or perforations to the rectum.
- Try to prevent constipation by doing the following: exercise regularly, eat enough dietary fiber, drink plenty of liquids, and establish a regular time for elimination.

water-soluble lubricant. Then, using a clean glove, the nurse will separate your buttocks and insert the tube 2 to 4 inches (5 to 10 centimeters) toward the navel. For a child, the tube is inserted only 2 to 3 inches (5 to 7.5 centimeters) and for an infant, 1 to 1½ inches (2.5 to 4 centimeters). The solution is infused slowly to avoid cramping. To obtain optimum flow, the solution is hung 12 to 18 inches (30 to 45 centimeters) above the adult's abdomen. A retention enema is administered at the slowest possible rate to avoid stimulating intestinal movement and to promote retention.

After most of the prescribed amount of solution has been administered, the tubing is clamped. The flow is stopped before the container empties completely to avoid introducing air into the bowel. The tube is then gently removed.

If an enema will be administered to clean out your bowels, you'll be instructed to try to retain the solution for 5 to 15 minutes, if possible, before emptying your bowels. If you'll be receiving a retention enema, you'll be advised to avoid defecation and retain the solution for 30 minutes or as otherwise prescribed; lying flat for the prescribed retention time will help to prevent stimulation of intestinal movement. When the solution has remained in the colon for the prescribed time or for as long as you can tolerate it, you'll be assisted onto the bedpan or to the commode or bathroom as needed.

A Harris flush enema is administered similarly, but the flow is stopped by lowering the solution container below bed level and allowing gravity to siphon the enema out of the colon. Raising and lowering the container continues until gas bubbles cease or the person feels more comfortable and abdominal distention ceases.

Commercially prepared small-volume enemas are administered according to the instructions provided with the package.

What are the possible complications?

Enema administration is usually a safe procedure. However, use of a solution containing too much soap may irritate the rectum. Improper administration may cause rectal abrasions or perforation. Enemas may also produce dizziness or faintness due to fluid and electrolyte loss or electrolyte imbalances, such as low sodium or potassium levels. An irregular heart rate may result from vascular reflex stimulation after insertion of the rectal catheter.

What happens after the treatment?

- You'll be provided with materials for anal cleaning and hand washing.
- The nurse will send specimens to the lab if ordered by your doctor. (See *Caring for yourself after an enema*).

REMOVAL OF INTESTINAL CONTENTS THROUGH A NASAL TUBE

Nasoenteric decompression (removal of intestinal contents through a tube inserted in the nose) involves passing a long tube through the nose and advancing it beyond the stomach into the intestine so that the contents can be suctioned out.

Why is this procedure done?

Intestinal contents are removed through a nasal tube to relieve acute intestinal blockage, to remove stomach contents for examination, and to prevent nausea, vomiting, and swelling of the abdomen with gas after surgery on the digestive tract.

This is the initial treatment for acute blockage of the intestine, along with fluid and electrolyte replacement. Blockage may result from polyps, scar tissue, impacted feces, twisting of the intestine, or localized cancer. Removal of the intestinal contents through a tube in the nose usually relieves the blockage, especially in the small intestine. However, if this treatment fails to relieve the blockage or if the person's condition worsens, bowel resection may be necessary.

Removal of the intestinal contents through a tube in the nose may also be performed to remove stomach contents for testing purposes or to prevent an upset stomach after abdominal surgery.

What happens before the procedure?

Your doctor or nurse will explain the procedure to you and you'll be told to expect mild discomfort as the doctor inserts and advances the tube. You'll receive a sedative if the procedure is difficult or painful.

What happens during the procedure?

A doctor or specially skilled nurse may perform the procedure. The doctor chooses the appropriate tube, basing the choice on the size of the person and of the nostrils, how long the tube will be in place, and the reason for the procedure. The tube is lubricated for easy insertion and is passed through the nostrils and advanced into the throat. When the tube is in the throat, the person is asked to swallow and is given small sips of water or ice chips to encourage swallowing so that the tube can enter the stomach. When the tube reaches the stomach, the person is then positioned on the right side until the tube enters the intestine, which usually takes up to 2 hours. After the tube progresses the necessary distance and an X-ray confirms correct placement, the tube is connected to intermittent suction.

When the tube is no longer necessary, it's removed.

What are the possible complications?

Common complications include inflammation of the mouth, nose, or esophagus and nasal or vocal cord ulcers. Rarely, incomplete filling of the lungs and pneumonia may result from the tube's presence in the esophagus and its interference with normal coughing. Excessive intestinal drainage can produce a chemical imbalance or displacement of the tube within the intestine.

What happens after the procedure?

- You'll have X-rays taken to confirm that the tube is in the right place.
- Your doctor or nurse will secure the tube to prevent further advancement and to prevent it from coming out.
- Your doctor or nurse will connect the tube to intermittent suction.
- The nurse will check the amount and nature of drainage from the tube.
- Your nurse will flush the tube with saline as ordered by the doctor.
- The nurse will check your vital signs and fluid and electrolyte status regularly.
- You'll be monitored for signs of the return of normal movement of the intestines. These include the presence of bowel sounds, which can be heard through a stethoscope; decreased abdominal swelling; passage of intestinal gas; or a spontaneous bowel movement.
- The doctor will give you instructions about your diet. You'll have to get enough fiber and drink enough fluids to promote normal bowel function.

STOMACH FLUSHING

This procedure involves flushing the stomach and removing ingested substances through a tube extending from the nose to the stomach. It requires insertion of the tube, the addition of flushing fluid, and the suctioning of stomach contents.

Stomach flushing with ice water or iced normal saline solution is an emergency treatment for gastrointestinal hemorrhage caused by stomach ulcers or the rupture of swollen veins in the esophagus or stomach. In some cases, continuous irrigation and the administration of drugs that constrict blood vessels may be used to control the bleeding.

Some experts question the effectiveness of using an iced solution for stomach flushing to treat gastrointestinal bleeding. The iced flushing solutions stimulate the vagus nerve, which triggers release of acid in the stomach. In turn, this stimulates spontaneous movement of the stomach, which can irritate the bleeding site.

Some doctors prefer using unchilled saline solution (which may prevent rapid electrolyte loss) or water if the person must avoid salt.

Why is this procedure done?

This procedure is performed to flush the stomach to remove ingested substances or to control bleeding in the upper gastrointestinal area. Stomach flushing may be done with lukewarm or ice water or with saline solution to treat people who have bleeding from swollen veins in the esophagus or stomach or who have a stomach ulcer. It's also used to treat a person who's been poisoned or who's taken a drug overdose.

When shouldn't this procedure be done?

Stomach flushing should not be performed after ingestion of a corrosive substance (such as lye, ammonia, or mineral acids) because the nasal tube may perforate the already damaged esophagus.

What happens before the procedure?

■ Your doctor or nurse will explain the procedure to you and your family and you'll be told that you may experience some discomfort during insertion of the tube.

Stomach flushing may be done with lukewarm or ice water or with saline solution to treat people who have bleeding from swollen veins in the esophagus or stomach or who have a stomach ulcer. It's also used to treat a person who's been poisoned or who's taken a drug overdose.

- You'll sit up in bed for the procedure and, if you have dentures, they'll be removed.

What happens during the procedure?

Stomach flushing is performed in an emergency department or intensive care unit by a doctor, a specialist such as a gastroenterologist, or a nurse; the tube is almost always inserted by a gastroenterologist. After the tube is inserted and correct placement has been verified, the flushing solution is instilled into the stomach and then removed. The flushing procedure is continued until the fluid that's removed is clear, indicating that the bleeding has stopped or the harmful substances have been removed. On completion of the procedure, the tube is removed or secured as ordered by your doctor.

What are the possible complications?

Complications of iced solutions used to flush the stomach are rare, but may be serious if untreated. The most common complication is inhaling material that's vomited. Other complications include fluid overload, electrolyte imbalance, or biochemical abnormalities, which are especially likely in elderly or sickly people. Slow heart rates may result from stimulation of the vagus nerve and lowered body temperature.

Additionally, because the tube has a large diameter, pressure from excessive suctioning may cause damage to the lining of the stomach.

What happens after the procedure?

- The nurse will monitor your vital signs regularly until your condition stabilizes.
- You'll be observed for signs of dehydration and intravenous fluids or blood transfusions will be administered as needed.

*T*UBE COMPRESSION OF THE ESOPHAGUS AND STOMACH

In this emergency treatment, insertion of a tube with subsequent inflation of its stomach and esophageal balloons helps to control severe bleeding of the esophagus or stomach resulting from the rupture of swollen veins. Tube compression requires close monitoring in an intensive care setting. Additional procedures to temporarily control bleeding may include flushing with lukewarm or iced saline solution and administration of a drug that constricts the blood vessels.

Why is this procedure done?

Tube compression is performed to provide temporary control of hemorrhage from the esophagus or stomach and to prevent excessive blood loss.

What happens before the procedure?

- Your doctor or nurse will explain the procedure to you (or to your family, if you're unable to communicate).
- The nurse will administer a sedative, as ordered by your doctor, to help you relax.

What happens during the procedure?

Ordinarily the doctor inserts and removes the esophageal tube, but a nurse may remove it in an emergency situation. The doctor inserts the tube through the person's nostril, or sometimes through the mouth, and then passes it through the esophagus into the stomach. Inflation of the tube's gastric and, depending on the type of tube, esophageal balloons exerts pressure on the swollen blood vessels and stops bleeding.

The esophageal balloon may be deflated after 24 hours. The tube may be left in place for another 12 to 24 hours to check for any renewed bleeding.

What are the possible complications?

Esophageal rupture, the most life-threatening complication associated with compression of the esophagus, can occur at any time but is most likely during insertion of the tube or inflation of the esophageal balloon. Balloon inflation for more than 24 hours may cause injury to the esophagus, which can produce further hemorrhage or perforation. Asphyxia may result if the balloon moves up the esophagus and blocks the windpipe. The lining of the nose may also be injured during insertion of the tube.

What happens after the procedure?

You'll be observed for signs of bleeding. When your condition is stable, you'll be discharged from the hospital.

INSERTION OF A CATHETER TO RELIEVE BILE DUCT OBSTRUCTION

Insertion of a catheter into the bile duct (the tube that carries bile to the intestine) to relieve obstruction of the flow of bile involves insertion of a catheter through the abdomen and liver into the bile duct. (This procedure is also known as *transhepatic biliary catheterization*.) The flow of bile may be reestablished into the the first part of the intestine, or it may be diverted outside the body to a drainage bag. Although not a cure, this procedure permits a more normal lifestyle.

Why is this procedure done?

Insertion of a catheter to relieve bile duct obstruction is done to relieve signs and symptoms of bile duct blockage and reduce the associated risk of infection of the bloodstream. The most common cause of bile duct obstruction requiring drainage is inoperable cancer of the liver, pancreas, or bile duct. This procedure may also be indicated to treat stones in the common bile duct, surgical injuries to the bile duct, or constriction of the bile duct resulting from inflammation.

What happens before the procedure?

- Your doctor or nurse will explain the procedure to you and your family. You'll be informed about what to expect before, during, and after the procedure. You'll be told that the procedure may take several hours and may cause pain and that pain medication will be available.
- Blood tests will be performed to make sure you don't have a bleeding disorder.
- You'll have nothing to eat or drink the day of the procedure.
- You or a responsible family member will sign a consent form.

What happens during the procedure?

Insertion of a catheter to relieve bile duct obstruction is performed by a radiologist, who inserts a needle through the skin and liver and into the bile duct. Using a guide wire, the radiologist inserts the catheter into the duct. If possible, the catheter is positioned in the duodenum to eventually reestablish downward bile flow. Drainage of bile outside the body may be necessary until swelling caused by the catheter subsides. With complete obstruction, the radiologist may position the end of the catheter above the obstruction and divert the bile

Insertion of a catheter to relieve bile duct obstruction is done to relieve signs and symptoms of bile duct blockage and reduce the associated risk of infection of the bloodstream. The most common cause of bile duct obstruction requiring drainage is inoperable cancer of the liver, pancreas, or bile duct.

drainage permanently into a collection bag outside the body. The catheter may be secured with stitches in the skin.

What are the possible complications?

The most common complication of insertion of a catheter to relieve bile duct obstruction is hemorrhage resulting from puncture of the liver, which has numerous blood vessels. Infection of the bloodstream may also occur when the bile duct is manipulated. The catheter may become blocked with debris or may be dislodged.

What happens after the procedure?

- The nurse will monitor your vital signs frequently to detect hemorrhage or infection.
- You'll stay in bed for at least 6 hours to reduce the risk of bleeding.
- The nurse will check the amount of drainage from the catheter and excessive bleeding will be reported to the doctor.
- You'll be observed for cramping, pain, or leakage of fluid around the catheter; this may indicate blockage of the catheter or displacement from the bile duct. (See *Catheter care at home*.)
- The nurse will flush the catheter every 8 hours, or as otherwise ordered by your doctor, to keep it open.
- The nurse will change the bandage over the catheter daily and check the skin at the catheter insertion site for signs of infection or irritation.

Widening of the bile duct sphincter

Widening of the bile duct sphincter (the muscle that controls release of bile into the intestine), also known as *endoscopic retrograde sphincterotomy*, is a procedure that widens the muscle in the bile duct to aid removal of retained gallstones after gallbladder removal. This procedure, which is performed with an endoscope (an instrument that permits visualization of the inside of the body) allows treatment without general anesthesia or a surgical incision, ensuring a quicker, safer recovery. And because it may be performed on an outpatient basis for some people, it's a cost-effective alternative to surgery.

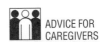
ADVICE FOR CAREGIVERS

Catheter care at home

Before leaving the hospital, a nurse will teach the family caregiver the proper method for irrigating the tube and changing the dressing. (The position of the catheter usually makes it difficult for the person to do alone.) Keep in mind the following guidelines.

Report any problems
You and the person with the catheter should stay alert for and report to the doctor the following signs of problems: fever and shaking chills, severe pain, excessive leakage around the catheter, and redness or tenderness around the catheter's insertion site. Also report an inability to flush the catheter or its accidental removal.

Other instructions
- Make sure the hospital has provided a referral to a home health care agency to supervise tube care.
- Make sure the person you're caring for keeps follow-up appointments with the radiologist to check the catheter's placement.

Caring for yourself after widening of the bile duct sphincter

After you've been discharged from the hospital, keep in mind the following:
- Follow your doctor's instructions and report to him any symptoms that may indicate a complication from the procedure, such as bloody stools, or a recurrence of bile duct obstruction, which is indicated by yellowish skin discoloration or pain.
- Keep follow-up appointments with your doctor.

Why is this procedure done?

Widening of the bile duct sphincter is performed to relieve obstructed drainage of bile. Originally developed to remove retained gallstones from the bile duct after removal of the gallbladder, it's now also used to treat people with certain diseases of the gallbladder and to make bile drainage possible for people with benign blockage of the bile duct.

What happens before the procedure?

- Your doctor or nurse will explain the procedure and reassure you that it should cause little or no discomfort.
- You'll lie on your left side on the X-ray table, with your left arm behind you. The nurse will administer a sedative, if ordered by your doctor.

What happens during the procedure?

After anesthetizing your throat, the doctor advances an endoscope through the stomach and duodenum (first part of the intestine) to the bile duct. Then the doctor passes a cutting wire, known as a *sphincterotome* or *papillotome,* through the endoscope and, under X-ray guidance, makes a small incision to widen the biliary sphincter. The stone may then drop out into the intestine so that it can be passed in stools; if not, the doctor may need to introduce (through the endoscope) another instrument to remove or crush the stone. An X-ray of the bile ducts confirms passage or removal of the stone. Alternatively, the doctor may introduce a prosthesis into the bile duct, through the endoscope to bypass a bile duct obstruction and restore normal drainage of bile. After the procedure, the doctor may insert a catheter through the nose to the bile duct for drainage of bile.

What are the possible complications?

Complications of endoscopic widening of the biliary sphincter include hemorrhage, inflammation of the pancreas or bile duct, and infection in the bloodstream.

What happens after the procedure?

- The nurse won't give you food or liquids until the local anesthetic wears off.
- Your vital signs will be checked frequently and you'll be observed for signs of hemorrhage.

- The nurse will also watch for signs and symptoms of other complications, which will be promptly reported to your doctor. (See *Caring for yourself after widening of the bile duct sphincter*.)

REMOVAL OF FLUID FROM THE ABDOMEN

This procedure (also called *paracentesis*) involves removal of accumulated fluid from the abdomen through a needle inserted into the abdominal wall.

Why is this procedure done?

Fluid is removed from the abdomen to obtain a specimen of fluid to diagnose the cause of fluid accumulation (such as cancer, inflammation of the abdominal wall, infectious organisms, or abdominal hemorrhage) or to relieve abdominal pressure and thereby ease associated abdominal and respiratory discomfort. Accumulated fluid is most commonly removed from the abdomen in people with cirrhosis of the liver, suspected abdominal hemorrhage from blunt trauma to the abdomen or duodenum, malignant lymphoma or other cancer, or other conditions that obstruct blood flow in the liver and cause fluid to collect in the abdomen.

When shouldn't this procedure be done?

People with markedly distended bowels should not be considered for this procedure because of the potential for tearing of the bowel.

What happens before the procedure?

- Your doctor or nurse will explain the procedure to you and your family.
- You or a responsible family member will sign a consent form.
- To prevent inadvertent puncture of the urinary bladder during this procedure, you'll be encouraged to urinate beforehand.
- The nurse will take your vital signs and measure the distance around your abdomen and your weight.
- You'll remain in a sitting position so that fluid accumulates in your lower abdominal cavity.
- The nurse may insert an intravenous catheter.

SELF-HELP

Caring for yourself after fluid removal

When you've been discharged from the hospital after removal of fluid from the abdomen, keep in mind the following:

- Be alert for the following symptoms: weight gain, increased abdominal size, breathing difficulty, swelling of the scrotum (in men), and abdominal discomfort. If these symptoms occur, report them to your doctor.
- Keep follow-up appointments with your doctor.

- You'll be told to stay as still as possible during the procedure to prevent injury from the needle.
- If the situation allows, your fluid intake will be restricted before the fluid is removed from your abdomen.

What happens during the procedure?

This procedure is typically performed under local anesthesia in your hospital room or in a special procedures room.

The doctor first makes a small incision and then inserts a spinal needle to remove the fluid. Typically, the amount of fluid removed at one time is limited to avoid circulatory complications. After removing the needle, the doctor stitches the incision. A dry, sterile pressure bandage is applied.

What are the possible complications?

Rapid removal of fluid may result in electrolyte imbalances (such as a low potassium level), protein depletion, and shock due to low blood volume. Other complications include perforation of abdominal organs by the needle, coma from decreased circulation, wound infection, and inflammation of the lining of the abdomen.

What happens after the procedure?

- The nurse will monitor your vital signs and check the dressing for drainage. You'll be observed for signs of shock, abdominal fluid leakage, and wound infection.
- The nurse will weigh you and measure the distance around your abdomen daily. Any increases will be reported to the doctor. (See *Caring for yourself after fluid removal.*)

4

TREATING NUTRITIONAL & METABOLIC DISORDERS

DRUGS FOR HIGH CHOLESTEROL

ANTILIPEMICS

High levels of fats (called lipids) in the bloodstream increase the risk of heart disease. High levels of cholesterol and triglycerides, in particular, increase the risk of heart attack and stroke.

Antilipemic drugs counteract high levels of these fats. The choice of drug depends on the type of fat that's elevated and certain characteristics of the person being treated (such as any other diseases he or she may have).

What are antilipemics used for?
These drugs further reduce levels of fats that do not respond to dietary restrictions, weight loss, or exercise.

What are some commonly used antilipemics?
- cholestyramine, known by the brand names Cholybar and Questran
- clofibrate, known by the brand name Atromid-S
- colestipol, known by the brand name Colestid
- dextrothyroxine, known by the brand name Choloxin
- gemfibrozil, known by the brand name Lopid
- lovastatin, known by the brand name Mevacor
- niacin, known by the brand names Niacin and Niacor
- pravastatin, known by the brand name Pravachol
- probucol, known by the brand name Lorelco
- simvastatin, known by the brand name Zocor

What are the possible side effects?
- Stomach upset, gas, worsening of preexisting digestive disorders, weakness
- Constipation (especially from cholestyramine and colestipol)
- Rash (especially from clofibrate)
- Weight gain (especially from clofibrate)

- Headache, skin flushing (especially from niacin or nicotinic acid)
- Hepatitis (especially from lovastatin, niacin, pravastatin, and simvastatin)

What are the guidelines for taking antilipemics?

- Remember to return for all follow-up blood tests. Frequent tests are necessary to check for the effectiveness of the drugs; they also permit early detection of side effects.
- If you're taking lovastatin, pravastatin, or simvastatin, be sure to tell your doctor about any flulike symptoms, muscle aches, or pains. They may be early signs of side effects.
- For maximum effectiveness, these drugs must be taken daily and you should continue to follow diet and exercise recommendations provided by the doctor.
- If you're taking cholestyramine or colestipol, your doctor may want you to take supplements that contain calcium and vitamins A and D because these drugs may interfere with the absorption of these vitamins.
- If you're taking colestipol or cholestyramine, constipation may be a problem. Eat plenty of fiber-rich foods and drink adequate fluids. If constipation persists, the doctor may prescribe a stool softener. Take these drugs 1 hour before or 2 hours after meals for maximum effectiveness.
- Heartburn, nausea, indigestion, and abdominal pain usually diminish during continued treatment.
- If you miss a dose of your medication, take it as soon as you remember unless it is almost time for the next dose. Never double the dose.
- Pravastatin or simvastatin may be taken with meals; lovastatin should be taken with dinner.

VITAMINS & MINERALS

VITAMIN SUPPLEMENTS

Vitamins are necessary for healthful living. Doctors often recommend vitamin supplements when a person's diet does not provide adequate nutrition. Because many are available without prescription, most vitamin use stems from self-medication by the public.

Vitamin supplements are widely promoted for the treatment or prevention of various conditions, ranging from the common cold to cancer. However, scientific studies haven't substantiated these claims. Although a number of conditions have been associated with vitamin deficiency, studies have yet to prove that taking excessive amounts of vitamins can improve a person's skin, make hair grow, strengthen eyesight, or lengthen a person's lifespan. In fact, vitamin supplements aren't necessary for well-nourished, healthy individuals. Excessive or inappropriate use, in fact, may cause loss of appetite, headache, nausea, and vomiting; it may even prevent doctors from diagnosing certain diseases.

What are vitamin supplements used for?
- To supplement dietary intake in people with poor diet
- To help correct vitamin deficiency
- To supplement dietary intake in people with increased nutritional needs, such as pregnant and breast-feeding women

What are some common brands of vitamin supplements?
- Gerimed
- Materna
- Prenate
- Vi-Daylin

What are the guidelines for taking vitamin supplements?
- Vitamin supplements are most commonly needed by pregnant and breast-feeding women, infants, strict vegetarians, elderly people, and those who are on calorie-restricted diets. Vitamin supplements are also

> *Although a number of conditions have been associated with vitamin deficiency, studies have yet to prove that taking excessive amounts of vitamins can improve a person's skin, make hair grow, strengthen eyesight, or lengthen a person's lifespan.*

used for postoperative patients and those undergoing treatment for cancer, alcoholism, digestive disturbances, or an overactive thyroid.

- Don't take excessive amounts of vitamins. Read the label; you do not need to take amounts that greatly exceed the recommended daily allowance (RDA). Vitamin supplements should contain 50% to 150% of the RDA for most vitamins; however, the intake of vitamins A, D, and folic acid shouldn't exceed the RDA. Therapeutic vitamin supplements, available by prescription only, may contain 300% to 500% of the RDA.
- Synthetic vitamins are no less effective than natural vitamins despite their lower cost.

MINERAL SUPPLEMENTS

These supplements correct mineral deficiency caused by poor diet, increased metabolic demands, or disease.

Minerals help build bone and soft tissue and form hair, nails, and skin. They also serve other physiologic purposes. Iron and copper, for instance, are necessary for the synthesis of hemoglobin and red blood cells. Other minerals help regulate muscle contraction and relaxation, blood clotting, and acid-base balance.

Mineral supplements are often sold in combination with vitamin preparations. They're most commonly prescribed for children, pregnant women, elderly people, and people with burns or other severe injuries. They're also given to people who are being fed intravenously.

What are mineral supplements used for?
- To correct mineral deficiencies or to help meet increased metabolic demands
- To offset poor mineral absorption

What are some commonly used mineral supplements?
Calcium
- calcium acetate, known by the brand names Phos-Ex and Phos-Lo
- calcium carbonate, known by the brand names Alka-Mints, Chooz, Dicarbosil, and Tums
- calcium citrate (generic)
- calcium phosphate tribasic, known by the brand name Posture

Potassium

- potassium bicarbonate, known by the brand names K+ Care ET, Klor-Con/EF, and K-lyte ET
- potassium chloride, known by the brand names Kaochlor, Kaon-Cl, Kay Ciel, Klorvess, and Slow-K
- potassium gluconate, known by the brand names Kaon and Kaylixer

Iron

- ferrous fumarate, known by the brand names Feostat, Ferranol, Fumasorb, and Hemocyte
- ferrous gluconate, known by the brand names Fergon and Ferralet
- ferrous sulfate, known by the brand names Feosol, Fer-In-Sol, Slow-Fe, and Fero-Grad

Zinc

- zinc chloride (generic)
- zinc sulfate (generic)

What are the possible side effects?

- Muscle spasms
- Numbness of the face, fingers, or toes
- Abdominal pain, constipation, and gastrointestinal upset (especially with iron)
- Hair loss
- Abnormal heartbeats
- Staining of teeth (iron supplements)

What are the guidelines for taking mineral supplements?

Calcium

- Calcium should not be used by people with a history of kidney stones without the consent of their doctor. Calcium supplements may enhance kidney stone formation.
- To prevent impaired absorption, don't take with dairy products, bran cereal, spinach, rhubarb, or corticosteroids.

Potassium

- Don't use potassium supplements if you are taking potassium-sparing diuretics, salt substitutes, angiotensin-converting enzyme inhibitors, or other potassium-containing drugs without first checking with your doctor.

- Take potassium supplements immediately after meals to help prevent an upset stomach.

Iron

- Don't use iron supplements if you have a history of digestive tract disorders, such as peptic ulcer, Crohn's disease, or ulcerative colitis, unless you check with your doctor first.
- Iron supplements should be taken with food to prevent stomach upset but not for at least 2 hours after eating dairy products, eggs, coffee, tea, or whole grain bread or cereals because these foods interfere with absorption. Liquid iron preparations may be diluted with orange juice or water but not with antacids.
- Stools may turn black because of unabsorbed iron. This effect, however, is harmless.
- If you miss a dose, take it as soon as you remember unless it's almost time for your next dose. Never double the dose.
- Watch for constipation. Check with the doctor if a laxative or stool softener is needed.
- To avoid staining the teeth, take iron elixir through a glass straw.
- Iron tablets are responsible for a number of fatal pediatric poisonings every year. Take every precaution to prevent children from ingesting iron tablets.

Zinc

Take zinc with meals but not with dairy products, which can decrease absorption.

All supplements

- Increase the amount of fiber in your diet and drink plenty of fluids to prevent constipation.
- Many drugs can interact with oral mineral supplements. Check with the doctor or pharmacist if you are taking other drugs with mineral supplements.

Mineral supplements are most commonly prescribed for children, pregnant women, elderly people, and people with burns or other severe injuries.

DIETS

CALORIE-MODIFIED DIET

If you say the word "diet" to most people, they'll tend to think of a calorie-modified diet, specifically, a low-calorie diet. These diets are among the most popular—and most abused—forms of self-treatment. In the United States, 25% to 50% of all adults are obese. They weigh 20% or more over the ideal weight for their height.

High-calorie diets are another type of calorie-modified diet. High-calorie diets are recommended for people who are malnourished or underweight. They are also used to prevent malnourishment in people who have higher than normal food energy needs, such as athletes or people battling serious illness.

Adhering to the calorie-modified diet is the major obstacle to its success. That's obvious for people requiring a low-calorie diet, but those who need a high-calorie diet may also find it difficult to stay on the diet.

Why is this diet recommended?

▪ Calorie-modified diets are used to help correct weight imbalances through balanced nutritional practices.

▪ Low-calorie modified diets are typically used for weight reduction and maintenance. They are recommended for people who are overweight or have mild, moderate, or morbid obesity.

▪ A high-calorie modified diet is typically recommended to people who have greatly increased food energy needs. Many of them are battling such diseases as cancer, overactive thyroid, physical wasting and malnutrition, cystic fibrosis, chronic lung disease, AIDS, severe stress, and trauma. Those involved in excessive activity such as athletic training may also need a high-calorie modified diet. Treatment of anorexia nervosa also includes a high-calorie diet.

What happens before the diet?

▪ Calorie-modified diets should be planned by a registered dietitian. In many cases, the U.S. food exchange system lists are used in formulating realistic calorie-modified diets. These lists are helpful in controlling calories and energy nutrients. Exchange lists consider proportions and portion sizes, which may be easier for the dieter than counting calories.

- You undergo a thorough medical exam.
- Your complete dietary history is taken. The dietitian asks what kinds of food you like and dislike and how they're prepared. The dietitian will also discuss eating habits with you; for example, whether you eat regular meals, skip some meals, or snack between meals. Then the dietitian will talk with you about food-related behavior, asking whether you sit down at a table to eat or eat while standing, driving, or watching TV. The dietitian will ask if you smoke and whether you're trying to quit. A person who's trying to quit smoking often has difficulty following a diet.
- If you're obese, the nurse or doctor will tell you about the benefits of exercise and the role of behavior modification, psychotherapy, and prescribed drugs in weight loss. They will encourage you to participate in a weight-loss support group. Reasonable weight-loss goals will be set. Slow, gradual reduction helps keep weight from returning.
- If you're underweight, a realistic goal for weight gain (typically about 1 pound [0.5 kilogram] per week) is set. Your doctor will recommend a hearty meal at breakfast and regular meals.
- The doctor or nurse weighs you before the diet begins and once weekly afterward to chart your progress. Daily weighings are not necessary once the diet begins because weight fluctuations are usually caused by fluid retention and can be misleading.

What happens during the diet?

- A low-calorie diet should provide sufficient calories to meet your metabolic needs and activity level. If followed, it will promote weight loss of about 1 to 2 pounds (0.5 to 1 kilogram) per week.
- The low-calorie diet includes foods from all four food groups but limits carbohydrates and restricts fats and alcohol. It also includes fiber to reduce caloric density and slow digestion. Your overall treatment plan for weight reduction should include diet, exercise, and behavior modification.
- Depending on your sex, weight, and activity level, a low-calorie diet may provide 1,000 to 1,800 calories per day, with about 20% of calories obtained from protein. For obesity, the doctor may recommend an extremely low-calorie diet — providing only 300 to 700 calories per day — that includes high-quality protein and few carbohydrates.

SELF-HELP

Staying on a calorie-modified diet

At home, try to follow these important guidelines.

Watch what you eat
- Plan menus and shopping lists for the week to prevent impulse buying and eating. Eat fish and poultry instead of red meat. Substitute polyunsaturated fats for saturated ones. Eat vegetables and fruits instead of sweets.
- If you're underweight, eat dried fruits and nuts for between-meal snacks because they're high in calories and nutritious. Eat bananas with breakfast and potatoes, pasta, noodles, or rice at least twice a day.
- Beware of fad and gimmick diets. These diets often severely restrict one or more food groups and may cause dangerous side effects.

Other instructions
- Enlist the support of your family. Their encouragement and cooperation are vital to your success with the diet.
- Don't abandon your diet simply because you sometimes cheat. Occasional cheating won't affect the long-term success of the diet. Set behavior goals for yourself, such as slowly reducing the number of cheating episodes per week.
- If you're underweight, you may need to reduce your activities.

- A high-calorie diet should have a high protein content and provide 500 to 1,000 additional calories with a goal for weight gain of about 1 pound per week for most people. Your fat intake should remain within normal limits to prevent appetite loss and nausea.
- High-calorie diets provide as many calories in as small a volume as possible. Between-meal snacking is often encouraged as an effective strategy for weight gain. Milk shakes, cream soups, peanut butter, and commercially prepared liquid supplements or powdered breakfast drinks are commonly used to increase caloric intake.
- High-calorie diets increase caloric intake gradually so that you can adjust to the added food amounts. Extra helpings, snacks, and concentrated supplements also help to increase caloric intake.
- You should keep a food diary and bring it to your follow-up office visits. Your doctor will review it and make suggestions that will help improve your diet. (See *Staying on a calorie-modified diet*.)

What are the possible complications?

- Severely restricted low-calorie diets can cause weakness, apathy, fatigue, and dehydration. If the calories and nutrients are inadequate for prolonged periods, protein and calorie malnutrition may result.

- High-calorie diets can result in high levels of lipids (fats) in the blood if you eat too many fatty foods.

What happens after the diet?

- A consultation with a dietitian may be recommended if you have a severe weight imbalance. A team effort—with doctor, nurse, dietitian, and therapist participating—may be necessary to help the person.
- Your doctor or dietitian will give you menus and other tips to help you stay on the diet.

FIBER-MODIFIED DIET

Fiber makes up a crucial part of the diet, and yet it's not completely digestible. The benefits of fiber are primarily mechanical: It promotes digestion and the elimination of body wastes.

Basically, a high-fiber diet substitutes high-fiber foods for low-fiber ones. A low-fiber diet, also called a low-residue diet, restricts dietary fiber and residue to eliminate or reduce mechanical stimulation of the digestive tract. Low-residue dietary restrictions range from mild to severe. Because low-fiber diets lack sufficient vitamins and minerals, they can be used for only a limited time.

Why is this diet recommended?

High-fiber diet

- To increase fecal bulk
- To increase movement of the intestinal walls
- To decrease pressure within the bowel
- To prevent and treat constipation, irritable bowel syndrome, Crohn's disease, and diverticulosis
- To help lower cholesterol levels in people with high cholesterol
- To help with weight loss in obesity, to improve sugar tolerance in diabetes, and in coronary artery disease. A high-fiber diet may reduce the risk of bowel cancer by reducing the number of cancer-causing agents in fecal matter.

Low-fiber diet

- To reduce stool bulk
- To slow transit time through the bowel

- To limit secretion of stomach acids
- To treat people with indigestion, nausea, dilated esophageal veins, stomach inflammation, diarrhea, bowel inflammation (as seen in the acute stages of diverticulosis, ulcerative colitis, and Crohn's disease), heart attack, and congestive heart failure
- To prepare people for bowel procedures.

What happens before the diet?

The dietitian explains and reviews the prescribed diet with you and, if appropriate, with the family.

What happens during the diet?

High-fiber diet

- Extra fiber is introduced gradually. If large amounts of fiber are introduced all at once, complications are more likely. If you're diabetic and on a high-fiber diet, you should consume 30 to 50 grams per day of fiber; if you're not diabetic, the diet is more flexible and should simply include as much fiber as is practical.
- Breads and other baked goods made from whole grains, especially bran, are included. You can add coarsely ground bran to cereals, muffins, or bread as an additional fiber supplement. Eat vegetables raw or cooked with minimal preparation. Those most helpful include carrots, peas, broccoli, corn, lettuce, dried peas, and beans. Fresh fruits should be eaten unpeeled (especially apples and pears). Other high-fiber fruits include berries, oranges, and stewed and dried fruits. Nuts and seeds are also considered high in fiber.

Low-fiber diet

- You eat soft, mild food. The diet excludes raw vegetables and fruits, nuts, seeds, coarse breads, and strong seasonings and limits fried foods and fats because they can cause a backup of stomach juices into the esophagus.
- This diet includes ground or well-cooked tender meat, fish, and poultry; eggs; up to 16 ounces (480 milliliters) of milk per day; and mild cheese. It may also include strained fruit juices, except prune juice; cooked or canned apples, apricots, white cherries, peaches, pears, and ripe bananas; strained vegetable juices; canned, cooked, or strained asparagus, beets, green beans, pumpkin, acorn squash, and spinach; white bread, toast, crackers, bagels, melba toast, and waffles; and refined cereals, such as Cream of Wheat, Cream of Rice, and puffed rice. Other foods permitted on the low-fiber diet include plain desserts made with soft, seedless foods; gelatin; candy, such as

Following a fiber-modified diet

At home, try to follow these important guidelines.

Drink plenty of water

- Drink at least six to eight 8-ounce glasses of water daily. If you don't have at least one soft stool per day, add a bran supplement to your diet.
- If you're a woman on a high-fiber diet, increase calcium intake to prevent osteoporosis. Drink at least two 8-ounce glasses of milk a day and eat cheese and yogurt. If you're trying to lose weight or have diabetes, drink skim milk and eat low-fat cheese.

Other instructions

- Because mineral and vitamin deficiencies may occur, you may need to eat a variety of foods. You may also need vitamin and mineral supplements.
- If you're on a high-fiber diet, eat iron-rich foods, such as liver. Also eat meat, nuts, beans, wheat germ, and cheese to increase your level of zinc.
- Take a list of high-fiber foods with you to the grocery.
- Schedule medical follow-ups so your progress can be evaluated and your nutritional status checked.

butterscotch, jelly beans, marshmallows, and plain hard candy; and honey, molasses, and sugar.

What are the possible complications?

- Intolerance for a high-fiber diet includes such symptoms as gas, abdominal distention, cramping, and diarrhea.
- Nutrient deficiencies—for example, iron deficiency or calcium deficiency—may occur in people on high- or low-fiber diets. Constipation can also occur because the low-fiber diet decreases stool bulk and slows the passage of stool through the bowel. Low-fiber diets may not provide enough calories if used for extended periods.

What happens after the diet?

Your doctor gives you instructions. (See *Following a fiber-modified diet.*)

PROTEIN-MODIFIED DIET

A high-protein diet can benefit people with increased tissue breakdown, nitrogen depletion caused by stress or increased secretions of hormones, or protein loss. Contrary to popular belief, the protein recommendation for athletes is the same as that for the general population. Athletes require more food because they use up more energy, but a balanced diet provides sufficient protein.

When a high-protein diet is necessary, its beneficial effects can be striking. In just a few weeks, the person's general health and well-being begin to improve. He or she gains weight and feels stronger; resistance to infection increases, and wounds heal faster.

Some people require a low-protein regimen. Protein restrictions may be necessary to keep a particular balance or to prevent the harmful accumulation of ammonia (urea). Typically, such people have illnesses that impair the body's ability to eliminate the by-products of protein breakdown, such as end-stage kidney disease or severe liver disease.

Why is this diet recommended?

High-protein diets are used:

- to meet the body's increased requirements for protein

- to treat people with protein-calorie malnutrition, severe stress, and high metabolic rate resulting from conditions such as burns, cancer, AIDS, or damaged kidneys that lose large amounts of protein
- to treat people with malabsorption syndromes, short-bowel syndrome, inflammatory bowel diseases, and celiac disease.

Low-protein diets are used to treat people with cirrhosis, hepatic coma, acute kidney disease, or chronic kidney disease not treated with dialysis. Some diseases, such as alcoholism, require different modifications of protein at different stages.

What happens before the diet?

- Protein-modified diets are usually prescribed by the doctor according to your condition. A registered dietitian frequently calculates allowed protein intake and reviews it with you. A nurse reinforces and works with you, your family, and a support team to promote the individualized plan.
- The dietitian or doctor reviews your diet history. If you require a high-protein diet, you'll need to eat plenty of carbohydrates; otherwise, your body simply burns protein as fuel.
- If you require a low-protein diet, the dietitian will develop an individualized plan for you. You'll need to limit the size of portions as well as the types of foods.

What happens during the diet?

- The goal of a high-protein diet is to provide approximately 1.5 grams of protein per kilogram of body weight and approximately 2,500 calories each day. You should select one-half to two-thirds of the day's protein allowance from complete proteins, such as milk and meats (vegetables, bread, and cereals contain incomplete protein), and divide the protein allowance as evenly as possible among the meals of the day. Nonfat dry milk may be added to regular milk and to casseroles to increase their protein content.
- A low-protein diet should provide 75% of the dietary allowance in the form of high-value protein, such as that found in eggs. A low-protein diet excludes meats and dairy products, which are high in protein. It includes beverages such as carbonated soft drinks, fruit drinks and punches, lemonade, and limeade; candies such as candy corn, fondant (made with egg white only), hard candies, gum, gumdrops, jelly beans, lollipops, marshmallows, and mints; flour products such as arrowroot, cornstarch, rice starch, tapioca, and wheat starch; certain sweeteners such as corn syrup, honey, jams, jellies,

SELF-HELP

Following a protein-modified diet

At home, try to follow these important guidelines:
- If you're on a high-protein diet, remember to increase protein and calorie consumption gradually.
- If you're on a low-protein diet, look for specialized low-protein breads and other low-protein foods that are commercially available.
- Continue taking your prescribed vitamin and mineral supplements at home.
- Make sure you return to your doctor for frequent checkups.

maple syrup, and confectioner's sugar; and most varieties of fruits and vegetables. Allowed fats include butter and margarine (unsalted), mayonnaise (without eggs), oils, and shortening. The protein allowance should be divided as evenly as possible among meals. Your diet should contain enough calories to meet energy requirements; it may include supplements to prevent amino acid deficiencies. (See *Following a protein-modified diet*.)

- If you are hospitalized and on a high-protein diet, you'll be weighed daily; other people on the diet are weighed weekly. You should aim for a weight gain of 1 to 2 pounds (0.5 to 1 kilogram) per week.

What are the possible complications?

A low-protein diet can lead to malnourishment if you do not receive adequate calories and nutrients. Amino acid deficiency can also occur.

LOW-CHOLESTEROL DIET

Diet represents the first line of defense against high cholesterol levels. It's an important part of the war against heart disease. However, a person with high cholesterol may also need to stop smoking, lose weight, and exercise more. If high cholesterol levels are hereditary, the person may require cholesterol-lowering drugs.

A low-cholesterol diet isn't a cure, so most people must remain on it permanently. Typically, results don't become apparent for at least 3 months.

Because cholesterol levels reflect overall fat intake, a low-cholesterol diet has much in common with a low-fat diet. But there are some differences because of the role that certain foods play in high cholesterol. For example, research has shown that cholesterol levels can be significantly reduced by substituting monounsaturated and polyunsaturated fats (such as olive oil, safflower oil, and canola oil) for saturated fats. Dietary fiber also lowers cholesterol levels, and some research suggests that leafy and root vegetables do so as well.

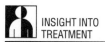

INSIGHT INTO
TREATMENT

Three ways to combat cholesterol

The American Heart Association recommends three diets for combating high blood cholesterol levels. These diets range from a slightly restrictive one, which aims to prevent excessive cholesterol intake, to a severely restricted one.

Accent on prevention

In the preventive diet, suitable for most people, about one third of the calories are evenly divided among the saturated, monounsaturated, and polyunsaturated fats. Carbohydrates — ideally, complex ones — make up half the calories, with protein making up the remainder. Total cholesterol intake doesn't exceed 300 milligrams per day.

This diet limits egg yolks to two weekly. Most organ meats are omitted. Soft margarine, vegetable oils and shortening, skim milk, and egg whites replace butter, lard, whole milk, and whole eggs. Beef may be eaten three times weekly.

Strictly lean

The American Heart Association's "phase 2" diet aims to correct mild high blood cholesterol. It contains the same distribution of fats, carbohydrates, and protein as the preventive diet but restricts cholesterol to 200 milligrams per day. It also limits the intake of milk, poultry, and seafood to 6 ounces (168 grams) a day, while emphasizing legumes, grains, fruits, and vegetables. Only extremely lean cuts of meats and skim-milk cheeses are permitted.

Lean and mean

The most restrictive diet is used for severe high blood cholesterol. Fats account for more than 25% of the calories consumed (again, equally distributed among saturated, monounsaturated, and polyunsaturated fats). Between 55% and 60% of calories come from carbohydrates. Meat, shellfish, and poultry servings are limited to 3 ounces (84 grams) daily.

Why is this diet recommended?

- To lower cholesterol levels and reduce the risk of heart disease
- To treat atherosclerosis, diabetes, high cholesterol, high blood pressure, and to prevent a heart attack

What happens before the diet?

- Your doctor usually prescribes a low-cholesterol diet. A registered dietitian may help you in menu planning.
- A health care professional will take a careful dietary history. For example, he or she will ask if you cook in animal fats, use butter or margarine, and typically bake, broil, or fry your food, and will note the number of eggs you eat every week.

What happens during the diet?

- Usually, the doctor will advise you to follow one of three diets recommended by the American Heart Association. Each of these

SELF-HELP

Following a low-cholesterol diet

At home, try to follow these important guidelines.

Be patient
Adapting to new eating patterns may take several months, so try mastering one part of the diet at a time. For example, limit your consumption of red meat before reducing the number of eggs you eat.

Watch what you eat
- When eating out, select salads and vegetables. Choose poultry over red meat. Avoid fried food, and choose simply prepared dishes instead of those with rich sauces or dressings. Vegetarian Chinese food and pasta are often good choices, except for pasta with large amounts of whole-milk cheeses.
- Use a cooking spray for frying and baking and tub margarine of a type that's high in polyunsatu-

rated or monounsaturated fat. Use a brand that shows vegetable oils first in the list of ingredients. Hydrogenated vegetable oils have more saturated fat than nonhydrogenated oils.
- Make soups or stews a day ahead and refrigerate them. Then skim off the hardened fat before reheating.

Other instructions
- Be sure to consume enough dairy products to make up for impaired calcium absorption, and eat beans and leafy vegetables to obtain iron and zinc.
- Use low-cholesterol substitutes for mayonnaise, salad dressings, hot dogs, egg noodles, ice cream, and many other foods.
- Ask the American Heart Association for pamphlets and recipe books for the low-cholesterol diet.

diets provides adequate nutrition. If necessary, calories can be reduced to help you lose weight, and salt may be restricted to curb high blood pressure. The low-cholesterol diet is phased in gradually. This makes it easier to follow, and it permits the doctor to check your response, which can vary greatly. (See *Three ways to combat cholesterol,* page 209.)

- Not all fats are the same. Saturated fats (which are often solid, such as butter or animal fat) contain cholesterol. You should try to maintain a diet in which the ratio of polyunsaturated to saturated fats is about 2:1 (in the typical American diet, this ratio is about 1:3).

- Low-density lipoprotein (LDL) carries cholesterol to the cells. High LDL can therefore promote the accumulation of cholesterol in the walls of arteries. High-density lipoprotein (HDL) is desirable because it helps to remove cholesterol from the blood and transport it to the liver for elimination.

- New, tasty foods can be exchanged for foods that are high in saturated fats. For example, beans provide an alternative source of protein. Whole grain cereal and bread, fruits, and raw vegetables can increase fiber content. Oat cereals and apples also help reduce cholesterol levels. (See *Following a low-cholesterol diet.*)

- You may need mineral supplements because high intake of dietary fiber may interfere with absorption of calcium, iron, and zinc.
- Levels of cholesterol and HDL, LDL, and very-low-density lipoprotein (VLDL) will be monitored to evaluate the effectiveness of the diet. Keep a chart of these values to provide positive reinforcement of the diet.

What are the possible complications?
The low-cholesterol diet doesn't typically produce complications.

Low-Fat Diet

Fat is a vital nutrient that supplies energy and fat-soluble vitamins. Unfortunately, most Americans eat too much of it—about 160 grams per day, on average, accounting for some 40% of their calories. Too much fat has been linked not only to obesity but also to heart disease and colon, prostate, and breast cancers.

Nutrition experts recommend that fats be limited to no more than 30% of total calories—that is, about 120 grams per day—including 10% from unsaturated fats and 8% from saturated fat. People with certain disorders may require even lower fat intake. A low-fat diet limits the daily amount to 50 grams per day; an extremely low-fat diet limits intake to only 25 to 30 grams per day.

Adhering to a low-fat diet is difficult. Simply reducing fat intake to 30% of ingested calories, for example, limits the person to three eggs a week and requires substitution of skim milk, margarine, and vegetable oils for whole milk, butter, and lard. More stringent diets, of course, are even more restrictive. (See *Foods with little or no fat.*)

Why is this diet recommended?
- To help prevent heart disease and breast, colon, or prostate cancer
- To help treat AIDS, blind-loop syndrome (depletion of vitamin B_{12} and fat malabsorption that results from bypassed intestinal segments), fatty stools, gallbladder disease, inflammatory bowel disease, liver disease, pancreatitis, short-bowel syndrome, celiac disease, topical sprue, radiation enteritis, and heartburn
- To help treat gout

Foods with little or no fat

- Coffee
- Tea (regular and herbal)
- Pasta
- French bread
- Rice
- Fruit juices
- All fruit except coconuts and avocados
- All vegetables
- Hot cereals
- Most cold cereals (check food labels for additives)
- All legumes (dry beans and peas)
- Air-popped corn
- Baked potatoes

Foods not permitted on a low-fat diet

Meats
- Sausage
- Lunch meat
- Spareribs
- Hot dogs
- Bacon
- Tuna packed in oil
- Salmon packed in oil

Dairy products
- Whole milk
- Whole-milk cheeses
- Yogurt (low-fat or nonfat is permitted)
- Ice cream

Fruits and vegetables
Buttered or au gratin, creamed, or fried vegetables

Breads and cereals
- Products made with added fat: biscuits, muffins, pancakes, doughnuts, waffles, and sweet rolls
- Breads made with eggs, cheese, or added fat

Miscellaneous
- Gravy
- Peanut butter
- Desserts
- Candy
- Any food containing chocolate or nuts

What happens before the diet?

- This diet is usually prescribed by your doctor; the dietician reviews it with you.
- A health professional will take your dietary history and will ask about food preferences and how often you eat in restaurants, especially the fast-food type.

What happens during the diet?

- The restriction of fat depends on the number of grams of fat permitted per day. Most low-fat diets eliminate whole milk and whole-milk cheeses; pastries, cake, and pies made with fat; and desserts and soups made from cream, chocolate, or nuts. (See *Foods not permitted on a low-fat diet.*)
- Your doctor will encourage you to substitute vegetables, fruits, rice, pasta, and bread and cereals without added fats for high-fat foods.
- Your doctor will advise you to limit your meat intake to 6 ounces (168 grams) of lean meat per day. Meat substitutes (such as eggs) are also limited because two medium eggs provide 10 grams of fat. Your intake of butter, margarine, oils, salad dressings, cream, and nuts also will be limited.
- A diet allowing 30 to 40 grams of fat per day excludes whole milk and its products and limits eggs to three per week. However, you may use skim milk and products made from it, and you can have 1 tablespoon of oil, lard, butter, or mayonnaise and 4 ounces (112 grams) of

SELF-HELP

Following a low-fat diet

At home, try to follow these important guidelines.

Use low-fat foods
- Learn how to shop for low-fat foods. For instance, look for dairy products made with skim milk and for pasta that doesn't contain eggs. Explore certain ethnic foods. Italian, Japanese, and Chinese foods are often low in fat and offer helpful variety to the diet. Stay away from Italian foods that contain cheese.
- Prepare foods properly to reduce dietary fat. For example, put baked meats or poultry on a rack away from the drippings. Remove skin and fat from foods before cooking them.
- Use fish, poultry, veal, and lean cuts of beef and pork as allowed. Remove visible fat and skin from meat. Broil, bake, or steam foods instead of frying them.
- Use egg whites for cooking.

Other instructions
- When eating out, order juice for an appetizer and use lemon juice or vinegar on salads. You must limit portions of meat; order foods that are broiled, baked, or poached. Omit sauces and gravies, and select ices or fruit for dessert.
- Buy some low-calorie cookbooks, which feature appealing low-fat recipes.
- Take vitamin supplements because a low-fat diet reduces your intake of fat-soluble vitamins.
- Substitute reduced-calorie, reduced-fat, and no-fat items for regular margarines, salad dressings, and mayonnaise.
- Check with your doctor to find out if your diet can include medium-chain triglycerides. These synthetic substances may be used in place of cooking oil.

lean meat daily. You should avoid such high-fat snacks as chocolate, nuts, cheese crackers, and potato chips. (See *Following a low-fat diet*.)

What are the possible complications?
Vitamin deficiencies can occur if you don't take vitamin supplements. Sometimes, you'll find it difficult to consume enough calories.

LOW-SALT DIET

The low-salt diet is one that people find difficult, often describing it as tasteless and bland. Most Americans typically consume over 5,000 milligrams of sodium (the main element in salt) per day. A low-salt diet may restrict sodium intake to as little as 250 milligrams per day.

SELF-HELP

Meal planning for a low-salt diet

Mild restrictions

Depending on a person's condition, the prescribed restrictions on salt intake may be mild or severe.

Sodium restricted to 4,000 to 5,000 milligrams per day

- Cook with a minimum of salt (up to ½ teaspoon per day).
- Use regular milk — limit buttermilk to once a week.
- Use fresh or frozen vegetables and low-salt vegetable juices. Avoid sauerkraut and other pickled vegetables prepared in brine.
- Eat fruits as desired.
- Beverages, sweets, and desserts may be taken as desired.
- Use regular bread, but avoid breads with salted tops.
- Use limited amounts of canned and dehydrated soups.
- Avoid any meat, fish, or poultry that is smoked, cured, or salted. Avoid lunch meat, hot dogs, sausages, sardines, anchovies, marinated herring, pickled meats and eggs, and processed cheese.
- Avoid salad dressing containing bacon fat, bacon bits, and salt pork.
- Avoid all seasonings or herbs labeled with the word SALT (garlic salt, celery salt, onion salt, and seasoned salt).
- Avoid commercially prepared potato, stuffing, and rice mixes.
- Avoid obviously salty foods, such as pickles and salted snacks.

Sodium restricted to 2,000 to 3,000 milligrams per day

- Cook food with a minimum of salt (up to ½ teaspoon per day) and don't use salt at the table.
- Avoid obviously salty foods, such as potato chips, pretzels, and snack crackers, and other high-salt foods, such as canned soups and vegetables, pre-

pared foods (such as TV dinners and frozen entrees), lunch meats, cheeses, or pickles, and any other foods preserved in brine. (Low-salt canned products may be included.)
- Avoid using canned tomatoes and tomato products, unless they are low-salt products.
- Avoid salted sauces or seasonings, such as chili sauce, mustard, catsup, and relish.
- Use unsalted meat, broth, soups, and butter.

Severe restrictions

Follow these same guidelines for all other levels of sodium restriction, but cook your food without salt.

Sodium restricted to 1,000 milligrams per day

- Regular milk, 1 pint
- Unsalted eggs
- Unsalted meat, 6 ounces, cooked
- Unsalted vegetables, three servings
- Citrus fruit, as desired
- Unsalted bread and its exchanges, as desired
- Regular bread, four slices
- Fats, sugars, and jellies without sodium preservatives

Sodium restricted to 800 milligrams per day

- Regular milk, 1 pint
- Unsalted eggs
- Unsalted meat, 6 ounces, cooked
- Unsalted vegetables, three servings
- Citrus fruit, as desired
- Unsalted bread and its exchanges, as desired
- Regular bread, one slice
- Unsalted butter, sugars, and jellies without sodium preservatives

Sodium restricted to 500 milligrams per day

- Regular milk, ½ pint
- Low-salt milk, ½ pint

Meal planning for a low-salt diet *(continued)*

Sodium restricted to 500 milligrams per day *(continued)*
- Unsalted egg, one (in place of 1 ounce of meat)
- Unsalted meat, 6 ounces, cooked
- Unsalted vegetables, three servings, but exclude beets, beet greens, carrots, kale, spinach, celery, white turnips, rutabagas, mustard greens, chard, and dandelion greens
- Citrus fruit, one serving
- Unsalted bread and its exchanges, as desired
- Fats, sugar, and jellies without sodium preservatives (no sherbet or gelatin)

Sodium restricted to 250 milligrams per day
- Low-salt milk, 1 pint
- Unsalted meat, 5 ounces, cooked (one unsalted egg can be substituted for 3 ounces meat)
- Unsalted vegetables, three servings (omit the same vegetables as those listed in the 500-milligram diet)
- Citrus fruit, three servings
- Unsalted bread and its exchanges, six servings
- Fats, sugar, and jellies without sodium preservatives

Why is this diet recommended?

- To restrict dietary salt, thereby preventing or correcting water retention and swelling
- To help correct a variety of disorders, including high blood pressure, congestive heart failure, some kidney diseases characterized by fluid retention and high blood pressure, and liver diseases characterized by fluid retention in the tissues and abdominal cavity, and to prevent heart attack. Low-salt diets may also be used in treating diabetes and coronary artery disease.

When shouldn't this diet be recommended?

- This diet should not be used in people with sodium-wasting kidney diseases, such as inflammation of the kidneys and polycystic kidney disease. When an obstruction causes the kidneys to distend with urine, it is best to avoid this diet.
- The low-salt diet should also be avoided in pregnant women, in people with severe cases of underactive thyroid, and in those with ileostomies.

What happens before the diet?

- A doctor usually prescribes the diet, and a dietitian assists in planning food choices. Depending on your condition, the prescribed restriction of salt can be mild or strict. (See *Meal planning for a low-salt diet.*)
- A nurse will ask you about your diet to estimate the salt content of your typical food choices as well as the amount of salt added at the table.

SELF-HELP

Following a low-salt diet

At home, try to follow these important guidelines.

Read labels carefully

- Learn to read food labels so you can determine sodium content. The sodium content is noted on the label (200 milligrams of salt equals 80 milligrams of sodium). Additives are listed in order of greatest quantity. Avoid a product if one of the following additives is among the first five listed: salt, sodium benzoate, sodium nitrate, or monosodium glutamate (MSG).
- Many over-the-counter medications, such as Alka-Seltzer, Di-Gel, Maalox Plus, Metamucil, Rolaids, and Vicks Formula 44 Cough Mixture, contain sodium. Consult your doctor or pharmacist about the sodium content of any over-the-counter medicine you want to take.
- To help make the diet more palatable, season foods with herbs and spices instead of salt. Avoid salt substitutes, unless your doctor approves. Some products advertised as low-sodium salt substitutes contain sodium chloride and may contain potassium or ammonium salts, which could be harmful if you have kidney or liver disease. Other products, classified as vegetized salts, use powdered dehydrated vegetables as a base and may contain considerable amounts of sodium.

Watch what you eat and how you prepare food

- When eating out, order baked, broiled, or roasted foods. Avoid gravies, soups, and cheesy dressings.
- Learn how to modify ethnic food practices. For example, if you like Southern cuisine, avoid cooking with bacon or salt pork.
- Jewish people who follow orthodox dietary laws regarding meat and poultry may need to make minor adjustments. To be kosher, ritually slaughtered meat and poultry must be salted for 1 hour to remove the blood. Although the meat or poultry is thoroughly washed before cooking, some salt is retained, increasing its sodium content by as much as 400%. Try using ammonium chloride instead of sodium chloride to draw the blood out. Also, boil the meat and discard the broth before serving.

- Use fresh tomatoes for soups and sauces. Use unsalted canned tomatoes, tomato paste, or tomato juice, and avoid or restrict your intake of olives, Italian cheeses, and Italian bread.
- Avoid seasoning food with MSG or soy sauce. A low-salt soy sauce is available but should be used carefully because it still contains a considerable amount of sodium.

Other instructions

- Know that low-salt milk, unsalted canned vegetables, unsalted butter and margarine, low-salt soups, and low-salt baking powder are available.
- Ask your dietitian for help in planning low-salt menus and methods for preparing foods at home. Dietitians use a system similar to counting calories for counting sodium milligrams. You can eat small portions of sodium-containing food as part of your daily salt allotment.
- Remember that bottled soft drinks may be high in salt, depending on the salt content of the water where they're manufactured.
- Be aware that eliminating dietary salt may place you at risk for iodine deficiency. Be sure to eat other foods containing iodine, such as seafood and vegetables grown in iodine-rich soil. You can have the iodine content of your garden soil analyzed. Your doctor may prescribe supplemental iodine tablets if the iodine content of your diet and local drinking water is inadequate. Contact the local water authority or have your well water tested to establish iodine content.
- Ask the American Heart Association for additional information about salt-restricted diets.

▪ The nurse will teach you how to identify dietary sources of sodium. Most people easily recognize salt because of its distinctive taste. But they may equate sodium solely with table salt (which is 46% sodium). Sodium is a natural component in many foods. Meat, fish, milk, and eggs usually contain more sodium than do whole grain cereals, fruits, and vegetables. Food additives such as monosodium glutamate and baking soda can significantly increase sodium content of food. Many food additives that add sodium do not give the food a salty taste.

What happens during the diet?

Low-salt diets that limit sodium intake to 250 or 500 milligrams per day should be used only briefly. If your sodium intake is limited to 250 milligrams per day, you must use distilled water for drinking and for making coffee, tea, and other beverages. All other diets allow 100 milligrams of sodium for 1,000 milliliters (1 quart) of tap water. (See *Following a low-salt diet*.)

What are the possible complications?

People restricted to 500 milligrams per day or less of sodium may develop low sodium and chloride levels.

GLUTEN-FREE DIET

A gluten-free diet helps prevent the bloating, projectile vomiting, diarrhea, weight loss, malnutrition, and poor growth patterns associated with celiac disease. In this disorder, which is usually first diagnosed in infancy or early childhood, the intestinal lining is damaged by the glutamine-bound fraction of protein (gliadin) in many grain products. Researchers aren't sure why celiac disease occurs.

A gluten-free diet can't reverse the intestinal damage of celiac disease, but it can usually prevent further damage, relieve symptoms, and correct malabsorption of nutrients. Children may show improvement after 2 weeks on a gluten-free diet; in adults, results take a little longer, typically a month or two.

Initially, the person's diet excludes sources of gluten but may include supplementary protein, calories, vitamins, and minerals to correct previous dietary deficiencies. After such deficiencies are cor-

Gluten-free diet guidelines

If your doctor puts you on a gluten-free diet, you must remain on it for the rest of your life. Follow these guidelines in preparing meals.

Meat and meat alternatives
All allowed except those that are breaded, prepared with bread crumbs, or creamed. Avoid sausage, hot dogs, and turkey injected with hydrolyzed vegetable protein.

Milk and milk products
All allowed except milk mixed with Ovaltine, commercial chocolate milk with a cereal additive, pudding thickened with wheat flour, or ice cream or sherbet containing gluten stabilizers.

Fruits and vegetables
All allowed except those that are breaded, prepared with bread crumbs, or creamed.

Grains
Allowed: Bread, cereal, or dessert products made from arrowroot, soybean flour, rice flour, potato flour, or gluten-free starch; gluten-free macaroni or porridge; tapioca; cornmeal, corn flakes, popcorn, and hominy; rice, creamed rice, puffed rice, and rice flakes; buckwheat products; and potato chips.

Not allowed: Bread, cereal, or dessert products made from wheat, rye, oats, or barley; commercially prepared mixes for biscuits, cornbread, muffins, pancakes, cakes, cookies, and waffles; bran, pasta, macaroni, and noodles; malt; pretzels; wheat germ; doughnuts; and ice cream cones.

Miscellaneous
Not allowed: Beer, ale, certain whiskeys (Canadian rye), cereal, beverages such as Postum, root beer, commercial salad dressings that contain gluten stabilizers, and soups containing any ingredient not allowed (such as barley).

rected, the person follows a diet that's normal except for its gluten content. The person must follow this diet scrupulously for the rest of his or her life. Eating even small amounts of gluten-containing foods may prevent remission or induce relapse. People who repeatedly go on and off the gluten-free diet may eventually fail to respond to it.

Why is this diet recommended?
The gluten-free diet is used to prevent complications of celiac disease.

What happens during the diet?
▪ The doctor commonly prescribes a gluten-free diet that must be followed for life. The dietitian outlines any specific restrictions of the diet and then assists the family with continued dietary management. (See *Gluten-free diet guidelines.*)

▪ A gluten-free diet eliminates all products containing wheat, rye, oats, barley, and malt. In their place, you may eat cereals and breads

SELF-HELP

Following a gluten-free diet

A gluten-free diet is difficult to follow because gluten is hidden in many foods—for example, in chocolate syrup, where it's used as a stabilizing and thickening agent. It's also in sausages, hot dogs, turkey injected with hydrolyzed vegetable protein, distilled white vinegar, and whiskeys.

Nevertheless, you must understand that this is a lifelong diet, and you'll need to keep in mind these important guidelines.

Precautions for parents

- If your child is put on a gluten-free diet, make sure you observe the child closely for improvement once the diet begins. Dramatic improvement is common within the first few days, and it will continue as long as the child follows the diet.
- Notify the doctor if your child ingests foods containing gluten.

Special foods

- Be aware that special foods are commercially available for people with celiac disease. So have your dietitian recommend appropriate brands.
- Rice and rice flour, often available in Asian food stores, are good choices. Health food stores also carry many of the appropriate foods.

Other points to remember

- Make sure you read food labels for gluten content. Many foods contain hidden gluten. Products that contain "hydrolyzed vegetable protein" or that have "vegetable protein added" must be avoided.
- When eating out, order broiled or boiled meat or fish, and avoid sauces, gravies, and breaded foods.
- Foods made with gluten-free flours may be less grainy if the flour is mixed with a liquid in a recipe. Boil the flour with the liquid and cool this mixture.
- See your doctor regularly so that he or she can evaluate your nutritional status.

made from rice, corn, soy, and potatoes. Initially, you should also avoid milk and milk products because intestinal damage often causes an intolerance to lactose. As your symptoms improve, these dairy products can be gradually reintroduced.

What are the possible complications?

Failure to follow the gluten-free diet causes complications of celiac disease: projectile vomiting, chronic diarrhea, and poor growth patterns. (See *Following a gluten-free diet*.)

LOW-PURINE DIET

This diet restricts foods such as liver, eggs, and sardines that contain preformed purines, which the body breaks down into uric acid. This diet used to be commonly prescribed to control gout and prevent kidney stones, but its use has recently become controversial. Because the body is now known to create purines, dietary measures alone will not control the uric acid level. The low-purine diet is now prescribed with a weight-control and exercise program to supplement therapy with drugs.

Why is this diet recommended?
- To lower uric acid levels while supplying adequate nutrients
- To help treat gout and kidney stones
- To treat people with increased uric acid levels that occur as a complication of obesity, high blood pressure, high levels of triglycerides in the blood, alcoholism, lead toxicity, pregnancy-induced high blood pressure, leukemia, high red blood cell count, psoriasis, or diuretic therapy

What happens before the diet?
- Your doctor prescribes this diet as part of your treatment. Usually, the dietitian explains it to you. It's only part of a comprehensive regimen.
- A nurse will review your dietary and medication history with you. The nurse will ask about your alcohol consumption, which can aggravate gout. Your use of medications is reviewed because hydrochlorothiazide, pyrazinamide, and other drugs can cause accumulation of uric acid in body tissues.

What happens during the diet?
- The low-purine diet contains limited amounts of fats, moderate amounts of protein, and plentiful amounts of complex carbohydrates. It also includes about 2 quarts (2 liters) per day of water and fruit juice to help promote uric acid excretion, decrease the risk of kidney stones, and prevent the dehydration associated with antigout medications. This diet also includes fruits and vegetables to increase the alkalinity of the urine and thereby increase the solubility of uric acid.

SELF-HELP

Following a low-purine diet

At home, try to follow these important guidelines.

Take special precautions
- Do not fast, follow low-carbohydrate diets, or lose weight rapidly. These will inhibit the excretion of uric acid. If you wish to lose weight, do it gradually.
- Don't drink alcoholic beverages, which can aggravate gout.
- Avoid aspirin and other salicylates. They can interact with certain antigout drugs to prevent uric acid excretion.

Other instructions
- Increase fluid intake by having soup or drinking a glass of water before each meal and at bedtime.
- Develop an exercise and weight-control program.
- Be aware that avoiding coffee, tea, and cocoa is no longer considered necessary.
- Keep a food diary and review it at follow-up visits.
- See your doctor regularly so that your progress can be monitored and the doctor can detect dietary deficiencies.

- The diet permits limited amounts of foods containing moderate amounts of purines, such as meats and dairy products and any food containing less than 150 milligrams of purines per 100 grams.
- Foods that are excluded include organ meats, such as liver, kidney, sweetbreads, brains, and heart; certain types of fish, including mussels, anchovies, sardines, fish roe, herring, shrimp, and mackerel; and certain other foods, such as mincemeat and yeast. (See *Following a low-purine diet.*)

What are the possible complications?
The low-purine diet doesn't usually cause complications.

LOW-PHENYLALANINE DIET

The low-phenylalanine diet, if begun shortly after birth and scrupulously followed, prevents mental retardation and neurologic damage in children with phenylketonuria. This is a congenital deficiency of the liver enzyme phenylalanine hydroxylase. (Most infants in the United States are screened for the disorder soon after birth.) Although the low-phenylalanine diet is effective, it is difficult to follow. Nevertheless, the child with phenylketonuria must begin to take responsibility for the diet at an early age—even before understanding the consequences of not doing so. Outside the home, the child may find that the diet sets him or her apart from other children.

Unfortunately, there is no safe age to discontinue the diet. Pregnant women with phenylketonuria must strictly follow the diet because excess phenylalanine can be transmitted to the fetus and cause congenital defects.

Why is this diet recommended?

The low-phenylalanine diet is recommended for all people with phenylketonuria. It reduces phenylalanine intake and prevents accumulation of excessive phenylalanine levels in the blood, while providing sufficient amino acids and nutrients for normal growth and development. A child can develop normally—physically and psychologically—only if the diet is followed scrupulously.

What happens before the diet?

- Your doctor will explain that this diet is essential for the developing nervous system of your child.
- A nurse will explain the diet thoroughly to you.

What happens during the diet?

When the child's blood level of phenylalanine is determined, the nutritionist establishes a diet that permits your child to maintain a tolerable blood phenylalanine level. The diet consists of two parts: milk substitutes for the infant's first food and guidelines for adding solid foods. The nutritionist continuously monitors and adjusts the diet according to the child's blood phenylalanine level, age, and weight.

To eliminate milk, which has a high phenylalanine content, you feed the infant a special formula containing casein hydrolysate products or elemental crystalline amino acids. Such formulas contain a limited amount of phenylalanine or are phenylalanine-free; all are balanced with fats, carbohydrates, vitamins, and minerals. You can add a small amount of milk or regular infant formula to the special formula to adjust the phenylalanine content and maintain an appropriate blood level.

As your infant grows, you can select solid foods from a list of phenylalanine food exchange groups or equivalents according to their phenylalanine content. Specially prepared beverages and other phenylalanine-free products are also used for growing children. (See *Caring for a child on a low-phenylalanine diet*.)

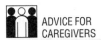

ADVICE FOR
CAREGIVERS

Caring for a child on a low-phenylalanine diet

If you're a parent with a child on a low-phenylalanine diet, try to follow these important guidelines.

Help your child adjust

- Don't be overly protective of your child or over-emphasize his diet. If you do, it can make the child feel limited socially and take all the pleasure out of eating for him. Treat your child as normally as possible. Family counseling may be necessary to help you and your child adjust to the diet regimen.
- The child must learn to become responsible for his own diet. Help him develop this responsibility early. For example, by age 3 or 4, children can learn that some foods are "no" foods and others are "yes" foods. Children can be taught to count out how many crackers they're allowed to eat.

Other points to remember

- Keep a daily food diary. It will be reviewed during follow-up visits to assess phenylalanine intake and overall nutrition.
- Tissue breakdown during illness can cause an accumulation of phenylalanine in the blood. The child may be restricted to clear liquids during illness. Reintroduce the formula or diet as soon as possible after the child recovers.
- There are specialty shops and mail-order firms that carry low-protein foods. You can also find cookbooks designed for a low-phenylalanine diet and vegetarian cookbooks that include dairy products.
- Be aware that Nutrasweet contains phenylalanine.

What are the possible complications?

The low-phenylalanine diet can cause stunted growth if the diet is not properly regulated and phenylalanine is eliminated totally from the diet.

LACTOSE-REDUCED DIET

A lactose-reduced diet is the only treatment for lactose intolerance (deficiency of the enzyme lactase), a common disorder that causes difficulty in digesting dairy products.

Beginning after age 4, nearly 70% of people develop some degree of lactose intolerance. The incidence of this disorder increases with age, perhaps because lactase activity decreases as a person grows older. Lactase activity is at its peak during infancy. For reasons not entirely understood, lactose intolerance is usually more pronounced among Blacks, Jews, Native Americans, and Asians. Rarely, complete lactose intolerance is present from birth. Secondary lactose intolerance may occur in people with such disorders as celiac disease, sprue, colitis, enteritis, cystic fibrosis, or malnutrition and in people who have undergone a gastrectomy (surgical removal of all or part of the stomach) or removal of a portion of the bowel.

Few people require a diet that's totally free of lactose. It depends on whether the person has a complete or partial lactase deficiency. Most people can tolerate some milk if it's carefully spaced throughout the day, and many can tolerate cheese or yogurt (in which lactose is broken down by the active cultures) as well as sweet acidophilus milk (which contains an enzyme that hydrolyzes lactose). Over-the-counter lactose enzyme tablets permit digestion of lactose-containing foods and benefit some people.

Because the lactose-reduced diet is somewhat flexible, it's easy to follow, and, unlike many other diets, it need not be permanent. Many people can gradually add dairy products without suffering ill effects. (See *What happens in lactose intolerance.*)

Why is this diet recommended?

The lactose-reduced diet is used to alleviate the gastrointestinal symptoms of lactose intolerance, such as abdominal cramps, bloating, gas, and diarrhea.

What happens before the diet?

- A nurse or doctor will explain why you have trouble digesting dairy products. This happens because undigested lactose is fermented by intestinal bacteria and it draws water into your intestine. The acids and gases formed by fermentation then combine with the excess water to cause bloating, cramping, and diarrhea. Because milk and milk products are the only sources of lactose, eliminating or limiting them can prevent gastrointestinal distress.
- Before prescribing this diet, your doctor will measure your ability to digest lactose by performing either of two tests: the lactose tolerance test or the lactose malabsorption test.
- After evaluating your ability to digest lactose, the doctor may recommend that you limit or eliminate consumption of milk and milk products or use lactose enzyme tablets.

What happens in lactose intolerance

Normal digestion

Carbohydrates typically reach the small intestine in disaccharide form. In normal digestion, lactose, one of these disaccharides, is broken down by lactase — an enzyme located in the intestine — before absorption takes place.

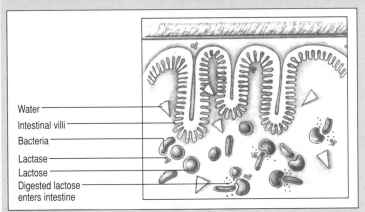

Water
Intestinal villi
Bacteria
Lactase
Lactose
Digested lactose enters intestine

Digestion in lactose intolerance

In lactose intolerance, the classic signs — bloating, gas, diarrhea, and malabsorption — result from undigested lactose in the small intestine (the undigested lactose is caused by a lactase deficiency). In the intestine, this lactose is attacked by bacteria giving off hydrogen as it's broken down. Lactose also draws water into the intestine by osmosis. The gas and increased fluid load trigger increased intestinal motility, which in turn inhibits absorption of other nutrients.

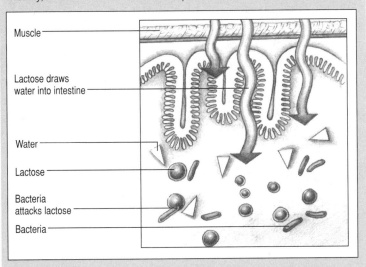

Muscle

Lactose draws water into intestine

Water

Lactose

Bacteria attacks lactose

Bacteria

SELF-HELP

Following a lactose-reduced diet

At home, try to follow these important guidelines.

Avoid milk and mild products
- Limit or eliminate the amount of ordinary milk and milk products you consume. For example, drink no more than half a cup of ordinary milk per day. Try substituting sweet acidophilus milk, eating small quantities of cheese or yogurt, and drinking small amounts of buttermilk. Doing so will break down or hydrolyze lactose.
- Avoid baked goods made with milk, sausages that contain milk solids, creamy sauces and gravies, and processed foods that contain other less obvious sources of lactose (chocolate, caramel, cocoa mixes, certain nondairy creamers, vitamins, instant potatoes, and frozen french fries).

Read food labels and use milk substitutes
- Read food labels carefully to detect the presence of milk, milk solids, whey, lactose, or casein.

- Substitute water or fruit juices for milk in recipes, and, when eating in restaurants, avoid foods prepared with sauces, gravies, or bread.
- Use calcium-fortified soy milk as a milk substitute.

Other instructions
- If your symptoms improve, try adding small amounts of dairy products at one meal. If you tolerate them well, you can gradually add more. Sometimes chocolate milk is tolerated better than regular milk. If you want to try adding cottage cheese to your diet, try different brands. The amount of lactose they contain varies widely.
- Try adding an enzyme preparation (such as Lact-Aid) to milk before drinking. The enzyme breaks down much of the lactose in milk.
- Be aware that other calcium-rich foods, such as dark green leafy vegetables and grains, may provide small amounts of available calcium, but calcium from these sources are not absorbed well by the body.

What happens during the diet?
- After the doctor makes this recommendation, you are taught the sources of lactose. With the help of a nurse or dietitian, you then find your level of tolerance. (See *Following a lactose-reduced diet.*)
- You may develop signs and symptoms of lactose intolerance, including cramping, bloating, and diarrhea. These are most likely to occur when you are establishing your level of tolerance, or when lactose-containing foods are gradually being reintroduced into your diet.

What are the possible complications?
Calcium deficiency can complicate the lactose-reduced diet as a result of reduced intake of milk and milk products.

OTHER TREATMENTS

TUBE FEEDINGS

A feeding tube delivers pureed food or a special liquid formula directly into the stomach or small intestine. The tube is most commonly inserted through the nose or through a surgical incision in the stomach or small intestine.

Why is this procedure done?

Tube feedings are given to provide necessary nutrition in people who are unable or unwilling to eat. If their gastrointestinal system is at least partially functioning, they may be candidates for a feeding tube. People who need this procedure include those with high metabolisms; those with oral or esophageal obstruction or injury; some people with neurologic disease, such as a stroke; unconscious people; and some people with psychological disorders.

When shouldn't this procedure be done?

- People at risk for pulmonary aspiration of stomach contents or those with severe vomiting or heartburn should not have a feeding tube inserted through the nose and into the stomach.
- People with stomach disease or who are at risk for aspiration should not have a feeding tube inserted nasally into the small intestine.

What happens before the procedure?

A nurse will explain why you need a feeding tube and how it will be provided.

What happens during the procedure?

- Feeding tubes deliver pureed foods or commercially prepared formulas. When tube feedings are started, the amount of nutrients delivered starts out slowly and is gradually increased as your tolerance allows. The feedings could be intermittent or continuous, although continuous feedings are most common.
- The nurse weighs you daily to assess the results of therapy.

If tube feedings are to continue after discharge, you or a family member will be given step-by-step instructions on how to administer the feedings at home.

▪ The nurse gives you meticulous mouth care. If a tube is in your nose, the nurse will also provide nasal hygiene daily. Skin care is provided if you have a surgically implanted feeding tube.

What are the possible complications?

Complications of a feeding tube may be mechanical, gastrointestinal, or metabolic. Fortunately, most can be managed without removing the feeding tube.

What happens after the procedure?

If tube feedings are to continue after discharge, you or a family member will be given step-by-step instructions on how to administer the feedings at home. Instructions will also include how the equipment works, how to care for it, how to troubleshoot any problems, and how to care for the insertion site.

NUTRITION THROUGH AN INTRAVENOUS LINE

People receiving nutrition through an intravenous line receive a nutrient solution containing dextrose, amino acids, fats, electrolytes, vitamins, micronutrients, and water. The nutrients are received through a catheter inserted in a central or a peripheral vein.

The intravenous line is inserted in a large, central vein for people who receive all of their nourishment in this manner. It's used to meet nutritional needs for a prolonged period and may be used as a preventive therapeutic measure. Nutrition from the intravenous line provides 2,000 to 5,000 calories daily and is used to replace nutrients in markedly malnourished people.

A direct central line puts a person at risk for a punctured lung but offers several advantages over a peripheral line. It's easily dressed and doesn't restrict activity. It permits the administration of any type of solution, regardless of density, and it eliminates the need for repeated venipuncture for blood testing.

Peripheral parenteral nutrition is administered through an intravenous line in the arm and supplies 1,400 to 2,000 calories daily. It's usually used for nutritional maintenance in people who've had nothing to eat by mouth for more than 3 days and who aren't expected to eat again for the next 10 to 14 days. Peripheral parenteral nutrition supplies the person's full caloric needs without the risks associated with central venous access. Because there are limits on what can be added to the solution, it can't meet full nutritional needs.

The type of solution used depends on the person's needs and condition.

Why is this treatment done?

- To provide essential nutrients for people who can't eat food through the mouth
- To provide supplemental nutrients for people with protein-wasting conditions
- To provide nutrition for people with severe Crohn's disease, intestinal fistulas, short-bowel syndrome, or ulcerative colitis, in whom gastrointestinal feeding is not possible or is ineffective
- To provide supplemental nutrition for malnourished and comatose people and for those with burns, trauma, or cancer

What happens before the treatment?

A nurse explains the treatment to you.

What happens during the treatment?

- The doctor inserts a special intravenous catheter into a large vein either at the bedside or in the operating room.
- The peripheral venous catheter, which is inserted into a vein in the arm, may be inserted by a specially trained nurse.
- The solution is connected to an intravenous line and then infused by a pump. The infusion begins at a slow rate, is gradually increased, and then is slowly tapered to discontinue. It may be given around the clock or as a nighttime feeding to allow greater freedom of movement during the day.

What are the possible complications?

Nutrition given through an intravenous line can cause potentially severe complications, such as infection, high blood sugar, and low blood potassium.

What happens after the treatment?

- The nurse weighs you every day at the same time, using the same scale, and with you wearing the same type of clothing.

Continuing intravenous nutrition at home

If intravenous nutrition will continue at home, a family member will be taught how to administer it before you leave the hospital. Make sure you follow these guidelines.

Store the solution properly

Be sure to store and refrigerate the solution properly. Each bag has an expiration date. Check the solution's date, composition, and appearance, and then, if the solution is OK to use, allow it to warm to room temperature first. For most people, the solution will be delivered daily or will have to be picked up from a local pharmacy.

Watch for possible complications

- You will be shown how to check urine sugar levels and how to monitor fluid intake and output. Watch for swelling of the arms, legs, hands, or feet, which indicates electrolyte imbalances, and be alert for signs of infection.
- Be aware of the potential complications of nutrition delivered through an intravenous line. And make sure you keep the telephone numbers of local police and fire department, ambulance company, hospital, and doctor within easy reach.

Other instructions

- Change the person's dressing whenever it becomes soiled or loose, at least once a week (for transparent polyurethane dressings) or every other day (for gauze dressings). A nurse will show you how to use the aseptic technique when changing the dressing.
- Inspect the catheter insertion site regularly for swelling, redness, or drainage. If you are inspecting your own dressing, use a mirror.
- Learn the techniques for cleaning the catheter and follow them regularly.
- The person should be weighed daily at the same time, on the same scale, and while wearing similar clothing.
- Know that it's a good idea to have a home health care nurse visit for at least the first week to be sure that the home infusions are being administered correctly.

- To prevent oral lesions and infections, you must brush your teeth and tongue frequently and use mouthwash and lip balm, as necessary. (See *Continuing intravenous nutrition at home*.)

REPLENISHING FLUIDS WITH INTRAVENOUS SOLUTIONS

Intravenous solutions are used to replenish water and electrolytes in the body. They are usually given when a person has a deficit in water or electrolytes.

To prevent heart failure from overload, people receiving fluid through intravenous solutions are monitored carefully if they have heart or kidney disease.

Why is this treatment done?
- To replace depleted body fluids
- To maintain blood flow to brain and vital organs
- To replace electrolytes
- To replace fluids when severe vomiting and diarrhea cause dehydration or when blood loss from trauma or surgery causes low blood volume

What happens before the treatment?
- The doctor will order the type of fluid and the rate of administration.
- The nurse may insert a urinary catheter.

What happens during the treatment?
- The nurse inserts one or two intravenous lines.
- The nurse takes your vital signs at regular intervals.
- You're monitored for fluid overload.

What are the possible complications?
- People receiving intravenous fluid solutions are at risk for fluid overload. This is especially true of people with heart or kidney disease.
- After blood replacement, the person is at risk for transfusion reaction and blood-borne diseases.
- Other complications are related to the specific type of infusion. Some may cause volume overload, congestive heart failure, and excess fluid in the lungs or brain. Others may cause allergic reactions, including fever, chills, and even anaphylactic shock.

What happens after the treatment?
You sometimes continue the treatment at home. If so, make sure you watch for early signs and symptoms of fluid depletion. Symptoms of dehydration include dry mouth, dizziness when you stand up, weakness, and fatigue. Notify your doctor if these occur. This is especially important for elderly people and children, who can quickly become dehydrated from vomiting and diarrhea.

SURGICAL TREATMENT OF OBESITY

Surgical treatment of obesity helps people lose weight and avoid life-threatening weight-related complications. Three commonly performed procedures are jejunoileal bypass, gastric bypass, and vertical banded gastroplasty. None of these procedures is totally effective or safe.

Jejunoileal bypass allows weight reduction by shortening the small intestine. Performed frequently in the 1970s, this procedure is now used less often because of postoperative complications. Gastric bypass (stomach bypass) and vertical banded gastroplasty are thought to produce weight loss by limiting the amount of food that can be ingested. These procedures are less likely than jejunoileal bypass to cause complications; however, their long-term effects are unknown.

Only people who weigh at least two times their ideal weight should be considered for weight-reduction surgery. Candidates for surgery include people who have tried conventional methods of weight reduction and have been approved for the procedure after a psychological consultation. This includes an examination of emotional stability and addictive behaviors. Candidates must be free of endocrine or metabolic disorders that can be treated effectively without surgery. They must also be free of liver, heart, inflammatory bowel, and kidney disease. And they must keep follow-up appointments and follow diet restrictions.

People with high blood pressure, diabetes, disabling bone disease, or extreme endocrine dysfunction may be considered for weight-reduction surgery without meeting the above criteria if the perceived benefits of surgery outweigh the risks.

Only people who weigh at least two times their ideal weight should be considered for weight-reduction surgery.

Why is this procedure done?
- To provide permanent weight loss in morbidly obese people who do not respond to traditional treatment
- To decrease the incidence of high blood pressure, degenerative arthritis, heart dysfunction, gallstones, Type II diabetes mellitus, and other disorders associated with morbid obesity

What happens before the procedure?
- The doctor reviews the purpose of the procedure and how it will be performed with you and your family.

SELF-HELP

Recovering from surgical treatment of obesity

After you've been discharged from the hospital, follow these guidelines.

Adjust your eating patterns
- Adhere to a daily multivitamin schedule and drink high-protein liquids.
- Eat slowly and chew food completely before swallowing. Stop eating if you sense fullness because overeating will cause vomiting.

Other instructions
- Follow the exercise instructions given by your doctor.
- Report any of the following signs and symptoms to the doctor: persistent nausea and vomiting, diarrhea, and temperature above 101° F (38.3° C).
- Keep your follow-up appointments, which are very important.
- Consider joining in a support group.

- You'll be asked to sign a consent form.
- The nurse will give you antibiotics to prevent infection.

What happens during the procedure?

- Jejunoileal bypass involves shortening the small bowel. This causes weight loss by decreasing the absorption of ingested nutrients.
- In the gastric bypass procedure, the doctor constructs a pouch that drains into a loop of the jejunum. It bypasses the lower stomach and small intestine and limits the amount of food ingested as well as the absorption of ingested nutrients.
- In vertical banded gastroplasty, the doctor creates a pouch in the upper stomach with vertically placed staples. This drastically reduces the amount that the stomach can hold.

What are the possible complications?

- Postoperative complications of these procedures include collapsed lung, deep vein thrombosis, vomiting, dehydration, bleeding, superficial and deep wound infection, pneumonia, and pulmonary embolus.
- Other complications can include vitamin B_{12}, iron, calcium, and potassium deficiencies; other fluid and electrolyte imbalances; and malnutrition. But these deficiencies are correctable with administration of oral and intravenous supplements. (See *Recovering from surgical treatment of obesity*.)
- Foul breath, body odor, gas, bloating, cramping abdominal pain, and diarrhea are common in malabsorptive conditions.

- Psychological problems that require treatment, sometimes with a stay in a hospital, often develop after surgery.
- Intra-abdominal abscess, bypass enteritis, perforation at the surgical site, intestinal obstruction, and symptomatic duodenal ulcers in the bypassed segment are sometimes noted. After jejunoileal bypass, diarrhea occurs in all people; migratory polyarthritis and liver and kidney dysfunction may also occur.

What happens after the procedure?

- The nurse administers antibiotics.
- You receive therapy to prevent the formation of blood clots.
- You receive medication for diarrhea.
- Your diet will progress from clear liquids to pureed foods. Some people may continue a liquid diet for 8 to 12 weeks.

5

*T*REATING BRAIN &
NERVOUS SYSTEM
DISORDERS

DRUG THERAPIES

ANTICONVULSANTS

Anticonvulsant drugs are used to prevent and treat seizures. Seizures can take many different forms. Generalized tonic-clonic, or grand mal, seizures are what many people think of when they hear the word *seizure,* but these disorders represent only a fraction of the different types of seizures that can occur.

Seizures result from abnormal electrical activity in the brain. The origin of this abnormal activity — referred to as a *focus* — can extend throughout the brain, causing a generalized seizure. Alternatively, the abnormal activity can remain relatively local, causing symptoms that relate to the location of the focus.

Because seizure disorders are complex, each anticonvulsant drug is used to treat specific seizure disorders. Frequently, these drugs are used in combination for complex or mixed seizure disorders.

What are anticonvulsants used for?
These drugs are used to reduce the frequency or severity of seizures.

What are some commonly used anticonvulsants?
Barbiturates
- phenobarbital (generic)
- primidone, known by the brand name Mysoline

Benzodiazepines
- clonazepam, known by the brand name Klonopin
- clorazepate, known by the brand name Tranxene
- diazepam, known by the brand name Valium

Hydantoins
- mephenytoin, known by the brand name Mesantoin
- phenytoin, known by the brand name Dilantin

Succinimides
- ethosuximide, known by the brand name Zarontin

Miscellaneous agents
- carbamazepine, known by the brand name Tegretol
- valproic acid derivatives, known by the brand names Depakene, Depakote, and Myproic Acid

What are the possible side effects?
- Respiratory depression (following overdose), difficulty breathing
- Blood disorders
- Drowsiness, fatigue, confusion, weakness, headache, dizziness, vertigo, fainting
- Euphoria, nightmares, hallucinations, slurred speech, insomnia, nervousness
- Dry mouth, taste alterations, loss of appetite, nausea, vomiting, diarrhea or constipation, abdominal discomfort
- Visual problems; rapid, uncontrolled eye movements
- Low blood pressure, abnormal heart rhythms
- Dental problems

Some anticonvulsants can cause tooth and gum problems that can lead to tooth loss. Regular visits to the dentist can help avoid these problems.

What are the guidelines for taking anticonvulsants?
- Anticonvulsants require careful monitoring of dosage for toxicity. You will need to have frequent blood tests to determine the correct dosage level and to detect early signs of toxicity.
- A family member should watch you for drowsiness, confusion, decreased attention span, and slurred speech; an elderly or young person may become very excitable. Typically, these reactions occur during the first 3 weeks of treatment. Avoid activities that require mental alertness, such as operating heavy machinery or driving a car. To avoid falls, be careful walking.
- Be wary of skin reactions, such as facial swelling, discoloration, itching, and skin rash or blisters. Call the doctor immediately if these occur.
- Regularly visit your dentist. Some anticonvulsants can cause tooth and gum problems that can lead to tooth loss. Regular visits to the dentist can help avoid these problems.
- Maintain a well-balanced diet even if you don't feel like eating. If vomiting is a problem, call the doctor. Taking the drug with meals may help minimize some of the drug's side effects on the digestive system.
- Be sure to tell the doctor about all of the other medications you are taking, including nonprescription drugs.

- Tell the doctor immediately about fever, sore throat, mouth ulcers, or easy bruising or bleeding.
- Never stop taking the drug suddenly. Doing so may place you at risk for severe seizures. If side effects are a problem, call the doctor, who may want to adjust the dosage or switch you to another drug.
- Avoid using alcohol or other central nervous system depressants.
- Follow the prescribed medication schedule closely. Take a missed dose as soon as you remember, unless it's time for your next dose. Never double the dose.
- Never break, crush, or chew extended-release capsules.
- Always report for regular physical exams and blood tests to evaluate the safety and effectiveness of therapy.
- Wear a medical identification bracelet or carry a card that specifies the name and dosage of the prescribed anticonvulsant drug.

BENZODIAZEPINES

The benzodiazepines are used to treat insomnia. People who have trouble falling asleep, staying asleep, or people who wake up too early in the morning may need one of these drugs. Because these drugs are safer, shorter acting, and react with fewer drugs, they're used more often than barbiturates for such sleep problems.

Benzodiazepines are also used to treat anxiety. Because of the dangers associated with the long-term use of these drugs, doctors prefer only to prescribe them for short-term use.

What are benzodiazepines used for?
- To treat insomnia
- To treat anxiety

What are some commonly used benzodiazepines?
To treat insomnia
- flurazepam, known by the brand name Dalmane
- quazepam, known by the brand name Doral
- temazepam, known by the brand name Restoril
- triazolam, known by the brand name Halcion

To treat anxiety
- alprazolam, known by the brand name Xanax
- chlordiazepoxide, known by the brand name Librium
- clorazepate, known by the brand name Tranxene
- diazepam, known by the brand name Valium
- halazepam, known by the brand name Paxipam
- lorazepam, known by the brand name Ativan
- oxazepam, known by the brand name Serax
- prazepam, known by the brand name Centrax

What are the possible side effects?
- Psychological and physical dependence with long-term use
- Excessive central nervous system depression when taken with other depressants such as alcohol
- Drowsiness, dizziness, light-headedness, unsteadiness, confusion
- Loss of appetite, dry mouth, abdominal discomfort, taste alterations, nausea, excessive thirst, constipation or diarrhea
- Suicidal thoughts, agitation, hyperexcitability, hallucinations, delirium, aggression, sleepwalking, other bizarre or abnormal behaviors, amnesia

What are the guidelines for taking benzodiazepines?
- Although benzodiazepines are effective and safe for short-term therapy, long-term use can result in psychological and physiologic dependence. And when taken in large doses with alcohol or other central nervous system depressants, the benzodiazepines can produce severe central nervous system depression and death.
- Benzodiazepine dependence occurs most commonly in people with a history of alcohol or drug abuse, and so their use should be avoided in such people, if possible. They should also be used cautiously in people with suicidal tendencies or in those whose history indicates that they may increase drug dosage on their own.
- Tell your doctor if you have kidney disease, respiratory disease, or glaucoma.
- Never increase the dose of a benzodiazepine on your own even if you feel the drug isn't working effectively. The drug's effects may not be apparent for 1 or 2 days.
- Avoid activities that require alertness and coordination, such as driving, until your response to the drug has been determined. You should understand that the drug's effects can linger into the day after you took the drug.

Although benzodiazepines are effective and safe for short-term therapy, long-term use can result in psychological and physiologic dependence.

- Avoid smoking. Tobacco apparently speeds the metabolism of benzodiazepines, thereby reducing their effectiveness.
- After you stop taking the drug, your body may take some time to adjust to withdrawal — from a few days to 3 weeks, depending on the dosage and the duration of therapy. Notify the doctor if you experience extreme irritability, nervousness, incoordination, or weakness. Rebound insomnia may be a problem for 2 or 3 nights.
- Seek alternative therapy to deal with the underlying cause of insomnia. Try relaxing with a warm glass of milk at bedtime, and avoid coffee, tea, and caffeine-containing soft drinks beginning in the late afternoon.

ERGOT ALKALOIDS

These drugs provide relief from vascular (migraine and cluster) headaches. When given early in a headache, these drugs constrict dilated blood vessels in the brain, reducing the blood flow and pressure around the brain, and relieve pain.

What are ergot alkaloids used for?
They're used to treat migraines and cluster headaches.

What are some commonly used ergot alkaloids?
- dihydroergotamine, known by the brand name D.H.E. 45
- ergotamine, known by the brand names Ergomar and Ergostat

What are the possible side effects?
- Swelling
- Itching; numbness and tingling of fingers, toes, or face
- Red or violet blisters on skin of hands or feet
- Pale or cold hands or feet, painful extremities
- Vision changes
- Anxiety, confusion
- Chest pain, heart rate changes
- Shortness of breath
- Nausea and vomiting, diarrhea, abdominal pain
- Fatigue, weakness in legs

What are the guidelines for taking ergot alkaloids?

▪ Take the drug during the prodromal stage of a headache or as soon as possible after its onset. Lie down in a quiet, darkened room, if possible.

▪ Don't increase the drug dosage without first consulting with your doctor.

▪ Try to identify the possible causes of your headache. Stress or drinking alcohol, for instance, can lead to headache. So can eating chocolate or drinking coffee, colas, or other caffeinated beverages.

▪ Call your doctor if your hands or feet hurt or feel cold, numb, or tingling. Also call your doctor if you have pain in your chest or on your side.

▪ Avoid overexposure to cold temperatures, which may worsen these side effects in the hands and feet.

▪ If you experience nausea, vomiting, or an upset stomach, take the drug with food or milk.

What else you should know

Ergotamine, considered the more effective of the two ergot alkaloids, is available in oral, inhalant, and sublingual (under the tongue) forms; the latter two forms provide more rapid action in treating acute episodes. Ergotamine also serves as an ingredient in products containing various mixtures of the belladonna alkaloids, phenobarbital, and caffeine.

Dihydroergotamine, which is administered by injection into a vein or muscle, produces fewer and less serious side effects on the digestive tract than ergotamine. It may be given to people prone to such side effects.

Because the ergot alkaloids constrict blood vessels, they shouldn't be used in people with high blood pressure, peripheral or occlusive vascular disease, coronary artery disease, phlebitis, or other debilitating diseases. People over age 40 should have a complete heart checkup, including an electrocardiogram, before starting ergot alkaloid therapy.

SURGERIES

CRANIOTOMY

A craniotomy creates an opening in the skull, thereby exposing the brain for various treatments. At one time, craniotomy was the treatment of choice for removing brain tumors, but it has been replaced by what are called superior radiologic techniques, which can localize brain lesions and enable neurosurgeons to use less invasive methods. These include laser surgery and stereotaxic surgery, which involves guiding a probe into the brain to remove sharply circumscribed, deeply embedded tumors. The method used will depend on the person's condition.

A craniotomy is a surgical procedure that creates an opening in the skull, thereby exposing the brain for various treatments.

Why is this procedure done?
- To expose the brain for surgery
- To create an opening for ventricular shunting, removal of a tumor or abscess, aspiration of a hematoma, or clipping of an aneurysm

What happens before the procedure?
- The person may receive anticonvulsant medication to reduce the risk of seizures after the operation.
- Steroids may be administered to prevent swelling of the brain.
- The person's hair is washed with an antimicrobial shampoo on the night before surgery.
- The person's legs will be wrapped with elastic bandages to improve circulation and reduce the risk of vein swelling and blood clots. A urinary catheter may be inserted.

What happens during the procedure?
Craniotomy is performed by a neurosurgeon using local or general anesthesia. Local anesthesia is used when the person's response to manipulation of the brain must be assessed during surgery. Electrocorticography (a test to measure electrical activity in the brain) may also be performed to help assess these response areas of the brain.

After making an incision through the scalp and stripping the muscle away from the scalp, the neurosurgeon drills several small burr holes into the skull, and then cuts the bone between them with a pneumatic drill or a wire saw. The bone flap is turned down or completely removed. The surgeon then proceeds with the indicated surgery. After closing the incision, the surgeon covers the site with a sterile dressing.

What are the possible complications?

- Increased intracranial pressure caused by brain swelling or bleeding is the major complication of intracranial surgery.
- Cardiac and respiratory complications, such as cardiac or respiratory arrest, can occur from damage to the brain stem's vital centers. Potential postoperative complications include infection, bleeding, pneumonia, cardiac irregularities, kidney and gastrointestinal disorders, and meningitis.

What happens after the procedure?

- The person awakes from surgery with a large dressing on his or her head to protect the incision. There may be a surgical drain implanted in the skull for a few days and the person will receive antibiotics to prevent infection.
- The person will probably have a headache and facial swelling for 2 to 3 days after surgery. Medication is given to reduce the pain. If all goes well, he or she should be out of bed within 2 to 3 days after surgery and the doctor will remove the sutures within 7 to 10 days. (See *Recovering from a craniotomy.*)

CEREBRAL ANEURYSM REPAIR

An aneurysm is an area of dilation or outpouching of a blood vessel wall. For cerebral aneurysm, surgical treatment is the only sure way to prevent initial rupture or rebleeding.

The surgeon can choose among several techniques for aneurysm repair, depending on the shape and location of the aneurysm. These techniques include clamping the affected artery, wrapping the aneurysm wall with a biological or synthetic material, or clipping (ligating) the aneurysm. Clipping is the treatment of choice.

The decision to perform surgery is based on many factors, such as the location of the aneurysm, the presence or absence of spasms in the blood vessel, and the general condition of the person.

 SELF-HELP

Recovering from a craniotomy

After you've been discharged from the hospital, follow these important guidelines.

Take your medication

- Continue taking prescribed anticonvulsants to minimize the risk of seizures. Depending on the type of surgery, you may need to continue anticonvulsant therapy for up to 12 months after surgery.
- Report any side effects of the drug, such as excessive drowsiness or confusion, and increased headache, sensitivity to light, or neck stiffness, which might indicate meningitis.

Other instructions

- Take proper care of your wound. You can allow shower water to run over the incision and wash it gently with soap, but don't scrub it. Keep the suture line dry.
- Regularly inspect the incision for redness, warmth, or tenderness and report such findings to the doctor.
- If you're self-conscious about your appearance, wear a wig, hat, or scarf until your hair grows back. As the hair begins to grow back, apply a lanolin-based lotion to the scalp—except for the suture line—to keep it supple and alleviate itching.

Techniques for repairing aneurysms

Using a metal spring clip, the surgeon can isolate a berry aneurysm (named for its shape) from the cerebral circulation. With other types of aneurysms, such as a fusiform aneurysm, the arterial wall is wrapped with biological or synthetic material for support.

CLIPPING A BERRY ANEURYSM

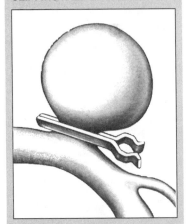

WRAPPING A FUSIFORM ANEURYSM

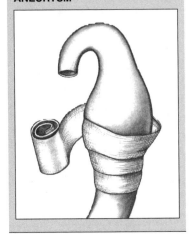

Why is this procedure done?

- To repair a cerebral aneurysm, preventing possible rupture or rebleeding and stabilizing cerebral blood flow
- To prevent initial rupture of a cerebral aneurysm or to stop bleeding associated with a rupture

What happens before the procedure?

- The person's activities and visitors are limited.
- Medications will be administered. These may include anticonvulsants to prevent seizures, corticosteroids to prevent brain swelling, stool softeners to prevent increased brain swelling caused by straining, and analgesics to relieve headache. If the person is receiving intravenous fluids, the intake and output will be monitored.
- The person must sign a consent form.
- The doctor orders a test called a *cerebral arteriography* to identify the location of the aneurysm and to rule out spasms in the blood vessels.

What happens during the procedure?

The surgeon will perform a craniotomy to expose the aneurysm. Because cerebral aneurysms usually occur in the internal carotid or middle cerebral artery, craniotomy is usually done in the back or front of the head. The surgeon visualizes the aneurysm with the aid of a microscope and then carefully frees the aneurysm from the brain tissue and wraps it with a biological or synthetic material. To clip the aneurysm, the surgeon opens a small, spring-loaded clip and slips it over the neck of the aneurysm or over its feeder vessel. (A large aneurysm may require more than one clip.) When the clip is in place, the surgeon releases it, letting it close and block blood flow to the aneurysm. The clip may simply be left in place or it may be secured with a liquid agent that quickly solidifies around the clip and the aneurysm. The surgeon then ligates and removes the sac of the aneurysm and closes the incision. (See *Techniques for repairing aneurysms.*)

What are the possible complications?

The complications of cerebral aneurysm repair are infection, bleeding, respiratory problems, and increased brain swelling. An additional risk is vasospasm, which can spread through the major cerebral vessels and cause ischemia and possible infarction of involved areas. The person's surgical risk depends on his or her preoperative condition and the complexity of the required surgery.

What happens after the procedure?

- A nurse monitors the person's vital signs as well as fluid and electrolyte balance and neurologic status.
- The person is encouraged to breathe deeply and is warned that coughing and sneezing may cause problems.
- The nurse will turn the person every 2 hours and will encourage him or her to do range-of-motion exercises every 2 hours. If the person can't perform active exercises, the nurse will help him or her to do passive leg exercises more often than every 2 hours to help prevent blood clots.
- The person's environment should be quiet and calm to minimize anxiety and help lower brain swelling. (See *Recovering from cerebral aneurysm repair.*)

REMOVING BLOOD FROM THE BRAIN AFTER AN INJURY

When a person suffers a blunt head injury, there may be bleeding and swelling in a part of the brain. This is called a *hematoma* or blood blister, and it usually requires lifesaving surgery to control the bleeding and reduce the pressure on the brain. Even if the person's life isn't in immediate danger, surgery is usually performed to prevent irreversible damage from a reduced flow of blood to the brain.

Epidural hematoma

An epidural hematoma is the accumulation of blood in the potential space between the skull and the outermost of the membranes surrounding the brain. About half of the people with this condition (usually children) experience a lucid interval followed by rapid deterioration and possible death or serious injury. Emergency surgery is usually required. The epidural hematoma is drained through burr holes, and the bleeding vessels are tied off. Early intervention usually allows complete recovery of neurologic function.

Subdural hematoma

A subdural hematoma is the accumulation of blood in the potential space between the layers of membranes surrounding the brain. Acute subdural hematomas produce symptoms within 24 to 48 hours. They are the result of a more severe underlying brain contusion. They require prompt surgery because the brain is unable to tolerate

SELF-HELP

Recovering from cerebral aneurysm repair

After you've been discharged from the hospital, follow these important guidelines:
- Gradually resume your normal activities.
- Take care of the wound as instructed in the hospital and examine the incision carefully.
- Continue taking prescribed medications, and report any side effects of the drugs.
- You can wear a wig, hat, or scarf if you feel self-conscious about your appearance.
- Make sure you return for scheduled follow-up exams and tests.

rapid compression. Because these lesions are of jellylike consistency, surgery is necessary to remove the clot. Less acute subdural hematomas produce symptoms within days of the injury. They are partially liquefied and may be removed through burr holes. Chronic subdural hematomas may not produce symptoms for weeks, perhaps for months. Such lesions are liquefied, and burr holes may be used to remove them, reducing the risks associated with more complicated surgery.

Intracerebral hematoma

An intracerebral hematoma involves bleeding in the brain itself. If the hematoma is accessible and the person's condition is deteriorating, it requires surgery.

Why is this procedure done?

This procedure removes an intracranial hematoma, relieving pressure on the vessels and tissues of the brain, and prevents reduced blood flow to the brain and brain damage.

What happens before the procedure?

The person or a responsible family member signs a consent form.

What happens during the procedure?

Depending on the type of hematoma, the surgeon gains access to the bleeding site by opening the skull or making burr holes.

If the hematoma is liquid, a twist drill is used to burr holes through the skull. The surgeon drills at least two holes to mark the extent of the clot and allow complete drainage. Once the surgeon reaches the clot, a small suction tip is inserted into the burr holes to remove the clot. The surgeon then inserts drains, which usually remain in place for 24 hours.

If the clot is solid (or, although liquid, can't be completely aspirated through burr holes), the surgeon opens the skull. This approach, called a *craniotomy*, is more common. After exposing the hematoma, the surgeon aspirates it with a small suction tip or uses a sodium chloride solution to wash out parts of the clot. He or she then ties off any bleeding vessels in the hematoma cavity and closes the bone and scalp flaps. (If brain swelling is severe, the craniotomy site may be left open and the flaps replaced only after swelling subsides.) The surgeon may place a drain in the surgical site.

SELF-HELP

Recovering from surgery to remove blood from the brain

After you have been discharged from the hospital, follow these important guidelines.

Take your medication

- Continue taking prescribed anticonvulsants to minimize the risk of seizures. Report any side effects of the drugs, such as excessive drowsiness or confusion.
- You may take Tylenol (acetaminophen) or another mild nonnarcotic pain reliever for headaches. Tell your doctor if the drug doesn't relieve your headache.

Other instructions

- You or a family member should take care of the sutures as you were shown in the hospital. Observe the suture line for signs of infection, such as redness and swelling. Report any such signs immediately.
- Watch for and report any neurologic symptoms, such as altered level of consciousness, sudden weakness, increased headaches, and visual disturbances.
- Wear a wig, hat, or scarf until your hair grows back. Use a lanolin-based lotion to help keep the scalp supple and decrease itching, but don't put any lotion on the suture line.

What are the possible complications?

Severe infection and seizures can occur, as well as breathing difficulties and increased swelling in the brain if a craniotomy is performed.

What happens after the procedure?

- The head of the bed is elevated about 30 degrees to promote drainage from the brain. For subdural hematomas, however, some doctors order that the person's head remain down for 24 hours after the operation in an effort to allow the brain to reexpand or to prevent a clot from reforming.
- The person is turned frequently and a nurse helps him or her perform passive range-of-motion exercises for all limbs. (See *Recovering from surgery to remove blood from the brain.*)

VENTRICULOSTOMY

A ventriculostomy is insertion of a catheter into the ventricle of the brain to help lower intracranial pressure while monitoring that pressure. A device known as a *subarachnoid screw* also provides intracranial pressure monitoring, but is less effective for lowering intracranial pressure.

Why is this procedure done?

- To lower intracranial pressure
- To provide access for monitoring that pressure
- To relieve pressure on the brain in conditions that produce it, such as hematomas, abscesses, tumors, aneurysms, and swelling of the brain and in conditions that increase blood volume inside the skull, such as hyperemia, hypercapnia (high carbon dioxide levels in the blood), and obstructions to venous outflow
- To provide drainage to relieve intracranial pressure in conditions such as communicating hydrocephalus and subarachnoid hemorrhage

What happens before the procedure?

- The person's head is shaved over the insertion site and a sterile dressing is placed over the site after the device is secured. This guards against infection.
- A sedative might be ordered.

What happens during the procedure?

The person receives a general anesthetic. The surgeon makes a burr hole in the person's skull, inserts an intraventricular catheter into the burr hole, sutures the catheter in place, and then connects the catheter to tubing filled with solution. Also connected is a machine that converts the brain pressure into electrical impulses that are relayed to the monitor. If fluids will be drained, stopcocks and a collection bag can be attached to the tubing.

What are the possible complications?

- Excessive fluid drainage is a potential complication of ventriculostomy and may result in collapsed ventricles, tonsillar herniation, and medullary compression. If the drainage stops, it may indicate that a clot is forming. If drainage is blocked, the person may develop signs of increased pressure on the brain.
- Infection, which can cause meningitis, is also possible.

What happens after the procedure?

- The person's room is kept softly lit and quiet. Bed rest is necessary. The person's head is raised 30 to 45 degrees to promote drainage.
- The person is told to exhale while moving or turning in bed and to not flex his or her neck or hips or push against the footboard.
- Usually, the device remains in place for 5 to 7 days; if the person needs it longer, it will be replaced by a new one.

VENTRICULAR SHUNT

Performed on both adults and children, this surgical treatment for hydrocephalus uses a catheter to drain cerebrospinal fluid into another body space, where the fluid is absorbed. The shunt extends from the cerebral ventricle to the scalp, where it's tunneled under the skin to the appropriate cavity.

There are various types of shunts that can drain fluid into the peritoneal sac, the ureters, the right atrium, or the pleural space.

A small percentage of people with congenital hydrocephalus outgrow the need for the shunt. Most hydrocephalic people, however, are dependent on the shunt for the rest of their lives.

Why is this procedure done?

Ventricular shunts relieve increased intracranial pressure by draining fluid from the ventricles of the brain.

What happens before the procedure?

- A nurse monitors the person's vital signs.
- The doctor or nurse explains the procedure to the person or the family.

What happens during the procedure?

Performed in an operating room with the person under general anesthesia, the procedure varies according to the type of shunt being inserted.

What are the possible complications?

- Infections such as ventriculitis and peritoneal infection may occur.

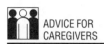
ADVICE FOR
CAREGIVERS

Caring for a child with a ventricular shunt

If your child has had a shunt inserted to remove excess fluid from his or her brain, you'll need to learn how to care for the shunt and your child at home to ensure the success of this treatment. Follow these important guidelines.

Caring for the shunt

Bathe the shunt incision line as you normally bathe your child's skin. When picking up your child, be sure to support the buttocks. This prevents the drainage tube from moving from its proper position.

Continue with your child's normal diet. To help prevent constipation, which can cause shunt malfunction, encourage the child to eat soft foods and drink plenty of liquids.

Be alert for signs of infection: rectal temperature above 101° F (38.3° C) for more than 6 hours, increased sleepiness, or warm, reddened skin at the incision site. Notify your doctor if you note any of these signs.

Keep in mind that reddened skin may be caused by lying on the shunt insertion side. Try to keep your child from lying on that side for prolonged periods.

Pumping the shunt

Your doctor may ask you to pump the shunt once or twice a day. If so, locate the pump by feeling for the soft center of the device under the skin behind the ear.

Now, depress the center of the pump with your forefinger and then slowly release it. Pump only as many times as your doctor has ordered (usually between 25 and 50 times, once or twice a day).

Checking for problems

Watch your child carefully for signs of shunt malfunction. Call your doctor immediately if you see bulging, tightness, and shining of the soft spots on your child's head. Also call the doctor if your child seems unusually fussy or sleepy, refuses to eat, vomits forcefully, or has difficulty grasping objects.

- Shunt malfunction can result if the shunt becomes blocked or kinked; this occurs most often in growing children and can result in increased intracranial pressure.
- Ventricular collapse from improper catheter placement or faulty pumping techniques can also occur. Complications of a ventriculoatrial shunt (which drains the fluid from the brain into the heart) involve the heart and blood vessels and can include irregular heartbeats, damage to heart valves with perforation of the heart from catheter migration, and blood clot formation.

What happens after the procedure?

- The person must lie flat for 3 to 5 days after shunt insertion, which will help the adjustment to lowered intracranial pressure. His or her head will be raised in stages, about 20 degrees at a time.
- The person's vital signs and neurologic status will be checked every 2 hours. (See *Caring for a child with a ventricular shunt.*)

CONGENITAL SPINAL DEFECT REPAIR

Also called *myelomeningocele,* this congenital spinal defect results from defective closure of the embryonic neural tube during the first trimester of pregnancy. The defect is a fragile saclike structure that protrudes over the spinal column and contains spinal membranes, cerebrospinal fluid, and a portion of the spinal cord. If the fluid leaks from this sac, it can cause infection and the infant may suffer permanent neurologic problems below the level of the sac. Most surgeons repair the defect within the first 24 to 48 hours after birth.

Early surgery can prevent infection and injury to the sac. It also prevents the further deterioration of nerve tissue that can be caused by enlargement of the sac. Some surgeons delay closure to evaluate the infant's neurologic function. However, surgery is usually delayed only when the infant is seriously debilitated or has associated defects that could complicate surgery.

Unfortunately, surgery can't reverse any existing nerve damage. It may, however, preserve existing function in the infant and prevent further deterioration.

Why is this surgery done?

This surgery repairs the congenital defect and prevents further nerve damage to the legs, bowel, and bladder.

What happens before the surgery?

- The nurse covers the fragile defect with sterile dressings and gently cleans and inspects it for signs of infection.
- The infant wears no clothing and is kept warm in an incubator.
- Parents hold their infant as often as possible to promote bonding.

What happens during the surgery?

- Under general anesthesia, the surgeon isolates the nerve tissue from the rest of the sac. After establishing this tissue's point of continuity with the spinal cord and nerve roots, he or she fashions a flap from the tissue. This flap protects the nerve junctions and eventually will become contiguous with the membranes surrounding the spinal cord.
- The surgeon then sutures the skin closed over the defect and covers the wound with a sterile gauze dressing and then a waterproof cover-

Caring for an infant after spinal surgery

Once your child has been discharged from the hospital after spinal surgery, follow these important guidelines.

Protect the baby's skin
- Watch for early signs of infection, such as redness or swelling. Keep the incision clean and dry and do frequent diaper changes and cleanings. The doctor will probably remove the sutures on the 10th day after surgery.
- Frequently reposition the baby. Massage and apply lotion to pressure points on the baby's skin to prevent irritation.

Other instructions
- If you're taught to manually express urine from the child's bladder, do so regularly. Begin bladder training when your child reaches age 3.
- If the doctor has prescribed an antibiotic, learn how to administer the drug and follow the dosing schedule.
- Arrange for a visiting nurse to provide periodic in-home care.
- Make sure your child receives regular neurologic assessments and physical exams to evaluate his or her development.
- You may need genetic counseling and may find it beneficial to join a local support group.

ing to protect the dressing from contamination by feces or urine. Because the defect is usually relatively small, skin grafts are rarely ordered for cosmetic repair.

What are the possible complications?
Infection (meningitis or ventriculitis), hydrocephalus (fluid on the brain), delayed wound healing, and increased intracranial pressure are the possible complications of congenital spinal defect repair.

What happens after the surgery?
- Sometimes the nurse does very gentle passive range-of-motion exercises on the infant's limbs.
- Before the infant goes home, the nurse teaches the parents how to care for the infant. (See *Caring for an infant after spinal surgery*.)

CORPUS CALLOSOTOMY

The corpus callosum is an area of fibers connecting the two cerebral hemispheres. A corpus callosotomy is a surgical procedure in which the corpus callosum is divided by a fine suction aspirator. It is performed to reduce disabling seizure activity.

A corpus callosotomy is typically done in two stages. Initially, the front two-thirds of the corpus callosum is divided. If seizure activity does not decrease after several months, the final one-third is divided in a second operation. Corpus callosotomy is performed in two steps to prevent acute disconnection syndrome, which causes apraxia (loss of ability to carry out familiar movements), mutism, apathy, confusion, and infantile behavior.

People are discharged approximately 12 to 14 days after surgery. They may be discharged with some neurologic deficits and may require physical, occupational, or speech therapy. Rehabilitation may be completed as an outpatient. Severe neurologic deficits may require rehabilitation in the hospital.

Corpus callosotomy decreases the number and severity of seizures, but is not a cure. Most people who are eligible for a callosotomy have severely disabling seizures.

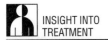

INSIGHT INTO
TREATMENT

Cortical resection

Cortical resection is a surgical procedure that removes epileptogenic tissue (tissue that acts as a focus for seizures) from the brain. Resection can remove any lobe, but most commonly the temporal lobe is removed. Cortical mapping (electrocorticography) is used during surgery to identify and remove the smallest possible area of the brain while still excising all epileptogenic tissue.

Testing before surgery
Before surgery, a test is done to identify the hemisphere of the brain that directs speech and memory.

The results will show whether the surgery will affect speech and memory and will dictate the size and area of resection.

Recovery period
Healing may take up to a year, and the person's seizure activity may continue during that time. Maintaining therapeutic blood levels of anticonvulsant drugs is important. If the person is free of seizures for 2 years and the electroencephalogram shows no epileptic activity, anticonvulsant drugs may be gradually discontinued.

Why is this surgery done?

- Corpus callosotomy is used to reduce the number of generalized seizures by interrupting the spread of epileptic discharges to the various hemispheres of the brain.

- Corpus callosotomy is considered only after trials of all appropriate anticonvulsant drugs have failed to control seizure activity, if seizure activity is disruptive to daily life, and if the seizure activity does not arise from a single area of the brain. If the diagnostic workup determines that the origin of the seizure activity is localized to a specific area of the brain, a cortical resection may be performed. (See *Cortical resection.*)

- People who have generalized atonic, tonic, or tonic-clonic seizures and those who have seizures with a frontal focus are considered the best candidates for this surgery. Electroencephalography (a test of the brain's electrical activity) usually shows multifocal or bilaterally synchronous abnormalities.

What happens before the surgery?

- The doctor orders a neurologic evaluation to establish the person's baseline status.
- Decadron is administered to help control cerebral swelling.
- The nurse gives the person a povidone-iodine shampoo the night before surgery.
- The neurosurgeon shaves the person's entire head before surgery.

SELF-HELP

Recovering from a corpus callosotomy

After you've been discharged from the hospital, follow these important guidelines.

Know what to expect

• Remember that you'll need to continue taking your anticonvulsant medication. It will probably be needed indefinitely.

• Because corpus callosotomy is not a cure, you will continue to have some seizures. Your seizures probably will become less frequent and less severe. Continued medical monitoring is necessary.

Other points to remember

• You can resume daily activities, but don't plan to return to work for at least 6 months. Avoid activities that might cause head injuries.

• Check your incision for signs of infection. Don't rub it during bathing.

What happens during the surgery?

With the person under general anesthesia, the neurosurgeon makes a vertex frontal craniotomy (opening of the scalp, skull, and dura) and divides the front two thirds of the corpus callosum. If satisfactory seizure control has not been obtained after several months, a second craniotomy is performed and the final third of the corpus callosum is divided.

What are the possible complications?

This surgical procedure has a low morbidity and mortality rate. Potential complications are those for any craniotomy: bleeding into the brain, neurologic deficits, infection, and death (rare). Mutism, lack of spontaneous speech, apathy, and infantile behavior have also been reported.

What happens after the surgery?

The person's vital signs are monitored. (See *Recovering from a corpus callosotomy.*)

RADIOSURGERY

Radiosurgery uses radiation instead of a scalpel or laser to treat a lesion. The radiation is applied to a small target, such as a brain tumor.

In conventional radiation therapy, the radiation is delivered through one to three openings. This limits the amount of radiation a person can receive to protect normal brain tissue from the effects of large radiation dosages. Radiosurgery can deliver high doses of radiation to the lesion and a relatively low dose of radiation to the surrounding normal brain tissue. Because of the delivery method, people who previously received the maximum conventional brain radiation treatments can receive an additional dose to the lesion using radiosurgery.

Why is this procedure done?

• To slow the growth of a brain tumor or possibly decrease its size

• To treat arteriovenous malformations that cannot be treated by conventional surgery because of the possibility of neurologic damage or the person's age. It is sometimes used with embolization procedures to treat arteriovenous malformations.

- To replace surgery when another medical condition poses a high surgical risk or because the person refuses surgery. In general, the lesion must be smaller than 3 centimeters for this procedure to be effective, although some centers have treated larger lesions.

What happens before the procedure?

The person undergoes a series of preoperative tests, fasts after midnight the night before the procedure, and takes a shower before the procedure.

What happens during the procedure?

The person is usually awake during the entire procedure. A head frame is placed on the person, followed by radiographic studies such as magnetic resonance imaging (MRI), a computed tomography (CAT) scan, or an angiogram. The three-dimensional coordinates of the lesion are determined through calculations based on those studies. The dosage plan is then calculated by a team consisting of the neurosurgeon, radiation oncologist, and radiation physicist. The radiation is then administered and the head frame removed.

What are the possible complications?

- Complications are rare but include vomiting or seizures.
- Complications that can occur 3 to 6 months after treatment are related to swelling and radiation. They can be controlled with corticosteroids.
- In people with arteriovenous malformations, complications are rare and are usually manifested as seizures. Malformations that are not totally obliterated may bleed, causing neurologic deficits.

What happens after the procedure?

- The person may go home following radiation or be monitored overnight in the hospital. (See *Recovering from radiosurgery,* page 256.)
- The person may be given analgesics for a mild to moderate headache after the head frame is removed.

SELF-HELP

Recovering from radiosurgery

After you've been discharged from the hospital, follow these important guidelines.

Know what to expect
- You'll be given a written schedule for follow-up radiographic studies. Usually, people with arteriovenous malformations will need an angiogram after 1 year. Persons with tumors will receive a follow-up CAT scan or MRI 1 to 3 months after the procedure and then every 3 to 6 months.
- The full effect of the treatment may not be known for up to 2 years, which is why close radiographic follow-up is important.

Report any problems
- Notify your doctor immediately of any changes in neurologic status, such as seizures or changes in your level of consciousness, behavior, vision, or muscle strength.

- Notify your doctor of continued headache or change in headache, severe nausea or vomiting, stiff neck, or sensitivity of eyes to light.
- Notify the doctor of any signs of infection at pin sites. Pin sites should be kept clean with soap and water.
- If you experience seizures, make sure you check with your doctor before you resume driving.

Other points to remember
- You may perform your normal daily activities, depending on how you tolerate them. There are no restrictions on diet or physical activity related to the radiosurgery procedure.
- If you have arteriovenous malformation, understand that the risk of bleeding will persist until the lesion is completely obliterated.

OTHER TREATMENTS

BLOCKING OFF AN ARTERIOVENOUS MALFORMATION

Arteriovenous malformations are clusters of defective, extraneous veins that result in abnormal blood flow. The size of the malformation varies from a few millimeters to a large tangled mass of arteries and veins. The arteriovenous malformation is surgically removed when possible. When that's not possible, the surgeon may inject small beads through a catheter into the feeder artery. This blocks all blood flow to the defective cluster. (See *How embolization of an arteriovenous malformation works.*)

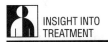

INSIGHT INTO
TREATMENT

How embolization of an arteriovenous malformation works

This illustration shows the feeder artery of an arteriovenous malformation. For embolization of the arteriovenous malformation, the surgeon injects small Silastic beads through a catheter placed in the malformation's feeder artery. These beads lodge in the artery, blocking blood flow to the malformation.

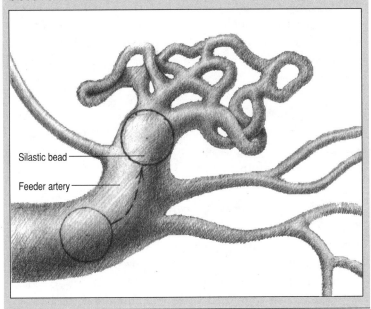

Silastic bead

Feeder artery

Why is this procedure done?

Blocking off an arteriovenous malformation is done to destroy it or to decrease its size by stopping the blood flow to it. This procedure is done in place of surgery for people at high risk or when the location of the arteriovenous malformation makes surgery impossible. It may also be used to decrease the size of large malformations before attempting surgery. This helps to reduce risks, especially bleeding, associated with surgery.

What happens before the procedure?

- The person must fast for 6 to 8 hours before the procedure.
- The nurse shaves the area around the catheter insertion site and cleans it with an antiseptic solution.

SELF-HELP

Recovering from embolization

Once you've been discharged from the hospital after the embolization procedure, make sure you follow these important guidelines:
- You or a family member should immediately report any abnormal symptoms, such as a severe headache, weakness in the extremities, or a deteriorating level of consciousness. These symptoms may indicate that the arteriovenous malformation is bleeding or increasing in size, which requires immediate medical attention.
- Make sure you keep your follow-up appointments.

- The person empties his or her bladder just before the procedure.
- The person or a family member signs a consent form.

What happens during the procedure?

- The doctor, using angiography, performs embolization therapy, in which a temporary or permanent substance is used to block blood flow to the arteriovenous malformation.
- The doctor usually performs the procedure under local anesthesia. He or she inserts a catheter in an artery in the person's thigh, then threads the flexible catheter to the malformation site and positions the tip as close as possible to the vessel cluster. The selected embolizing substance (for example, small Silastic beads) is injected and carried by blood flow to block the arteriovenous malformation. A calibrated-leak balloon may be used instead to release embolizing material.

Two or more procedures may be required to shut off the malformation adequately. Using several procedures instead of attempting to embolize a large arteriovenous malformation in a single procedure decreases the incidence of associated complications. A second procedure is typically performed several weeks after the first.

What are the possible complications?

The major complication of treatment to block a malformation is neurologic deficit caused by blocking off of normal vessels by the substance intended to block only the arteriovenous malformation. If the substance passes into the systemic circulation, a clot in the lungs may occur. Other complications include intracranial bleeding, inflammation, infection, and complications related to angiography (such as allergic reaction, blood clots in the femoral artery, and bleeding at the catheter insertion site).

What happens after the procedure?

- The person must remain on bed rest for 24 hours.
- The affected leg is extended and immobilized for 12 hours after the procedure.
- The person's room must be kept quiet, and few visitors are allowed. (See *Recovering from embolization*.)

BARBITURATE-INDUCED COMA

An induced coma is a treatment method that uses high intravenous doses of a short-acting barbiturate (such as pentobarbital or thiopental) to produce coma. It is only used when swelling of the brain has not subsided after such conventional treatment as surgical decompression, osmotic diuretics, fluid restriction, steroids, hyperventilation, and cerebrospinal fluid drainage.

Why is this treatment done?
■ To reduce the person's cerebral metabolic rate and cerebral blood flow, which relieves pressure on the brain and prevents brain tissue damage
■ To treat people with rapidly deteriorating neurologic status who are unresponsive to other treatments

What happens before the treatment?
The doctor establishes a reliable neurologic baseline via an electroencephalogram, which measures the electrical activity in the brain; a computed tomography (CAT) scan; and possibly brain stem auditory-evoked response testing. The coma should only be induced in an intensive care setting. The person is placed on mechanical ventilation, and intracranial, central venous, pulmonary artery, cardiac, and intra-arterial pressures are monitored. The person also requires an indwelling urinary catheter and a feeding tube that runs from the nose to the stomach.

What happens during the treatment?
As soon as the tests are completed and the monitoring equipment is in place, the doctor induces the coma according to the hospital's policy. This is done by administering a loading dose of the barbiturate and then establishing an hourly maintenance dose that will keep the barbiturate at the level required to decrease swelling in the brain.

When the person's swelling has stabilized within acceptable limits, usually in 24 to 36 hours, or if the person shows signs of progressive neurologic impairment, therapy is discontinued. Withdrawal from barbiturate therapy should occur over 24 hours to several days because abrupt withdrawal can cause seizures.

> *Barbiturate coma carries some serious risks, related mainly to the small margin between therapeutic and toxic doses. A high dose is needed to induce coma, but toxicity can produce severe, possibly fatal, central nervous system and respiratory depression.*

What are the possible complications?

Barbiturate coma carries some serious risks, related mainly to the small margin between therapeutic and toxic doses. A high dose is needed to induce coma, but toxicity can produce severe, possibly fatal, central nervous system and respiratory depression. Even a therapeutic dose can cause such complications as low blood pressure and irregular heartbeat. Abrupt withdrawal may cause seizures or delirium. In addition, these people are also susceptible to infection and such complications of immobility as bed sores and muscle contractures.

What happens after the treatment?

As the person emerges from the coma, the nurse watches him or her for signs of returning neurologic function. Only after withdrawal from the coma is complete and the person is fully conscious can the doctor determine the extent of damage to his nervous system.

PLASMAPHERESIS

Plasmapheresis, also known as therapeutic plasma exchange, is the removal of plasma from withdrawn blood and the reinfusion of formed blood elements.

Plasmapheresis techniques were first used routinely in the 1960s. Through this exchange treatment, 50% to 90% of unwanted plasma factors can be removed. These factors may include autoantibodies, immune complexes, metabolites, or unknown mediators of disease.

The procedure can take up to 5 hours and may be performed as often as four times a week in acutely ill people but is otherwise limited to about once every 2 weeks.

Why is this procedure done?

- To remove disease mediators or toxic substances from circulating blood
- To treat people with kidney disease, too-thick blood, and the bleeding disorders thrombotic thrombocytopenic purpura and idiopathic thrombocytopenic purpura
- To treat certain neurologic disorders, such as Guillain-Barré syndrome, MS, and especially myasthenia gravis, in which it is used to

remove circulating antiacetylcholine receptor antibodies; successful treatment may relieve symptoms for months, with varying results

What happens before the procedure?

- The doctor or nurse tells the person to report any sensations of numbness or tingling.
- The person may eat lightly before treatment and should drink milk before and during treatment to help reduce the risk of too little calcium in the blood.
- The person must empty his or her bladder.

What happens during the procedure?

Plasmapheresis is performed under a doctor's supervision. It requires a specially trained technician or nurse to operate the cell separator and a primary nurse to monitor the person and provide supportive care. It can be performed in the hospital or in another setting.

During this treatment, which can last 5 hours, blood is removed from the person's vein and flows into a cell separator. There it's divided into plasma and formed elements.

The plasma is collected in a container for disposal, and the formed elements are mixed with a plasma replacement solution and returned to the person through a vein.

In a newer method, automated pheresis, the plasma is separated out, filtered to remove a specific disease mediator, and then returned to the person.

Whichever method is used, people tend to do well if fluids are replaced to equal the amounts that were removed.

What are the possible complications?

- Infection around the puncture site
- Allergic reaction to the ingredients of the replacement solution
- A calcium deficiency in the blood
- A magnesium deficiency in the blood after repeated plasmapheresis, producing severe muscle cramps; tetany; and numbness, tingling, or prickling sensations
- Irregular heartbeats because of plasmapheresis-induced electrolyte imbalances
- Complications of low blood volume, such as dizziness and low blood pressure
- Symptoms of myasthenic crisis (in the patient with myasthenia gravis), such as difficulty swallowing, drooping of an eyelid, and

SELF-HELP

Caring for yourself during plasmapheresis treatments

During the course of your plasmapheresis treatments, make sure that you follow these important guidelines.

Get enough rest
You may feel tired for a day or two after plasmapheresis. And during repeated treatments, you may develop chronic fatigue. Therefore, make sure you rest frequently and avoid strenuous activities during this period.

Other points to remember
- Maintain a high-protein diet and take a multivitamin with iron daily, unless your doctor advises you otherwise.
- If you're undergoing repeated plasmapheresis, you may require transfusions of fresh-frozen plasma to replace the normal clotting factors lost.
- Because the treatment can suppress your immune system, stay away from people with colds or other contagious viruses.
- Watch for and report any signs of hepatitis, such as fever, yellowing of the skin and whites of the eyes, and itching skin.

double vision, because of the removal of antibodies or antimyasthenic drugs from the blood
- Rare, life-threatening complications, including hemolysis and blood clots

What happens after the procedure?

The person may feel tired for a day or two after the procedure. (See *Caring for yourself during plasmapheresis treatments.*)

6

TREATING MUSCLE & BONE DISORDERS

DRUG THERAPIES

ANTIMYASTHENICS

Myasthenia gravis is a disease characterized by progressive muscle weakness. Antimyasthenics, also called *cholinesterase inhibitors,* have been one of the primary treatments for this disorder for many years.

Patients with myasthenia gravis have a disorder in the transmission of the signal between skeletal muscles and the nerves that serve them. The neurotransmitter acetylcholine is released from the nerve, but the receptors on the muscle are either diminished in number or incapable of responding. Antimyasthenics amplify the signal from the nerve by blocking the breakdown of acetylcholine. The amplified signal improves muscle strength.

What are antimyasthenics used for?
- To treat myasthenic symptoms by inhibiting the destruction of acetylcholine, thus increasing muscle strength
- To aid in diagnosis of myasthenia gravis (edrophonium)
- To decrease urine retention after surgery
- To reverse the effects of certain drugs used during anesthesia

What are some commonly used antimyasthenics?
- ambenonium, known by the brand name Mytelase
- edrophonium, known by the brand names Enlon, Reversol, and Tensilon
- neostigmine, known by the brand name Prostigmin
- pyridostigmine, known by the brand names Mestinon and Regonol

What are the possible side effects?
- Headaches, weakness
- Sweating
- Abdominal pain, nausea and vomiting, diarrhea, excessive salivation
- Difficulty breathing

To maximize the effectiveness of the antimyasthenic you're taking, schedule your largest doses before usual periods of fatigue, such as the late afternoon and before meals, and schedule rest times for such periods.

What are the guidelines for taking antimyasthenics?

- Make sure your doctor knows about all other medications you are taking, including nonprescription drugs.
- Drug dosage must be carefully adjusted to obtain optimum results. However, the symptoms of excessive drug dosage closely resemble the symptoms associated with worsening of the disease (muscle weakness). Report any signs of muscle weakness immediately.
- To maximize the effectiveness of the antimyasthenic you're taking, schedule your largest doses before usual periods of fatigue, such as the late afternoon and before meals, and schedule rest times for such periods.
- Evaluate and record variations in muscle strength. Keep a diary of these variations, correlated to the time of day and medication schedule, to help the doctor evaluate therapy.
- During adjustment to therapy, take the drug with food or milk to minimize gastrointestinal distress. Scheduling a dose 30 minutes before meals may improve your ability to swallow food.
- Because even a minor respiratory infection can aggravate myasthenic symptoms, avoid contact with all persons with infections.
- Wear a medical identification bracelet or carry a card indicating your condition and current drug regimen.

SKELETAL MUSCLE RELAXANTS

These drugs are often used to help people with painful muscle spasms resulting from minor strains, sprains, or fractures. Some people with moderate to severe muscle spasms from illnesses such as MS or spinal cord injury may also benefit from therapy.

Most of these drugs are also potent central nervous system depressants. Diazepam (known by the brand name Valium) is often used as a skeletal muscle relaxant; however, it is also a potent antianxiety drug and sedative.

What are skeletal muscle relaxants used for?

- To reduce muscle spasms and relieve pain
- To decrease muscle spasticity caused by nerve damage

What are some commonly used skeletal muscle relaxants?

- baclofen, known by the brand name Lioresal
- carisoprodol, known by the brand names Rela and Soma
- chlorzoxazone, known by the brand name Parafon Forte
- cyclobenzaprine, known by the brand name Flexeril
- dantrolene, known by the brand name Dantrium
- methocarbamol, known by the brand name Robaxin

What are the possible side effects?

- Drowsiness, dizziness, tremor, nervousness, confusion, depression, hallucinations
- Nausea, dry mouth, constipation
- Rapid heart rate, low blood pressure

What are the guidelines for taking skeletal muscle relaxants?

- These drugs often cause moderate to severe drowsiness and dizziness. Avoid hazardous tasks such as driving or operating heavy machinery until the side effects of the drug on the central nervous system are known.
- Dry mouth is a common problem. Use ice chips or sugarless gum or hard candy to relieve dry mouth. If it persists, the doctor may prescribe a saliva substitute. Because dry mouth increases the risk of dental problems, call the doctor if this problem persists beyond 2 weeks.
- If you miss a dose, take it as soon as you remember, unless it's time for the next dose. Never double the dose.
- Avoid alcohol and other central nervous system depressants such as antihistamines while taking skeletal muscle relaxants. Combining these drugs can cause severe depression of the central nervous system.
- Don't take any other drugs, including nonprescription drugs, without first checking with your doctor.
- To minimize stomach upset, take these drugs with food or milk. If swallowing large tablets is a problem, check with the pharmacist, who may be able to substitute a liquid form of the drug or issue guidelines for crushing the tablets.
- Methocarbamol may turn your urine green, black, or brown; chlorzoxazone may turn the urine orange or purple. These are normal effects of the drug and not harmful to you.

- After prolonged use of these drugs, they should be discontinued gradually. Be sure to follow your doctor's guidelines for discontinuing therapy.
- Don't stop taking the drug if side effects are a problem; discuss these effects with your doctor, who may switch you to another drug or change the dosage.

SURGERIES

AMPUTATION

Amputation, the partial or complete removal of a body part or organ, may be performed as an elective surgical procedure in severe disease such as malignant bone tumors, or it can occur traumatically as the result of an accident. In traumatic amputation, surgery is required to care for the resulting wound.

As an elective surgical treatment, amputation is performed to preserve function in the remaining body part or, at times, to prevent death. In most cases, amputation is really a reconstructive surgery that attempts to improve the person's quality of life by relieving symptoms and improving function.

Why is this surgery done?
Elective surgical amputation may be necessary because of complications of diabetes, congenital deformity, malignant tumors, frostbite, or gangrene. Peripheral vascular disease is the cause of most lower limb amputations.

Common causes of traumatic amputation include crush and thermal injuries, power tool and motor vehicle accidents, gunshot wounds, and household injuries.

What happens before the surgery?
- Because you may find the loss of a body part emotionally devastating, the nurse will provide emotional support and discuss with you the type and level of amputation to be performed.
- You'll be taught and encouraged to perform range-of-motion and strengthening exercises before and after surgery to maintain muscle

strength and tone, prevent contractures, and promote mobility and independence.

- Before lower limb amputation, especially leg amputation, the nurse and the physical therapist will prepare you for getting around and will teach you transfer techniques. The sooner you get out of bed after surgery, the better your chances for successful rehabilitation.
- If appropriate, the nurse will help you plan for the disposal of the amputated part in accordance with your religious beliefs.

What happens during the surgery?

The two basic forms of surgical amputation are the closed or flap technique, the most commonly performed type, and the open technique, a rarely performed emergency procedure. In either technique, you'll receive a general or a spinal anesthetic (or perhaps a local anesthetic for a finger or toe amputation).

The *closed or flap technique* is appropriate when there is no infection. In this procedure the surgeon cuts the tissue to the bone, leaving enough tissue to cover the stump. Then, after the bone is removed, the skin flap is sutured over the bone stump; small drains may be inserted to promote wound healing.

The *open technique,* commonly used to treat an infected septic wound, consists of two separate operations. First, the surgeon makes an incision through the bone and all the tissue, leaving the wound open to drain and sometimes applying traction. After bed rest and antibiotic therapy resolve the infection, the surgeon completes the repair and constructs a stump.

What are the possible complications?

Complications that may follow amputation include bleeding (the most life-threatening complication), severe pain, infection, necrosis (tissue death), bursting open of the wound, skin irritation from dressings or drainage, contractures, and phantom sensations. (See *Understanding phantom sensations.*)

What happens after the surgery?

- The nurse will rewrap the stump three or four times a day.
- The nurse may also provide analgesics and other pain-control measures (such as heat application or whirlpool).
- The nurse will help you change position every 2 hours. You'll be instructed to avoid positions that would encourage contractures. For example, don't let the stump hang over the edge of a bed or chair for

---

Understanding phantom sensations

Phantom sensations — sensations in the missing limb as if the limb were still part of you — are a real, not an imagined, complication of amputation. People describe these sensations as an itching, a tingling or, most often, as a pain that is acute, crushing, cramping, burning, or throbbing.

Causes: Two theories
No one knows exactly what causes phantom sensations, but one theory holds that remaining nerve tracks still send messages to the brain. According to another theory, suppressed anger, denial, depression, and grief over the amputation contribute to the sensation.

Exacerbations and remissions
Phantom sensations usually feel more severe immediately after the amputation and generally subside with time. However, exacerbations and remissions of phantom itching and tingling can occur for years.

Phantom sensations have been treated with analgesics, anti-inflammatory drugs, distraction, early ambulation, transcutaneous electrical nerve stimulation, nerve block, and psychotherapy.

How to care for the amputation site

If you think you'll require additional help at home, have the nurse make appropriate referrals to home health care agencies before you're discharged. Then, once you leave the hospital after the surgery, follow these important guidelines.

Report any problems
- Report signs of infection, such as fever and chills.
- Carefully check the amputation site for swelling, redness, skin changes (rashes, blisters, or abrasions), excessive drainage, and increased pain. Report any of these signs to your doctor.

Other instructions
- Keeping the stump meticulously clean by frequently changing dressings can speed healing. As the wound heals, you'll need to change the dressing less often.
- Make sure to follow carefully the nurse's instructions for wrapping the stump or applying a stump shrinker; otherwise, you run the risk of impairing circulation.

a prolonged time. (See *How to care for the amputation site* for more details.)
- You and your family will be provided with information about available prostheses. If this was not done before surgery, a consultation with a prosthetist and a meeting with a well-adjusted amputee will be arranged.
- If you're unable to maintain a positive outlook, you may receive psychological counseling to help you adjust to your loss.
- If necessary, the social services department will help you deal with lifestyle changes and financial, family, and social problems after discharge.

OPEN FRACTURE REDUCTION

Open fracture reduction is the surgical restoration of the normal position and alignment of bone fragments or a dislocated joint. It is followed by insertion of internal fixation devices — pins, screws, nails, wires, rods, or plates — to maintain positioning until healing occurs. When closed reduction of a fracture or dislocation is impossible or inadvisable, open reduction and internal fixation may be necessary.

This procedure is most often performed in adults and adolescents. It's usually avoided in children because the handling of bones and placement of fixation devices can disrupt normal bone growth and development.

Timing is critical to the success of this operation. Best results are obtained when the bones are set and fixation performed as soon as possible after injury, before the bones have had a chance to set improperly. If necessary, skeletal traction may precede open reduction and fixation to reduce severe muscle spasm and help realign grossly angulated fracture fragments or dislocations. Typically, a cast or splint is applied after surgery to immobilize the injury site and aid healing. (See *Recovering from open fracture reduction* for self-care activities to be carried out at home.)

Why is this surgery done?
Open reduction with internal fixation is performed to restore normal alignment to bone segments and maintain positioning during heal-

SELF-HELP

Recovering from open fracture reduction

By following the guidelines listed below, you can help ensure a complete recovery.

Know what to expect
- The doctor will restrict your activity and instruct you not to place weight on the affected limb for a time.
- If required to so do by the nurse, you'll have to demonstrate the correct use of crutches before discharge.
- To maintain muscle tone and promote mobility, you'll need to perform the prescribed exercises.
- Because pain in the affected bone may persist for several months, your doctor may prescribe analgesics.

Report any problems
- Watch for and report signs of wound infection, including fever, fatigue, increased pain at the incision site, redness, pus-filled drainage, or separation of wound edges.
- Watch for signs of skin irritation around the cast edges. Report severe irritation, foul odor, or discharge.
- Immediately report signs of impaired circulation, such as numbness or coldness.

Other instructions
- If you are discharged with a cast in place, make sure you understand how to care for it before you leave the hospital.
- Do not get the cast wet or insert objects under it to scratch itching skin.
- If you are discharged with a removable splint, make sure you know how to apply and remove the device.
- Maintain a balanced diet with generous amounts of protein, calcium, and vitamin C. Also, drink plenty of fluids.

ing with screws, rods, pins, plates, or other fixation devices. This procedure should be performed for compound fractures, comminuted fractures (with the bone shattered into three or more fragments), impacted fractures (with one bone fragment), or a fracture or dislocation that has caused serious nerve or circulatory impairment.

When shouldn't this surgery be done?
If severe tissue damage accompanies fracture or dislocation, application of a cast may be inadvisable and skin or skeletal traction may be used instead.

What happens before the surgery?
- The fracture site will be immobilized, if appropriate, to reduce pain and swelling.
- You may have to have X-rays to visualize the fracture.
- The nurse will administer narcotic analgesics, sedatives, and antibiotics as ordered.

- The procedure will be briefly explained to you as time permits.
- Your food intake will be restricted after midnight on the night before surgery.

What happens during the surgery?

While you are under general anesthesia, the surgeon makes an incision through the skin and soft tissue, spreads the muscle to expose the fragments or dislocated joint segments, and then inserts one or more screws or another type of fixation device to immobilize the fragments in proper alignment. Next, the surgeon closes the incision and applies a cast, a splint, or traction, if necessary, to protect the surgical site and maintain alignment. (See *Understanding internal fixation methods.*)

What are the possible complications?

Potential complications associated with open reduction and internal fixation include infection, reduced blood volume, compartment syndrome, and fat embolism. A person with a severe open fracture of a large bone, such as the femur, is at particular risk for shock from loss of blood. Fat embolism is a potentially fatal complication that follows the release of fat droplets from the bone marrow; these can lodge in the lungs or the brain. They typically develop within 24 hours after a fracture but may be delayed up to 72 hours.

What happens after the surgery?

- The affected body part will be maintained in proper alignment, and, if possible, supported and elevated to reduce swelling and the risk of circulatory impairment.
- If you've suffered a major fracture that requires long-term immobilization with traction, you'll be repositioned often to prevent bed sores and enhance comfort. The nurse will encourage coughing and deep-breathing to prevent pulmonary complications and adequate fluid intake to prevent urinary stagnation and constipation.
- As instructed by the doctor or physical therapist, the nurse will assist with active or passive range-of-motion exercises to prevent loss of muscle and muscle function. The nurse will encourage you to get out of bed and move about as soon as possible after surgery and will assist with walking as necessary.

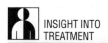

INSIGHT INTO
TREATMENT

Understanding internal fixation methods

Choice of a specific fixation device depends on the location, type, and configuration of the fracture.

In a trochanteric fracture, the surgeon may use a hip pin or nail with or without a plate. A pin or plate with extra nails stabilizes the fracture by approximating the bone ends at the fracture site.

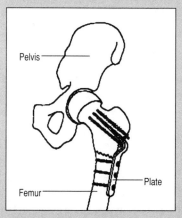

In an uncomplicated fracture of the femur, the surgeon may use a rod, as shown. This device permits early ambulation with partial weight bearing.

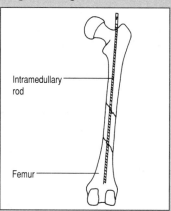

Another choice for fixation of a long-bone fracture is a screw plate, shown here on the tibia.

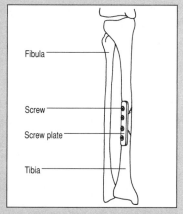

In an arm fracture, the surgeon may fix the bones with a plate, rod, screw, or nail. Most radial and ulnar fractures may be fixed with plates, whereas humeral fractures may be fixed with rods.

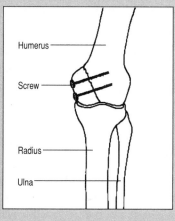

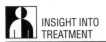
INSIGHT INTO TREATMENT

Reconstruction alternatives

Arthroplasty is a surgical technique intended to restore motion to a stiffened joint. Joint replacement is one option; other options include joint resection or interpositional reconstruction.

Joint resection
Joint resection involves careful excision of bone portions, creating a ¾-inch (2-centimeter) gap in one or both bone surfaces of the joint. Fibrous scar tissue eventually fills in the gap. Although this surgery restores mobility and relieves pain, it decreases joint stability.

Interpositional reconstruction
Interpositional reconstruction involves reshaping the joint and placing a prosthetic disk between the reshaped bony ends. The prosthesis used for this procedure may be composed of metal, plastic, fascia, or skin. However, after repeated injury and surgical reshaping, total joint replacement may become necessary.

JOINT REPLACEMENT

Total or partial replacement of a joint with a synthetic prosthesis aims to restore mobility and stability and to relieve pain. Recent improvements in surgical techniques and prosthetic devices have made joint replacement increasingly common. Some centers now specialize in custom joint replacement; in this technique, a mold is taken of the person's joint, which is then replicated within 99% of the original using computer techniques. All joints except the spine can be replaced with a prosthesis; hip and knee replacements are the most common. The benefits of joint replacement include not only improved, pain-free mobility but also an increased sense of independence and self-worth. (See *Reconstruction alternatives*.)

Why is this surgery done?
This procedure is performed to replace a joint that has been diseased or damaged by arthritis, other degenerative joint disorders, or extensive joint trauma. If performed correctly, this surgery restores or improves joint function and eliminates or reduces pain.

What happens before the surgery?
- The doctor or nurse will inform you about postoperative measures, such as positioning, transfer techniques, assisted walking, and an exercise regimen. The exercise program begins shortly after surgery, even while you're still confined to bed.
- Either you or a responsible family member will be required to sign a consent form.

What happens during the surgery?
Surgery is performed using general anesthesia. The details of the joint replacement procedure vary slightly depending on the joint and its condition. In a total hip replacement, for instance, the surgeon replaces the head and neck of the femur (thigh bone) and the acetabulum (socket into which the joint fits) with a prosthesis. Several prostheses are available, but the femoral component is typically constructed of stainless steel or vitalium; the acetabular component, of polyethylene with metal backing. The surgeon may secure the device in place with methyl methacrylate adhesive, which fills the gap between the prosthesis and the bone. Prosthetic components may also

be made of ceramic materials or porous coated metals that do not require adhesives. Bone ingrowth and repair allow fixation of these prostheses.

To prevent infection, special precautions are taken during surgery. Blood loss is usually large and is monitored carefully. Large amounts of fluids are commonly infused intravenously, and whole blood or packed-cell transfusions are usually administered.

For total knee replacement, the surgeon replaces the affected bones with a prosthesis. As with total hip replacement, the surgeon may either use methyl methacrylate adhesive to secure the prosthesis or allow bone ingrowth to fixate prostheses that do not require adhesives. Strict infection precautions are needed; a tourniquet may be used to control blood loss. (See *Living with a joint replacement*, page 276.)

What are the possible complications?

Complications of joint replacement include shock from loss of blood, inflammation of the veins and formation of blood clots, infection, dislocation of the prosthesis (with hip replacement), and the need for eventual revision.

What happens after the surgery?

- Surgery may not relieve pain immediately; pain may actually worsen for several weeks. Analgesics will be available as needed.
- You'll be kept on bed rest for the prescribed period after surgery.
- The nurse may use pillows or traction to maintain the affected joint in proper alignment.
- Antiembolism stockings will be applied.
- The nurse will reposition you often to enhance comfort and prevent bed sores. Frequent coughing and deep-breathing will be encouraged to prevent pulmonary complications and adequate fluid intake to promote urination and prevent constipation.
- You'll be encouraged to implement the recommended exercise program. (Some doctors routinely order physical therapy to begin on the day of surgery.) The doctor may prescribe continuous passive motion, which involves use of a machine or a system of suspended ropes and pulleys or a series of active or passive range-of-motion exercises. (For further details, see "Range-of-Motion Exercises," pages 289 to 293.)
- The nurse will assist you to walk and will make certain that you obtain and can correctly use prescribed supportive equipment, such as crutches, walker, or cane.

SELF-HELP

Living with a joint replacement

To prevent some of the possible complications of joint replacement surgery, follow the guidelines outlined below.

Protect the prosthesis
- If you have had hip replacement, you must be careful to keep your hips abducted and not to cross your legs when sitting. This will reduce the risk of dislocating the prosthesis. Avoid flexing your hips more than 90 degrees when rising from a bed or chair and sitting in low chairs or in a bathtub. Sit in chairs that have high arms and a firm seat; sleep only on a firm mattress.
- If you have had shoulder joint replacement, you will need to keep your arm in a sling until swelling goes down. You may then slowly begin the prescribed exercise program when healing is complete, usually about 6 weeks after surgery.
- You may need preventive antibiotics for minor surgical procedures or dental procedures to prevent bacterial infection.
- Do not let anyone perform magnetic resonance imaging studies on you because the metal in the prosthesis will interfere with the reading.

Know when to call your doctor
- Promptly report signs of possible infection, such as persistent fever and increased pain, tenderness, and stiffness in the joint and surrounding area.

- Remember that infection may develop even several months after joint replacement. Make sure to report suddenly increased pain or decreased function, because they may indicate that the prosthesis has become dislodged.

Other instructions
- Adhere to the exercise schedule prescribed by the doctor and physical therapist. Do not rush rehabilitation, no matter how well you feel.
- Depending on the location and extent of surgery, the doctor may order you to avoid bending or lifting, extensive stair climbing, or sitting for prolonged periods (including long car trips or plane flights).
- Make sure not to overuse the joint—especially if it is a weight-bearing joint.
- If you have had knee replacement, you may be instructed to wear a knee brace or an immobilizer. If this is the case, make sure you know how to apply the device correctly.
- Report for follow-up evaluation and testing as necessary.

CARPAL TUNNEL RELEASE

Carpal tunnel syndrome is a relatively common, painful disorder caused by compression of the nerve within the carpal tunnel of the wrist by the overlying carpal ligament. This syndrome may develop after strenuous or repetitive use of the hands or may follow wrist injuries, such as fractures, dislocations, or bruises. Often, however, the person has no history of significant trauma.

If rest, splinting, and corticosteroid injections fail to relieve carpal tunnel syndrome, surgery may be necessary. This surgery involves cutting the entire carpal tunnel ligament and may include freeing nerve fibers as well. Surgical division of the ligament gives lasting relief from pain. However, muscle strength returns slowly, and complete recovery is unlikely if the muscle has pronounced deterioration.

Why is this surgery done?

Carpal tunnel release is performed to decompress the nerve within the carpal tunnel, thereby relieving pain and restoring function. It should also be performed on people who experience pain and loss of function of the affected wrist and hand, when noninvasive therapies have proven ineffective.

What happens before the surgery?

- The nurse shaves and cleans the affected arm.
- The nurse teaches you rehabilitative exercises, such as range-of-motion exercises of the wrist and fingers, which will be recommended after surgery if you can tolerate them.

What happens during the surgery?

This procedure is performed in the operating room, usually with a local anesthetic. The surgeon can choose from several techniques, each of which involves cutting across the carpal ligament to relieve pressure on the median nerve. Depending on the extent of nerve compression, he or she also may have to free nerve fibers from the surrounding tissue.

What are the possible complications?

This relatively simple surgery is generally risk-free, but certain complications may arise. These include infection, painful scar formation, and inflammation of the tendon sheath. (See *Recovering from carpal tunnel release* for further tips on having an uncomplicated recovery.)

What happens after the surgery?

- Your hand will be kept elevated to reduce swelling and discomfort.
- The nurse will assess for pain and provide analgesics as needed.
- You'll be encouraged to perform exercises daily to improve circulation and enhance muscle tone. If these exercises are painful, you'll

 SELF-HELP

Recovering from carpal tunnel release

Take the following steps to ensure complete recovery from carpal tunnel release and to protect against a recurrence of carpal tunnel syndrome.

Keep the incision site clean

- Keep the incision site clean and dry. You may need to cover it with a surgical or rubber glove when immersing it in water for exercises or when bathing.
- You must change the dressing once a day until healing is complete.
- Notify the doctor of any redness, swelling, pain, or persistent or excessive drainage at the operative site.

Continue daily exercises

- Continue daily wrist and finger exercises. However, be careful not to overuse the affected wrist or lift any object heavier than a thin magazine.
- If your carpal tunnel syndrome is work-related, you should consult an occupational counselor to find more suitable employment.

perform them with the wrist and hand immersed in warm water. (You'll be made to wear a surgical glove if the dressing is still in place.)

FASCIOTOMY

Fasciotomy is a surgical incision into the tissue called the *fascia* when swelling creates increased pressure within a muscle compartment. This increased pressure causes pain, numbness, tingling or prickling, paralysis, pallor, and pulselessness in the involved area.

Fascia is a sheet or band of inelastic fibrous tissue that encloses muscles, nerves, and circulatory structures of the musculoskeletal system; fascia separates these structures into compartments that have entrance and exit points large enough to permit only the passage of blood vessels and nerves.

Fasciotomy is usually considered an emergency procedure because it must be performed within 6 to 12 hours of the onset of symptoms to prevent deficiency of blood supply in the affected area. If performed within this time, the prognosis is good for functional return to the affected limb. If performed after this time, the risk of complication is higher and functional return is less likely.

Why is this surgery done?
Fasciotomy is primarily used as emergency treatment for compartment syndrome. It relieves pressure in the involved compartment, reducing swelling and increasing blood flow. The musculoskeletal compartments in which the syndrome most commonly occurs are those located in the legs and the arms, but the syndrome can also develop in the shoulder, hand, buttocks, foot, and thigh.

What happens before the surgery?
▪ If compartment syndrome occurs in an extremity, the nurse will position the extremity no higher than the heart.
▪ All splints and constricting dressings will be loosened or removed. If you have a cast, the cast and the padding will be split to relieve pressure. The extremity will then be immobilized with nonconstricting splints.

What happens during the surgery?

The orthopedic surgeon makes an incision through the skin and into the fascia that encloses the involved compartment and extends the incision the length of the compartment to relieve pressure in all the tissues involved. The surgeon removes any dead tissue or masses of blood that are found. The incision is then left open, covered only by a sterile dressing, until swelling has subsided (usually 3 to 7 days). After the swelling has subsided, the skin is closed by stitches or skin grafts.

What are the possible complications?

Complications of fasciotomy can include soft-tissue and bone infections resulting from an open wound, amputation of the limb because of extensive muscle death and compromised blood flow, kidney failure, loss of function of the involved area, and death resulting from toxic blood infection.

What happens after the surgery?

- The nurse will reassure and support you and your family because the incision is left open and bed rest must be maintained.
- The nurse will teach you signs and symptoms of complications that you should report to your doctor. (See *Recovering after a fasciotomy*.)
- The affected extremity will be placed at heart level to ensure adequate circulation.

Arthroscopy

Arthroscopy is a surgical procedure that uses a specially designed fiber-optic tubular instrument called an *arthroscope* for visual examination of the interior of a joint. The procedure is performed under local, spinal, or general anesthesia, depending on the anticipated length and complexity of the procedure.

Arthroscopy is most commonly used to examine the knee but is increasingly being used for other joints (the shoulder, elbow, ankle, wrist, and hip). Arthroscopy is a useful diagnostic aid only after a thorough clinical workup and conservative treatment have failed to remedy the joint problem.

 SELF-HELP

Recovering after a fasciotomy

Take the following precautions to help avoid complications after a fasciotomy.

Report any problems
- Notify the doctor immediately if any of the following signs and symptoms of infection occurs: redness, drainage, fever, warmth at the incision site, or swelling.
- Report numbness and tingling to the doctor.

Other instructions
- At discharge, your wound will be closed either by sutures or skin graft. Care for the graft or suture as recommended by the surgeon.
- You'll be responsible for monitoring your pulse in the affected extremity. Do so as instructed by the doctor and report any abnormalities.
- Take antibiotics exactly as prescribed, even if you feel better before you've finished taking the entire course.

Why is this procedure done?

- To detect, monitor, and diagnose joint-related diseases
- To remove loose fragments from joint cavities
- To allow diagnostic viewing of joints

What happens before the procedure?

- The doctor or nurse describes the procedure to you.
- The nurse explains expected outcomes and the usual rehabilitative course, including teaching you and your family how to perform the prescribed exercises after surgery.
- You'll be reminded to report any skin abrasions on the affected extremity or any new medical problems.

What happens during the procedure?

This procedure is performed in the operating room under local or general anesthesia. After inserting a large-bore needle into the joint, the surgeon injects sterile 0.9% sodium chloride solution to distend the joint and then introduces the arthroscope into the joint through a small incision in the skin. The surgeon then empties the joint of blood and debris using irrigation and suction. When the joint is clear, the surgeon examines the cartilage and ligaments for abnormalities. The surgeon may then make a small incision at another place on the limb and use this new entry site to insert small instruments to facilitate manipulation of anatomic structures and to allow certain repairs. These small incisions cause little or no scarring.

When the exam and procedure are finished, the arthroscope is removed and the joint is irrigated. Adhesive strips are applied over the incision sites, and a compression bandage is applied over the surgical site.

What are the possible complications?

Arthroscopy rarely causes complications. The most common complications are infection and inflammation and clots in blood vessels, but even these occur in fewer than 1% of patients. Blood in the joint cavity, stiffness, and delayed wound healing may occur. Damage to the blood vessels leading to loss of the limb is possible when arthroscopic instruments damage arteries, but this is rare. There also is a small risk of instrument breakage within the joint.

SELF-HELP

Recovering after arthroscopy

Take the following steps to minimize the risk of complications after arthroscopy.

Know what to expect
- You may begin to resume a normal diet with clear liquids; if no nausea develops over several hours, you may resume your regular diet.
- You should avoid alcoholic beverages for at least 24 hours.
- You should avoid driving and other hazardous tasks that require alertness and good coordination.
- Follow the surgeon's directions regarding restricted activities. If your activity is not restricted, your surgeon may put you on a physical therapy regimen as early as 2 days after surgery.
- You may be required to keep the affected extremity elevated.

- You may apply ice for 24 to 48 hours after the procedure.

Other instructions
- Take prescribed medications as directed. Analgesics will relieve the pain, allowing you to participate more easily in prescribed exercises.
- Follow the surgeon's instructions for performing all exercises correctly, even if you have to enlist the help of family members to perform the active or active-assistive maneuvers.
- Make sure to keep the dressing clean and dry.
- Do not change your own dressing. The surgeon will change it during your first follow-up visit.
- Inform the surgeon of any loss of sensation, coldness, blueness, swelling, or rash, or if the dressing is uncomfortable or tight.

What happens after the procedure?
- The nurse will apply an ice pack to the affected extremity.
- Typically, you'll be discharged from the same-day surgical department after several hours in the recovery room. After a more extensive procedure such as arthrotomy, you may need to stay overnight in the hospital, primarily for pain control. (See *Recovering after arthroscopy* for other self-care measures.)

LAMINECTOMY AND SPINAL FUSION

In laminectomy, the surgeon removes one or more of the bony laminae (the flattened portions on either side of the vertebra's arch) that cover the vertebrae.

After removal of several laminae, spinal fusion—grafting of bone chips between vertebral spaces—is often performed to stabilize the spine. Spinal fusion also may be done apart from laminectomy in

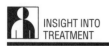

Alternatives to laminectomy

Microsurgical diskectomy, percutaneous automated diskectomy, and chemonucleolysis are alternative treatments for a herniated disk.

Microsurgical diskectomy

This treatment involves use of microsurgical techniques. Through a small incision, the involved area can be visualized and herniated disk material can be cut out. Extruded fragments may also be removed. Blood loss is minimal, complications are less frequent, and the postoperative course is generally less painful.

Percutaneous automated diskectomy

In this technique for removal of lumbar herniated disks, the doctor uses a nucletome, an instrument with cutting and aspiration capabilities, to gently aspirate (through a small skin incision) only the disk portion that is causing pain. Typically used for small,

less severe disk abnormalities, the procedure can be performed on an outpatient basis using local anesthesia. It's not effective for people who have disk extrusion or fragments in the spinal canal.

Chemonucleolysis

This treatment involves injection of the enzymes chymopapain or collagenase that reduce the nucleus pulposus of the herniated disk. Usually performed with radiographic visualization, it eliminates the need for major surgery. However, it has risks. Studies indicate disk space narrowing after chemonucleolysis, leading to irreversible osteoarthritis-like changes. Anaphylactic reactions are also possible.

---

some patients with vertebrae weakened by trauma or disease. (See *Alternatives to laminectomy*.)

Why is this surgery done?

Laminectomy

This procedure is most commonly performed to relieve pressure on the spinal cord or spinal nerve roots resulting from a herniated disk. It may also be done to treat a compression fracture, dislocated vertebrae, or spinal cord tumor; to repair spinal cord defects; to provide spinal cord stimulation; and to allow insertion of infusion pumps for pain control.

Spinal fusion

Spinal fusion may be needed to treat traumatic disruption of the vertebrae as well as ruptured disks that have resulted in unusual instability. The end result of spinal fusion is to strengthen and stabilize the spine. Commonly, this procedure is performed when more conservative treatments prove ineffective.

What happens before the surgery?

- The nurse will explain the procedure and answer your questions.
- The nurse will explain that you'll return from surgery with a dressing over the incision and will maintain bed rest for the time prescribed by the doctor. You'll be turned often to prevent bed sores and pulmonary complications. The nurse will show you the logrolling method of turning and the correct way to rise from a bed or chair.
- You must sign a consent form.

What happens during the surgery?

To perform a laminectomy, the surgeon makes a midline vertical incision, strips the muscles and membranes from the bony laminae, and then removes one or more sections of laminae to expose the spinal defect. For a herniated disk, the surgeon removes part or all of the disk. For a spinal cord tumor, he or she cuts through bone, explores the cord for cancer cells, and then dissects the tumor and removes it, using suction, forceps, or dissecting scissors.

To perform spinal fusion, the surgeon exposes the affected vertebrae and then inserts bone chips obtained from the hip or, rarely, from a bone bank. To restore optimal strength to the vertebral column, the surgeon wires these bone grafts into several vertebrae surrounding the area of instability.

What are the possible complications?

Complications may include recurrence of herniation, nerve root injury causing motor and sensory deficits, injury to blood vessels, and urine retention or paralysis of the intestine.

What happens after the surgery?

- Your back pain won't be relieved immediately and may even worsen after the surgery. Pain will be relieved only after chronic nerve irritation and swelling subside, which may take up to several weeks. Analgesics and muscle relaxants will be available during recovery should you need them.
- After lower back laminectomy, you'll be made to lie flat for the prescribed period, with 6-inch (15-centimeter) blocks to elevate the head of your bed. You won't be allowed to sit up or raise your head. When you're able to assume a side-lying position, make sure you keep your spine straight, with your knees flexed and drawn up toward your chest. The nurse will insert a pillow between your knees to relieve pressure on the spine and will use logrolling to turn you.

SELF-HELP

Recuperating from spinal surgery

Your recovery will proceed more smoothly if you take the following precautions.

Guard against infection

- Keep the incision site meticulously clean.
- Report signs of infection immediately.
- Reduce your chances of getting an infection by avoiding tub baths until healing is complete. Instead, shower with your back away from the stream of water.

Protect your back

- Minimize sitting to decrease pressure on the disk space; support your lower back when sitting; bend at the knees, not the waist.
- Allow rest periods between activities.
- Wear a fitted corset or brace for 6 to 8 weeks postoperatively, as instructed.
- Avoid lifting or pulling heavy objects.
- Perform daily stretching exercises as directed.
- Maintain normal weight.
- After lumbar laminectomy, gradually increase your activity.

- After laminectomy around the neck area, you should avoid extreme movements of the neck and should wear a soft cervical collar.
- If you don't urinate within 8 to 12 hours after surgery, a urinary catheter may be inserted to relieve urine retention. If you can void normally, the nurse will assist you in getting on and off a bedpan while maintaining proper alignment.
- The nurse will encourage you to perform prescribed exercises. (See *Recuperating from spinal surgery* for more information on ensuring an uncomplicated recovery.)

COTREL-DUBOUSSET SPINAL INSTRUMENTATION

Cotrel-Dubousset spinal instrumentation was developed in France in 1984. Used to treat spinal instability or deformity, this technique involves placing a series of rods and hooks to distract, compress, and derotate the spine. Cross-linking devices serve to further stabilize the spine. Because the surgeon attaches this device to so many points of the spine, the person may not need to wear a brace after the operation. Eliminating the need for a brace sets the Cotrel-Dubousset technique apart from other types of spinal instrumentation, such as the Har-

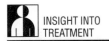
INSIGHT INTO
TREATMENT

Types of spinal instrumentation

The type of instrumentation you'll receive will be selected from the list of options below.

Luque rod instrumentation

The surgeon uses Luque rod instrumentation for people with neuromuscular curves. Unlike Harrington rod
instrumentation, Luque rods are custom-contoured
and are segmentally fixated with sublaminar wires
that are threaded at each vertebral level. An advantage of Luque rods is that postoperative casting and
bracing are avoided. The main disadvantage is a
higher neurologic risk because wires must be threaded under the vertebral laminae near the neural elements.

Harri-Drummond instrumentation

Harri-Drummond instrumentation uses a Harrington
rod on the concave side of the curve and a con-
toured Luque rod on the convex side. It achieves the
segmental fixation capabilities of the Luque rod without increasing the incidence of neural complications.
A disadvantage of this instrumentation is the need
for postoperative casting or bracing.

Cotrel-Dubousset instrumentation

This technique involves placing a series of rods and
hooks to distract, compress, and derotate the spine.
Cross-linking devices provide further stability. This
apparatus can be adapted to normal sagittal spinal
alignment and lumbar lordosis. Because the surgeon attaches it to many points, you may not need to
wear a brace after the operation.

Zeilke instrumentation

Similar to Cotrel-Dubousset instrumentation in con-
struction and function, Zeilke instrumentation may be
used alone or combined with the second stage of
the operation to treat a double spinal curve. If this is
the instrumentation you'll receive, you'll be advised
that you may have to wear a brace for about 7
months after this surgery.

The Kaneda device

This is a new type of spinal instrumentation. It provides
a treatment option for thoracolumbar burst fracture. It
addresses such potential problems of spinal injury as
the treatment of bone fragments in the spinal canal and
repair of anterior decompression of the spine followed
by posterior fusion with extensive surgery.

rington rod and Zeilke instrumentation. (See *Types of spinal instrumentation.*)

Why is this surgery done?

Cotrel-Dubousset instrumentation is used when the spinal column is
considered unstable because of tumor, infection, fracture, or increasing deformity. The installation of the Cotrel-Dubousset device stabilizes the spinal column during spinal fusion.

When shouldn't this surgery be done?

Cotrel-Dubousset instrumentation should not be performed in people who have significant osteoporosis.

Cotrel-Dubousset instrumentation

Cotrel-Dubousset instrumentation involves placing a series of rods and hooks to distract, compress, and derotate the spine. Cross-linking devices are added to provide further stability.

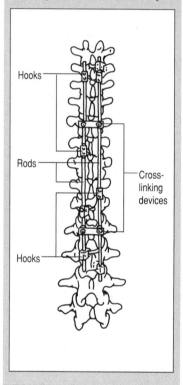

Hooks

Rods

Cross-linking devices

Hooks

What happens before the surgery?

■ The doctor or nurse explains the surgery and postoperative course to you and your family.

■ The nurse will demonstrate mobilization techniques to be used after the surgery. These include logrolling, sitting, and standing.

What happens during the surgery?

Cotrel-Dubousset spinal instrumentation is used by an experienced spinal surgeon and staff. Typically, the surgeon makes a midline incision in the back. He or she performs a spinal fusion by stripping the muscles from the area to be fused and by peeling away the surface layer of bone. Then the surgeon obtains a bone graft — usually from the hip — and places it along the area to be fused.

After the spine is prepared, multiple Cotrel-Dubousset hooks are placed at the previously determined levels and two Cotrel-Dubousset rods are placed into the hooks; then, two cross-linking devices are added to provide greater stability. Any remaining bone graft is then placed along the length of the fusion and the back wound is closed (See *Cotrel-Dubousset instrumentation*).

What are the possible complications?

Pain, inflammatory reaction due to foreign body, local wound infection, and inflammation of the spinal cord membrane may complicate the person's recovery. There is also the risk that the instrumentation may loosen or break and require repair. Although the Cotrel-Dubousset instrumentation does not increase the incidence of complications, all spinal surgery carries a risk of neurologic deficit and paralysis.

What happens after the surgery?

■ You'll be transferred to the orthopedic unit for rehabilitation within 24 to 48 hours.

■ The nurse will instruct you on respiratory care, such as coughing and deep-breathing exercises. (See *Recovering from Cotrel-Dubousset instrumentation*.)

SELF-HELP

Recovering from Cotrel-Dubousset instrumentation

Follow these guidelines to enhance your recovery after the procedure.

Take special precautions
- Notify the doctor if you have a temperature over 101° F (38° C) for more than 24 hours, local redness, a swollen or inflamed wound, or any wound drainage.
- If you have fixation to the sacrum, avoid prolonged sitting.
- Avoid heavy lifting and strenuous activity, as well as bending at the site.
- Gradually resume normal activity.

Watch what you eat
- Eat a well-balanced diet to promote bone growth, muscle strength, and return to normal bowel function.
- The doctor may recommend a high-fiber diet to counteract the constipating effects of pain medication and iron. In addition, you should avoid straining during elimination.

Other points to remember
- Make sure to provide wound care as recommended by the doctor.
- You will be prescribed narcotic analgesics to manage the pain. These will be gradually withdrawn and nonnarcotic medication will be substituted.

HARRINGTON ROD

The Harrington rod is a form of spinal instrumentation that involves the surgical placement of one or two (twin) metal rods to straighten or stabilize the spine through internal fixation. This rigid instrument contains hooks that attach to the flattened area on either side of the vertebra at designated levels above and below the curvature. (See *Types of spinal instrumentation,* page 285.)

The major advantage of using the Harrington rod is its longstanding proven reduction of lateral curvatures of the spine. Other advantages include the relative simplicity of application and a low rate of complications. A major disadvantage is that it requires prolonged casting after surgery. Like other spinal implants, the Harrington rod should not be implanted in people who have significant osteoporosis. (For more information about another technique, see "Cotrel-Dubousset Spinal Instrumentation," pages 284 to 287.)

Why is this surgery done?

The Harrington rod is inserted to maintain alignment of the vertebrae after fusion of the spinal column. Harrington rod placement should be performed for a spinal curvature too severe for correction

SELF-HELP

Recovering after Harrington rod insertion

Your recovery will be a lot smoother if you take the time to learn what to expect from spinal instrumentation.

Know what to expect

• Confinement in a Risser body cast will last for 6 months; you'll spend an additional 3 to 6 months in a brace.

• Be aware that muscle aches and pains will decrease with increased activity.

• You can increase physical activity after the cast is removed, but you must avoid contact sports and gymnastics.

• It is important that you place and wear the brace as instructed.

Other instructions

• Care for your cast as instructed and be alert for all complications.

• Do not make sudden position changes.

• Eat a well-balanced diet to promote bone growth, muscle strength, and return to normal bowel function.

• Notify the doctor of fever over 101° F (38.3° C) that persists longer than 24 hours; increased pain, redness, swelling, or drainage; or numbness or tingling of extremities.

by a brace, an angle of the spinal column greater than 60 degrees, or conditions for which a brace is not a feasible alternative.

A Harrington rod is the standard treatment for scoliosis (commonly called *spinal curvature*). The rod may be used for correction of other deformities. It is also used for spinal tumors and spinal injuries.

What happens before the surgery?

• The nurse will explain the procedure to you. If you're an adolescent, the nurse will also provide an opportunity for you to speak with someone your own age who has undergone the same procedure to minimize fear and anxiety about the surgery and the cast you'll have to wear afterward.

• During the preoperative period you may have your upper body in traction or in an upper body cast to stretch contracted muscles. If so, you'll need assistance with activities of daily living.

• You'll be offered pain medication, as prescribed, to diminish discomfort.

• The doctor will order X-rays to assess spinal and respiratory status.

• The nurse will give you an enema to clear the lower bowel.

• An indwelling urinary catheter will be inserted.

What happens during the surgery?

An orthopedic surgeon places the Harrington rod in the concavity of the spinal curve from the lowest to the highest vertebra to be fused and bends it to conform to the curvature. The rod is attached to the vertebral column. The rod then is fixed in two areas and may be used on both sides of the vertebral column. The rod maintains alignment, which allows the bone grafts to heal and the vertebra to fuse solidly.

What are the possible complications?

Complications after placement of a Harrington rod may include pain, inflammatory reaction (due to a foreign body), local wound infection, and meningeal infection (infection of the membranes covering the spinal cord and brain).

Surgical intervention may be required if the spinal attachments holding the rods move or if the instrumentation breaks and requires repair. Prolonged use of the body cast or brace or surgical intervention may be necessary if the bone grafts, required for correction of the curvature, do not unite solidly. Although the risk of neurologic complications is low with Harrington rod placement, all spinal surgery carries some risk of neurologic deficit and paralysis.

What happens after the surgery?

- Immediately after the operation, you are placed in a Risser cast for 6 months and afterward you must use a brace for another 3 to 6 months, depending on your healing ability.
- On the first day after surgery, you'll be kept in flat position and logrolled every 2 hours to prevent the development of bed sores.
- Your activity level will be gradually increased as recommended by the doctor and as tolerated. You'll be encouraged to perform self-care and range-of-motion exercises for arms and legs. (See *Recovering after Harrington rod insertion.*)
- The nurse will instruct you about coughing and deep-breathing.
- You'll be given clear liquids to start and then your diet will be advanced as tolerated to prevent nausea and vomiting.

EXERCISE & MOVEMENT

RANGE-OF-MOTION EXERCISES

Range-of-motion exercises are isotonic exercises that contract and shorten muscles. (See "Strengthening Exercises," pages 293 to 295, for a complete description of isotonic exercise.) They are designed to move the person's joints through as full a range of motion as possible. Each joint of the body has a normal range of motion. When they're performed properly, range-of-motion exercises help to improve or maintain joint mobility, improve circulation, enhance muscle tone, and prevent contractures and subsequent deformity.

Range-of-motion exercises may be active, active-assistive, or passive. The active exercises are performed by the person himself. Active-assistive exercises are performed by the person with the assistance of a nurse or physical therapist. Passive range-of-motion exercises are performed manually by a nurse, a physical therapist, a member of the person's family, or another caregiver or with the aid of a continuous passive motion machine. (See *Understanding continuous passive motion,* page 290.)

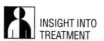

INSIGHT INTO
TREATMENT

Understanding continuous passive motion

Continuous passive motion uses an electrically powered machine to automatically move a joint through its normal range of motion for an extended time. Continuous passive motion is most commonly used in people recovering from total hip or knee replacement, internal fixation of knee or ankle fractures, or removal of the synovial membrane in the knee or other major joints. The use of the continuous passive motion machine prevents the development of scar tissue and enhances rehabilitation. However, it may cause bleeding in some people, especially if used immediately after surgery.

Performing continuous passive motion therapy
- The nurse will attach the machine to your bed and set the prescribed degree of flexion and extension and cycles per minute.
- Your extremity will be securely fastened in the frame. Sheepskin padding will be used to protect your skin.
- The nurse will remain with you for at least one cycle and double-check the degree of flexion and extension.
- The therapy will be continued for the prescribed time, which varies from continuously to 8 to 20 hours per day.

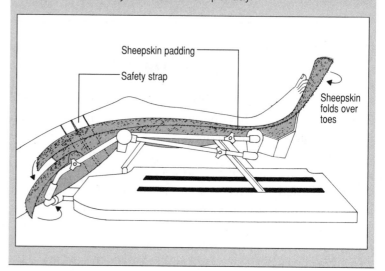

Sheepskin padding

Safety strap

Sheepskin folds over toes

Why is this therapy done?

Range-of-motion exercises should be performed during prolonged physical inactivity, provided that there are no medical reasons why the person should not perform them. They are performed to maintain or restore normal joint movement and muscle tone, prevent stiffness and contractures, improve circulation, and, possibly, speed return of function.

Active range-of-motion exercises should be performed by people who have good neuromuscular function. Passive range-of-motion exercises should be performed for people with temporary or permanent loss of function, paralysis, or decreased level of consciousness.

When shouldn't this therapy be done?

Range-of-motion exercises should not be performed by people with severe arthritic joint inflammation, recent trauma with possible concealed fracture or internal injuries, blood vessel inflammation or clots, severe pain, and a stiff or immovable joint. Forced passive stretching—movement of a joint that's immobile because of disuse, disease, or injury—must be specially ordered and performed by a doctor or physical therapist.

What happens before the therapy?

- The nurse will explain the exercises to you or whomever will be your primary caregiver after discharge.
- If you are to perform active range-of-motion exercises, the nurse will instruct you to perform the exercises at least twice a day, but warn you not to overextend or overexert yourself, which can lead to complications.
- Before passive range-of-motion therapy, the nurse raises your bed to a comfortable working height and positions you properly—if possible, flat on your back, without a pillow, with hands at your sides and your feet together.

What happens during the therapy?

Depending on the type, mobility, and condition of the joints being exercised, range-of-motion therapy will include some or all of the following movements: flexion and extension, internal and external rotation, abduction and adduction, supination and pronation, dorsiflexion and plantar flexion, and eversion and inversion. (See *Pictorial glossary of joint movement,* page 292.)

To perform passive range-of-motion exercises, your health care provider (who may be a doctor, nurse, or physical therapist) will support the extremity at the joint and move the joint slowly, smoothly, and gently through its normal range of motion. If the joint is painful to the touch, as in arthritis, the extremity will be supported as close to

Pictorial glossary of joint movement

Below is a guide to the joint movements produced during range-of-motion exercises.

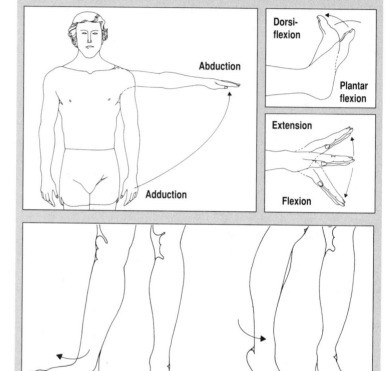

Abduction

Adduction

Dorsi-flexion

Plantar flexion

Extension

Flexion

External rotation

Internal rotation

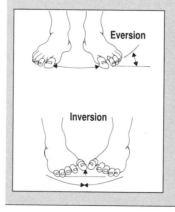

Eversion

Inversion

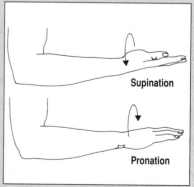

Supination

Pronation

the joint as possible without causing pain. To help prevent complications, only one extremity at a time will be exercised, no movement will be forced, and the exercise will be stopped at once if you complain of pain.

To perform active range-of-motion therapy, you must understand the prescribed exercises and their recommended frequency. You must move the involved joints slowly and smoothly through their range of motion and must stop and report any unusual pain or stiffness. Move each joint through its range of motion, typically about three to five times twice daily.

Because you will continue these exercises at home, you should consult your nurse for clarification of any confusing details before discharge. (See *Performing range-of-motion exercises at home*.)

What are the possible complications?

Potential complications of active range-of-motion exercises include exacerbation of inflammation from overmanipulation and joint or muscle injury from forced or excessive movement. Possible complications of passive range-of-motion therapy include joint instability from hyperextension and joint dislocation or bone fracture from excessively vigorous exercise.

What happens after the therapy?

- The nurse will position you comfortably in bed and encourage you to relax after passive range-of-motion exercises.
- You'll be given analgesics, as needed, if pain develops.

STRENGTHENING EXERCISES

Using exercise to strengthen weakened muscles is probably one of the most commonly used rehabilitation procedures. *Strength* is defined as the maximum force that can be exerted by a muscle. Significant muscular inactivity can result in weakness, and forceful muscular activity can lead to strength gains. Exercises to increase strength depend on muscular contraction. Three different modes of exercise are commonly used to increase muscle strength — isotonic, isometric, and isokinetic exercise.

 SELF-HELP

Performing range-of-motion exercises at home

Take the following steps to improve your chances for a smooth recovery.

Learn the exercises

- Before discharge, make sure that you and a family member or caregiver understand each aspect of the prescribed exercise program and the need for performing each exercise exactly as instructed. The nurse may provide written, illustrated, or tape-recorded instructions to make it easier for you to understand what's expected of you.
- To demonstrate that you understand the instructions and can do the exercises, you or your caregiver should perform each aspect of prescribed range-of-motion therapy for the nurse before discharge.

Other instructions

- You or your caregiver should report any complications associated with range-of-motion exercise, such as increased joint or muscle pain, stiffness, or immobility.
- Make sure you keep all scheduled follow-up appointments so the doctor can evaluate your progress and the effectiveness of the exercise program.

Isotonic exercise is the movement of a fixed load through the allowed joint range of motion. This is the most common form of strengthening exercise and usually involves the use of simple equipment, such as weights and pulleys, as well as specialized exercise units.

Isometric exercise involves the contraction of muscle without joint movement. In contrast to isotonic and isokinetic exercises, which are dynamic forms, isometrics are a static form of exercise. Isometric exercise may be used to help maintain strength when a joint is immobilized.

Isokinetic exercise is movement performed at a fixed speed against resistance supplied by specialized equipment that accommodates to the specific force exerted by the individual muscle. This accommodation extends throughout the entire range of motion, making this form of strengthening exercise the most efficient. It allows the maximum amount of muscular exertion that can be performed throughout the joint's range of motion. However, this method involves the use of expensive equipment. Isokinetic equipment is also used for testing muscle groups.

Why is this therapy done?

Strengthening exercises are done to increase muscle strength, endurance, and power and to improve functional ability.

Virtually everyone can benefit from a properly designed strengthening exercise program. Rehabilitative strengthening exercises are often prescribed for individuals with muscle weakness associated with inactivity due to disease, injury, or lifestyle habits, provided there are no reasons why the exercises would be inadvisable.

When shouldn't this therapy be done?

Strengthening exercises should not be performed after certain surgical procedures, such as skin grafting, in which the body part may need to be immobilized for a time. They also should not be performed in the presence of muscle or joint inflammation or pain during exercise. Strengthening exercises may also be inadvisable or may require careful adjustment and close supervision for people with unstable chest pain, recent heart attack, uncontrolled heartbeat irregularities, congestive heart failure, inflammation and clotting of blood vessels, or obstruction of the pulmonary artery, among other conditions.

What happens before the therapy?

The doctor or nurse will assess which muscles need to be strengthened.

What happens during the therapy?

Strengthening exercise programs may be designed by doctors, physical therapists, occupational therapists, or athletic trainers. These individuals, as well as nurses and physical therapy assistants, may administer these exercise programs. Strengthening programs are frequently conducted and supervised in hospitals, therapy clinics, and athletic training facilities.

An effective strengthening program must be individually designed to meet the person's needs. Consideration must be given to the method of exercise to be used. Isotonic exercise, the most common form, may use several different approaches. The person may exercise with the maximal weight that can be used for 5 to 10 repetitions, commonly using barbells, pulleys, and cuff-strap weights.

For isometric exercise, the person will contract the muscle, hold for 6 seconds, and then relax and repeat. This is performed while keeping the affected part in a fixed position.

Isokinetic exercise involves the use of specialized equipment that supplies resistance. However, unlike isotonic exercise, this resistance is able to accommodate to the force exerted by the individual muscle throughout the entire range of motion.

What are the possible complications?

Complications may include muscle soreness and fatigue. Heart and blood vessel complications are possible.

What happens after the therapy?

- The exercise program will be modified as needed. (See *Performing strengthening exercises at home.*)
- The nurse may provide written and illustrated instructions to make following the exercise program easier.

 SELF-HELP

Performing strengthening exercises at home

To get the maximum benefit from strengthening exercises, follow these guidelines:
- Make certain to perform each exercise accurately, according to the instructions given by the nurse.
- Remember to breathe during exercise activity and to exhale during the exertional phase of each maneuver.
- Don't overexercise.
- Contact the physical therapist if problems or questions arise.

OTHER TREATMENTS

CLOSED FRACTURE REDUCTION

Closed fracture reduction is manual manipulation of a fractured bone into alignment without breaking the skin barrier. A closed reduction should be attempted as soon as possible because swelling, which tends to increase for 6 to 12 hours after injury, can inhibit adequate reduction.

Because complete anatomical reduction is virtually impossible without actually visualizing the bone, an open reduction with internal fixation may be necessary after a closed reduction has been attempted.

The advantage of a closed reduction is that the skin barrier remains intact. The fracture site therefore is less likely to develop infection, inflammation, or delayed union; local tissue damage also is kept to a minimum.

Maintaining alignment after closed reduction can be achieved by several different methods: Casting and splinting stabilize the joint above and below the fracture; traction maintains alignment by creating a continuous pull on the limb to hold the fragmented ends in place and decrease muscle spasms; and percutaneous pinning involves inserting a pin below the skin surface and using wire to maintain alignment.

Why is this procedure done?

This procedure is performed to realign a fractured bone while keeping the skin over the site intact. Closed reduction of a fracture should be performed when the bone is displaced and can be realigned with external manipulation.

What happens during the procedure?

After examining an X-ray of the fracture, the orthopedic surgeon manually manipulates the site to align the fragments of the fractured bone. This is achieved by applying pressure to the long axis of the bone and reversing the mechanism that initiated the fracture. Because the main obstacle to achieving adequate reduction is muscle spasm, the person usually receives pain medication or anesthesia.

X-rays are repeated throughout the procedure to assess alignment of the bone.

What are the possible complications?

The usual complication of closed reduction is increased bleeding into the tissue around the fracture site caused by the manipulation of the bone.

Specific complications are associated with each method of maintaining alignment. With percutaneous pinning, infection can occur at the insertion sites. The use of skin traction may result in skin damage to the area when the adhesive tape is removed. Casting is associated with several complications: Bed sores may form from either the initial trauma or folds in the cast padding, and joint stiffness may result from immobilization of the joints above and below the fracture.

What happens after the procedure?

- The limb with the fractured bone will be elevated and ice will be applied to decrease swelling.
- The nurse will assist you with activities of daily living as needed.
- Prescribed pain medication will be administered to keep you comfortable.
- Your position will be changed every 2 hours to ease muscle fatigue and relieve pressure point areas. (See *Recovering after closed fracture reduction* for more details on taking care of yourself.)
- Before leaving the hospital, the nurse should refer you for physical therapy.

 SELF-HELP

Recovering after closed fracture reduction

To ensure that the closed fracture reduction results in a properly set bone, observe the following precautions:
- Report fever, increased drainage or pain, or a change in sensation (numbness or tingling) or temperature of the affected extremity.
- Use prescribed analgesics as instructed.
- Keep the cast or splint dry to prevent it from deteriorating.
- Follow the nurse's instructions for how to do range-of-motion exercises. They will keep joints flexible and maintain muscle tone.

ARTHROCENTESIS

Arthrocentesis involves insertion of a needle into a joint space to suction off synovial fluid or blood or to instill anti-inflammatory drugs. It also may be performed to obtain a specimen for diagnostic testing.

Arthrocentesis is most commonly performed on the knee, less often on the elbow, shoulder, or other joints. It's often combined with two related procedures: arthroscopy, which allows visualization of the joint, and arthrography, an X-ray showing joint tissue and structure.

Why is this procedure done?

Arthrocentesis is commonly used to relieve the pain, distention, and inflammation resulting from accumulation of fluid within a joint. It's also performed to administer local drug therapy, especially when other routes of administration have been unsuccessful. As a diagnostic aid, arthrocentesis is performed when an infection or other inflammatory joint disease (such as rheumatoid arthritis) is suspected.

When shouldn't this procedure be done?

Arthrocentesis should not be performed if there is bacteria in the blood, if there is any local infection around the joint structure, or if the skin around the site is not intact. The presence of bacteria makes this procedure dangerous because insertion of the needle almost always causes some breakage of small blood vessels and leakage of blood into the joint fluid, which contaminates the joint fluid. This procedure should also not be performed in the weight-bearing joints of people with osteoarthritis, except in rare cases, because the benefits for these people are short-lived and frequent injections result in joint destruction.

What happens before the procedure?

- The nurse makes sure that you understand the procedure.
- The nurse will inform you that a local anesthetic will be given, but that you may feel some pain as the needle is introduced into the joint space.
- If you are having arthrocentesis to withdraw a sample of synovial fluid for analysis, your food or fluids may be restricted for 6 to 12 hours before the procedure.

What happens during the procedure?

Throughout the procedure, the joint must be kept motionless. Depending on the approach used and the site, the joint is stabilized in extension or flexion. Using sterile technique, the doctor prepares the site, injects or sprays a local anesthetic at the site, and then inserts the appropriate needle and siphons off 10 to 15 milliliters of synovial fluid. To administer medication into the joint, the needle is left in place while the fluid-filled syringe is detached and replaced by the drug-filled syringe. Then the drug is injected.

What are the possible complications?

Although rare, complications of arthrocentesis may include joint infection, damage to the cartilage, hemorrhage leading to accumulation of blood within the joint, tendon rupture, and temporary nerve palsy.

What happens after the procedure?

- The affected limb will be elevated and the nurse will apply ice or cold packs to the joint for 24 to 36 hours to decrease pain and swelling.
- To minimize the risk of infection, the puncture site will be kept clean.
- The nurse will teach you which steps to take to care for yourself during the recovery period. (See *Recovering after arthrocentesis.*)

BONE GROWTH STIMULATION

Bone growth stimulation involves the application of a mild electric current to bone fracture fragments to help stimulate new bone growth and speed healing.

Three methods of electrical bone growth stimulation are currently used, one noninvasive method and two types of invasive bone growth stimulators, which are partially or fully implantable. Each method requires 3 to 6 months of therapy to be effective. (See *Methods of stimulating bone growth*, page 300.)

The invasive devices are direct current stimulators. They produce a fixed electrical field that runs a constant direct current into the fracture site to produce bone regeneration 24 hours a day. The noninvasive pulsating electromagnetic fields device stimulates with electromagnetic forces. These devices are applied for from 3 to 10 hours daily, depending on the manufacturer's recommendations.

Selection of a bone growth stimulator depends on such factors as the fracture's type and location, the doctor's preference, and perhaps most important, the person's ability to comply with treatment. The fully implanted system requires little or no intervention from the person being treated; the semi-implanted and pulsating electromagnetic fields systems require that the person manage his or her own treatment schedule and maintain the equipment.

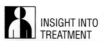

INSIGHT INTO
TREATMENT

Methods of stimulating bone growth

Placement of electrical bone growth stimulators may be invasive or noninvasive.

Invasive system

An invasive system, shown at right, involves placement of a spiral-like cathode inside the bone. A wire leads from the cathode to a battery-powered generator, also implanted in the local tissues. The person's body completes the electrical circuit.

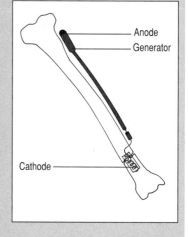

Noninvasive system

A noninvasive system, shown at right, may include a cufflike transducer that wraps around the person's limb at the level of the injury. Electric current penetrates the leg.

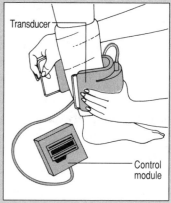

Why is this treatment done?

Bone growth stimulation is reserved for people with fractures that fail to heal within 6 to 9 months of injury (about 5% of all skeletal fractures).

Studies continue on new applications for this electrical treatment. Researchers hope eventually to use it to reverse osteoporosis and even to heal soft tissue injuries, such as pressure ulcers, bruises, and other skin ulcers.

When shouldn't this treatment be done?

These devices should not be used if the gap in the fractured bone is larger than half the diameter of the bone at the level of the fracture.

What happens before the treatment?

▪ The nurse will explain the procedure to you. If you'll be receiving a percutaneous stimulator or a pulsating electromagnetic fields device, you'll be responsible for managing your own schedule and maintaining the equipment.

▪ You'll also be instructed in cast care. If you'll have a pulsating electromagnetic fields device, you must not place any weight on the involved limb until healing is completed.

▪ If you have a lower extremity fracture, you won't be able to bear weight on the affected leg for the length of the therapy.

What happens during the treatment?

For invasive device

Before implantation of an invasive device, you'll receive spinal or general anesthesia.

The fully implantable direct current stimulator consists of a power generator (a small battery pack), titanium cathode, and lead wires. The cathode is implanted in the fractured bone and the generator in nearby deep muscle fascia. The generator is connected to the cathode by a lead wire that is tunneled through the tissue. The device runs 24 hours a day.

The semi-implantable percutaneous stimulator uses several Teflon-coated cathode pins, an external anode skin pad, and battery pack. Cathodes are implanted just inside the margin of each bone at the fracture site. The cathode wires are brought out to the skin surface, and the surgical area is covered with cast padding. The cathode wires are attached to the battery pack. The anode pad is applied to the skin and attached to the battery pack with a lead wire, and a non–weight-bearing cast is applied to the site over the battery pack.

For noninvasive device

The noninvasive pulsating electromagnetic fields device uses external wire coils and a generator to produce the therapeutic electric current. You are first fitted with a snug plaster cast. The doctor then measures the cast's circumference at the fracture site. This measurement guides the distance between the electromagnetic coils placed on either side of the injured area as well as the amount of voltage required for the

Enhancing bone-growth stimulation

Follow these guidelines to enhance the effectiveness of bone-growth stimulation therapy.

Take special precautions
- Report any signs of infection at the treatment site.
- Make sure you understand how to care for the cast before leaving the hospital.
- Do not put weight on the affected leg until after X-rays have confirmed complete healing.

Other points to remember
- If you have a pulsating electromagnetic fields device, wear the coils 3 to 10 hours a day (depending on the manufacturer's instructions) for intervals no shorter than 1 hour. Wearing the coils while you sleep will provide a long period of uninterrupted therapy.
- Make sure to test the unit regularly and to call the doctor if it doesn't work properly or if the generator alarm signals.
- Keep all scheduled follow-up appointments. These exams are needed to evaluate therapy and healing.

generator. The coils are placed on the cast and are held in place with a Velcro strap or a cufflike transducer. X-rays confirm proper coil placement in relation to the fracture.

What are the possible complications?

Complications after implantation of the direct current stimulator or the percutaneous stimulator include infection and discharge at the implantation site. Few complications are seen with the pulsating electromagnetic fields device, probably because it does not require implantation.

What happens after the treatment?

- If you have an implanted or semi-implantable device, the nurse will check your vital signs and assess the status of nerves and blood vessels in the affected limb.
- For all types of devices, the nurse will reinforce the doctor's instructions regarding any weight-bearing restrictions you'll have to observe. (See *Enhancing bone-growth stimulation*.)

IMMOBILIZATION

Commonly used to maintain proper alignment and limit movement, immobilization devices also relieve pressure and pain. These devices include plaster and synthetic casts, splints, slings, skin or skeletal traction, braces, and cervical collars. All types of immobilization devices help heal injured bones and surrounding soft tissue. (See *Understanding types of immobilization* for details on common devices.)

Why is this treatment done?

Immobilization is used to maintain alignment, limit movement, or provide support in management of musculoskeletal injuries or disorders.

Immobilization devices are used for various skeletal injuries. Casts are applied after closed or open reduction of fractures or after other severe injuries; splints are used to immobilize fractures or dislocations (partial and complete); slings are used to support and immobilize an injured arm, wrist, or hand, to support the weight of a splint, or to hold dressings in place; skin or skeletal traction, with a system of weights and pulleys to reduce fractures, is used to treat

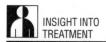
INSIGHT INTO
TREATMENT

Understanding types of immobilization

Use the following table as a guide to immobilization devices and their care.

TYPE	DESCRIPTION	PURPOSE	SPECIAL CONSIDERATIONS
Braces	Braces are support devices made of metal, leather, and hard plastic and are typically worn externally.	• To limit movement and enhance stability of an injured or weakened joint • To help correct neuromuscular defects in people with cerebral palsy, other spastic disorders, and scoliosis (spinal curvature)	• Keep an eye on the skin under the brace for abrasions. • Be aware that any fluctuation in your weight may change the fit.
Casts	Casts are made of plaster or synthetic material and may be applied to any body part, covering a single finger or the whole body; types of casts include the Minerva jacket, hip-spica, and extremity fixation with plaster of paris.	To maintain correct alignment and immobilization during healing; casts are used for traumatic injuries and correction of congenital deformities, including severe ligament rupture, limb or spinal fractures, club foot, and congenital hip deformity; if necessary, may be used with traction to enhance immobilization	You'll be asked to report extreme pain or pressure beneath the cast to your health care provider. Also report any drainage or fever, which may point to infection under the cast.
Collars	Made of soft foam or metal and plastic components, collars fit around the neck and under the chin; common types include the Philadelphia collar, doll's collar, Camp Victoria collar, and soft or hard cervical collar.	To support an injured or weakened cervical spine and maintain alignment during healing	• The nurse will regularly inspect the skin under the collar for abrasions and breakdown. • Because the collar will restrict your head movement, you may need assistance with eating and other activities. • A Philadelphia collar will be removed one half at a time while you are lying flat.
Skeletal traction	Skeletal traction involves placing a pin through the bone to which the traction apparatus is attached; common types include the halo vest and pin placement through the long bones of the legs and arms.	To immobilize bones and allow healing of fractures, correction of congenital abnormalities, or stabilization of spinal degeneration	• You'll be taught how to use the trapeze to lift yourself off the bed if permitted. • You'll be taught how to walk with an altered center of gravity, and shown how to adapt your clothing to fit over the vest. Do not bend over, but use an assistive device for reaching. You'll be required to change the vest liner as necessary.

(continued)

Understanding types of immobilization *(continued)*

TYPE	DESCRIPTION	PURPOSE	SPECIAL CONSIDERATIONS
Skin traction	Applied to the skin and soft tissue, skin traction indirectly pulls on the skeletal system and typically consists of weights, ropes, pulleys, and slings.	• To relieve muscle spasms • To restrict movement and provide correct alignment in cervical disk disease, pelvic fractures or fractures of the extremities, and spinal deformities	The nurse will show you how to move in bed without disturbing the traction.
Slings	Slings are composed of a soft fabric material or elastic adhesive fabric.	• To support an injured arm, hand, or wrist • Used with other types of immobilization to treat other upper extremity problems, such as shoulder dislocation	• It's important that you wear the sling for the prescribed period to prevent further injury or delayed healing. • Regularly perform passive range-of-motion exercises, as ordered.
Splints	Splints are made of leather, metal, and hard plastic components.	• To provide support for injured or weakened limbs or digits • To help correct deformities • To help treat spinal tuberculosis, hip dislocation, long-bone fractures, scoliosis, footdrop, and inflammatory lesions of the hip, spine, or shoulder	• Frequently inspect the splint for proper fit, cleanliness, and overall condition. • Regularly assess for skin breakdown under the splint. • Clean the leather components of the splint daily with saddle soap to keep them soft and supple.

dislocations, correct deformities, or decrease muscle spasms; braces are used to support weakened or deformed joints; and cervical collars are used to immobilize the neck, decrease muscle spasms and, possibly, relieve pain.

What happens before the treatment?

▪ The nurse will explain to you the purpose of the immobilization device the doctor has chosen, and, if possible, will show you the device before application and demonstrate how it works. The nurse will also tell you approximately how long the device will remain in place.

▪ Your initial discomfort will resolve as you become accustomed to the device.

▪ If you are in pain, the doctor may prescribe analgesics and muscle relaxants.

SELF-HELP

Managing with an immobilization device

Take the following precautions to ensure that immobilization achieves the desired effects.

Learn to use the equipment

- Make sure you and your caregiver know how to care for the immobilization device.
- If you have a removable device, such as a knee immobilizer, make sure you know how to apply it correctly before leaving the hospital.
- If you're using crutches, make sure you understand how to use them.

Other instructions

- If you need assistance with daily activities, ask your caregiver to help you.
- Promptly report signs of complications, including increased pain, inability to move fingers or toes, drainage, or swelling in the involved area.
- Restrict your activities while the immobilization device is in place to prevent it from becoming dislodged.
- Reduce your chances of falling by making sure your environment is safe.
- Keep scheduled medical appointments so that your doctor or nurse can evaluate healing.

What happens during the treatment?

The doctor usually applies the immobilization device. In certain situations, a nurse may apply a splint. Slings and braces may also be applied by a nurse or other trained individual. Application procedures vary depending on the type of immobilization device.

What are the possible complications?

Damage to the nerves and blood vessels is the major complication related to immobilization devices and can result in loss of a limb or limb function. Traction, casting, and splinting may result in loss of sensation in the perineal area, and compartment syndrome (see "Fasciotomy," pages 278 to 279). Additionally, complications of long-term immobility may include constipation, vein inflammation with blood clot, urinary stagnation, pneumonia, and depression. Skin irritation or breakdown may also occur with any device. Osteomyelitis (bone inflammation) is a complication of skeletal traction.

What happens after the treatment?

- To enhance comfort and prevent bed sores, the nurse will frequently reposition you if you're in traction or require long-term bed rest. Maintain proper body alignment. (See *Managing with an immobilization device.*)

- The nurse will also assist you with active or passive range-of-motion exercises to maintain muscle tone and prevent contractures.
- Regular coughing and deep-breathing will be encouraged to prevent pulmonary complications and adequate fluid intake to prevent urinary stasis (stagnation) and constipation.
- You will be given analgesics as needed.

FOOT CARE

An effective foot care regimen restores or maintains skin integrity and enhances circulation to rejuvenate or maintain sensory function and, if necessary, to aid healing.

Why is this therapy done?
Foot care should be performed for people with peripheral blood vessel disease, diabetes-related nerve disorders, traumatic injury, or prolonged immobilization. Additionally, it promotes cleanliness, controls odor, prevents infection, and improves circulation in the feet.

What happens before the therapy?
- The doctor or nurse will discuss the purpose of foot care with you, and explain all the steps. If you'll be performing foot care at home, pay close attention and ask questions.
- Your feet will be inspected for blisters, bruises, cracks, open lesions, corns, calluses, and areas of dry, reddened skin.

What happens during the therapy?
If you're in bed, the nurse will place a pillow under your knees to provide support and position the edge of a towel over the rim of a basin to cushion your lower legs. Then, the nurse will immerse one of your feet in water, wash it with soap, and allow it to soak for 5 to 10 minutes. If you're permitted to sit up and dangle your legs over the side of the bed, you may place your foot in a basin on a small footstool or the floor. Then the foot will be rinsed, removed from the basin, and patted dry. (Rubbing could damage the skin.) The nurse will apply lotion or oil to the foot immediately after drying to prevent evaporating water from drying the skin. If moisture remains

SELF-HELP

Taking care of your feet

To help restore or maintain skin integrity, take the following measures.

Protect your feet
- Always test the temperature of the water before immersing your feet. This is particularly important to remember if you have poor peripheral circulation: You could immerse your feet in water hot enough to cause burns without feeling pain.
- Do not soak your feet for longer than 10 minutes because this may increase the risk of infection and skin damage.
- Avoid using heating pads and hot-water bottles to warm cold feet. Instead, wear warm, dry socks and use an extra blanket in bed.

- Wear well-fitting and protective footwear (leather shoes).
- Do not wear tight shoes or tight-fitting socks or garter belts because they reduce the circulation to the feet.
- Avoid going barefoot.

Other precautions
- Use an extra sheet in place of the bath blanket and a plastic bag to protect your bed linens.
- Check the skin of your feet daily for cuts, cracks, blisters, or red, swollen areas.
- See your podiatrist regularly.

between the toes, a mild foot powder will be applied to that area. The procedure is repeated on the other foot.

Next, the nurse will clean the toenails with a cotton-tipped applicator or cotton ball. He or she will gently remove dirt or debris from under the nails with an orangewood stick to avoid injuring the delicate skin. The toenails are trimmed if necessary by cutting straight across (to prevent ingrown nails) and then filing the nails even with the ends of the toes. Special care is taken with diabetic persons and other persons who have reduced sensation in the feet.

What are the possible complications?
Potential complications include damage to the nailbeds and cuticles as well as infection. Diabetic people and others with reduced sensation in the feet may be at higher risk for complications.

What happens after the therapy?
- If you'll be performing regular foot care at home, you'll be asked to demonstrate all the steps of foot care before discharge. (See *Taking care of your feet* for further details.)

HYDROTHERAPY

Hydrotherapy is the external use of water to promote relaxation, increase circulation, alter body temperature, strengthen muscles, improve joint mobility, and aid the cleaning of wounds. The beneficial effects of water are well-known, and it has been used as a therapeutic modality for thousands of years. The buoyancy of water allows the person to achieve greater range of motion and to have fuller use of the extremities with less discomfort. Hydrotherapy can be performed in whirlpools, tanks, Hubbard tanks, and swimming pools.

The benefits of whirlpool therapy are derived from the increase in tissue temperature and mechanical stimulation produced by the agitation of the water. The Hubbard tank allows immersion of the entire body; smaller tanks are used for treating extremities or for immersion of the lower body.

Why is this therapy done?

Hydrotherapy is performed for various conditions. Whirlpool and Hubbard tank treatments are most commonly administered for wound cleaning. The therapeutic swimming pool may be used to promote relaxation and relieve pain. People with arthritis, chronic pain, low back pain, and other painful conditions typically enjoy the pool for these sedative effects and for the ease of performing (muscle) strengthening and (joint) mobility exercises. The buoyancy of the water may be used to assist with exercises for weakened muscles. Conversely, strengthening exercises may be performed in the pool, using the water to provide resistance to specific muscles. The buoyancy of the water can be used to aid gait training, especially for people with painful joints or significant weakness.

Finally, the therapeutic swimming pool can be psychologically and physically beneficial for people with spinal cord injuries. The buoyancy of the water allows them some control of body movement that is impossible out of water.

When shouldn't this therapy be done?

Hydrotherapy may be inadvisable depending on the form of hydrotherapy selected and the condition for which it is used. Water temperature should not exceed 95° F (35° C) for people with poor circulation. People with heart problems may not be candidates for therapeutic activities in the swimming pool or may need to have close monitoring. People who are incontinent or have open draining wounds should not use the swimming pool to avoid bacterial cross-contamination, nor should people with excessively high, low, or unstable blood pressure. People with MS may react adversely in warm, humid conditions and will need close monitoring.

Hydrotherapy also should not be performed if the person's status reflects sudden changes, such as fever, electrolyte or fluid imbalance, or unstable vital signs. Immersion isn't recommended for people with mending fractures, respiratory aids, or for people with skin grafts less than 5 days old.

What happens before the therapy?

A member of your health care team will determine which exercises should be performed in the water and will provide you with clear instructions.

What happens during the therapy?

Hydrotherapy is usually administered by a physical therapist or a physical therapy assistant in a hospital setting or physical therapy clinical setting. Other health care professionals who can provide hydrotherapy include athletic trainers, recreation therapists, occupational therapists, and nurses. Hydrotherapy treatments are usually performed in whirlpools, Hubbard tanks, or swimming pools.

Most whirlpool treatments are performed with water temperature at 98° to 104° F (36.6° to 40° C). If the therapy involves total immersion, you'll be slowly lowered into the tank by a hoist. You are positioned so that your head is supported by a headrest. Smaller tanks may be used if only one body part, such as an arm or leg, requires therapy. During immersion, certain other treatments can be accomplished, such as removing dead tissue from wounds and passive or active range-of-motion exercises. Hydrotherapy usually lasts 20 minutes, after which you'll be slowly removed from the tank, dried, and covered with a warm sheet or blanket.

What are the possible complications?

Cardiac or respiratory arrest are possible complications of hydrotherapy if water temperature is not given careful consideration. High water temperatures and humid conditions place a significant demand on the heart and blood vessels and on the pulmonary system. Therefore, people with cardiac and pulmonary disorders need close assessment to evaluate the risk of hydrotherapy. Thermal injury (scalding) is also a potential complication of hydrotherapy; to avoid it, water temperature should never exceed 110° F (43° C).

Infection is another complication of hydrotherapy. To prevent it, antibacterial agents must be added to the water.

TRACTION

Mechanical traction exerts a pulling force on a part of the body — usually the spine, pelvis, or long bones of the arms and legs. Either skin or skeletal traction may be used. Skin traction is applied directly to the skin and thus indirectly to the bone. In skeletal traction, an orthopedic surgeon inserts a pin or wire through the bone and attaches the traction equipment to the pin or wire to exert a direct, constant, longitudinal pulling force.

Why is this therapy done?
Traction devices are used to repair fractures, treat dislocations, correct or prevent deformities, improve or correct contractures, or decrease muscle spasms. The type of traction is determined by the doctor according to the person's condition, age, and weight as well as the condition of the skin, the duration of traction, and the purpose of traction.

When shouldn't this therapy be done?
Skin traction should not be performed in severe injury with open wounds and in people with an allergy to tape or other skin traction equipment, circulatory disturbances, dermatitis, or varicose veins. Infections such as osteomyelitis (bone inflammation) also make skeletal traction inadvisable.

What happens before the therapy?
- Your doctor explains the purpose of traction to you and your family. The doctor emphasizes the importance of maintaining proper body alignment.
- You'll be taught how to use an overhead trapeze to assist with position changes.

Traction devices are used to repair fractures, treat dislocations, correct or prevent deformities, improve or correct contractures, or decrease muscle spasms.

INSIGHT INTO TREATMENT

Comparing types of traction

Traction therapy restricts movement of a person's affected limb or body part and may confine the person to prolonged bed rest. The limb is immobilized by pulling with equal force on each end of the injured area — an equal mix of traction and countertraction. Weights provide the pulling force. Countertraction is produced by using other weights or by positioning the person's body weight against the traction pull.

Skin traction

This procedure immobilizes a body part intermittently over an extended period through direct application of a pulling force to the person's skin. The force may be applied using adhesive or nonadhesive traction tape or other skin traction devices such as a boot, belt, or halter. Adhesive attachment allows more continuous traction; nonadhesive attachment allows easier removal for care.

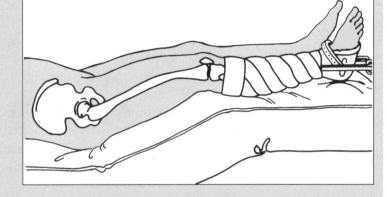

Skeletal traction

This technique immobilizes a body part for prolonged periods by attaching weighted equipment directly to the person's bones. This may be accomplished with pins, screws, wires, or tongs. Skeletal traction allows more prolonged traction with heavier weight than skin traction.

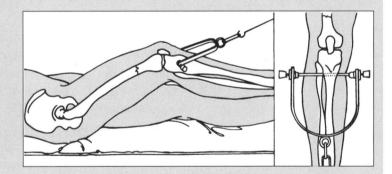

What happens during the therapy?

Skin traction

The surgeon may use skin traction or skeletal traction, depending on the injury or condition. Skin traction may be applied at the bedside. It is usually used when a light, temporary, or noncontinuous pulling force is required. The amount of weight most often used is 5 to 10 pounds (2.2 to 4.5 kilograms). Types of skin traction include Buck's traction, pelvic traction with pelvic belt, and cervical traction with cervical halter. (See *Comparing types of traction.*)

Skeletal traction

Skeletal traction involves placement of wires, pins, or tongs into or through the bones; these may be inserted under local, general, or spinal anesthesia in aseptic conditions. Skeletal traction is most often used for fractures of the thigh, upper arm, larger bone of the lower leg, or neck. The usual amount of weight is 25 to 40 pounds (11.3 to 18 kilograms). Types of skeletal traction include balanced skeletal traction, overhead arm traction, and cervical traction with tongs (for the neck). Skeletal traction may be kept in place 3 to 4 months. Pads, slings, or pushers may be combined with the traction to reduce the fracture.

Once the surgery is completed, a nurse will support you and show you how much movement you're allowed. He or she will instruct you not to readjust the equipment and to report any pain or pressure from the traction equipment.

About every 2 hours, the nurse will check you for proper body alignment and reposition you as necessary. You'll be encouraged to do coughing and deep-breathing exercises. The nurse will also be assist you with range-of-motion exercises for unaffected extremities and apply elastic support stockings as appropriate.

Remember that traction must be continuous to be effective, and that you should perform as much self-care as possible to reestablish a positive self-concept.

What are the possible complications?

Immobility during traction may result in bed sores, destruction of muscle, weakness, contractures, and osteoporosis; it can also cause gastrointestinal disturbances, such as constipation; urinary problems; respiratory problems; and circulatory disturbances. Prolonged immobility, especially after traumatic injury, may promote depression or other emotional disturbances. Skeletal traction may cause osteomyelitis (bone inflammation) originating at the pin or wire sites. Nonunion or delayed union, as well as pin breakage, may occur.

7

TREATING KIDNEY & URINARY TRACT DISORDERS

DRUG THERAPIES

Antispasmodics

For most people, symptoms of urinary tract problems — including pain, frequent urination, bladder spasm, and loss of control over urination — are troublesome and are the reason they visit the doctor. If the problem is caused by bacteria in the urinary tract, the doctor will prescribe an antibiotic. Unfortunately, it may take a few days before the antibiotic is effective, and most people desire relief immediately.

Antispasmodics are prescribed by doctors to relieve these urinary tract symptoms.

What are antispasmodics used for?
- To relieve symptoms of bladder problems
- To increase bladder capacity (oxybutynin)

What are some commonly used antispasmodics?
- flavoxate, known by the brand name Urispas
- oxybutynin, known by the brand name Ditropan

What are the possible side effects?
- Constipation
- Urine retention
- Visual disturbances, such as eye pain, blurred vision, and light sensitivity
- Rapid heart rate
- Fever
- Rash, itching
- Mental confusion, memory loss, behavioral changes

What are the guidelines for taking antispasmodics?
- Tell the doctor about any other medications you're taking, including nonprescription drugs.
- Be sure to tell the doctor if you have glaucoma, digestive problems, or a known urinary tract disease.
- If you get a rash, start to itch a lot, or have visual problems, call your doctor immediately. You may be having a reaction to the drug.

- Be sure to drink plenty of fluids to promote adequate urine flow and prevent constipation.
- Take Ditropan or Uripas with milk or food to help reduce stomach problems. You may take these drugs with water on an empty stomach if you don't experience any discomfort.
- If you miss a dose, take it as soon as you remember unless it's time for the next dose. Never take a double dose.

What else you should know

- Because antispasmodics can cause dizziness or drowsiness, don't drive or perform activities that require alertness, coordination, and clear vision until response to the drug has been determined.
- Don't use alcohol and depressant medication (such as tranquilizers), which can increase the drug's sedative effects.
- These drugs interfere with the body's normal mechanisms for controlling temperature. Avoid prolonged exercise or strenuous activity, especially in hot weather, to prevent drug-induced heatstroke.
- Use sugarless gum, hard candy, or ice chips to relieve dry mouth and throat. Report excessive dryness that lasts longer than 2 weeks.
- Wear sunglasses on bright days to minimize your sensitivity to light.

Because antispasmodics can cause dizziness or drowsiness, don't drive or perform activities that require alertness, coordination, and clear vision until response to the drug has been determined.

CHOLINERGICS

Cholinergic drugs are used to treat urine retention after surgery. They cause emptying of the bladder. They're also used to enhance contraction of the small intestine, preventing postoperative obstruction.

What are cholinergics used for?

These drugs are used to treat urine retention after surgery.

What are some commonly used cholinergics?

- bethanechol, known by the brand names Duvoid, Urabeth, and Urecholine

What are the possible side effects?

- Dizziness, confusion, hallucinations, nervousness
- Muscle weakness

- Difficulty breathing, asthmatic attacks
- Nausea, vomiting, excessive salivation, belching
- Involuntary defecation, diarrhea
- Urinary urgency
- Skin flushing or heat sensation
- Slow heart rate

What are the guidelines for taking cholinergics?

Stop using the drug immediately and contact the doctor if excessive salivation, diarrhea, or muscle weakness develops.

SURGERIES

NEPHRECTOMY

Nephrectomy is the surgical removal of one (unilateral) or both (bilateral) kidneys. Unilateral nephrectomy, the more commonly performed procedure, usually doesn't interfere with kidney function as long as the kidney that remains is healthy. Bilateral nephrectomy requires lifelong dialysis or transplantation to support kidney function.

Three major types of nephrectomy are performed: partial nephrectomy, involving removal of only a portion of the kidney; simple nephrectomy, removal of the entire kidney; and radical nephrectomy, removal of the entire kidney, the surrounding fatty tissue, and the entire ureter.

Why is this surgery done?

Nephrectomy is the treatment of choice for advanced kidney cancer or for kidney cancer that doesn't respond to chemotherapy and radiation; it's also indicated as the primary treatment for other kidney lesions. Nephrectomy may also be performed to treat kidney injury, infection, high blood pressure, and other lesions when conservative treatments fail. This procedure is also used to harvest a healthy kidney for transplantation.

What happens before the surgery?

- The nurse will reinforce the surgeon's explanation of the surgery, and describe the care you'll receive before and after surgery.
- The nurse also will ensure that you or a responsible family member has signed a consent form.
- If you're having one kidney removed, the doctor will reassure you that one healthy kidney provides adequate function. The remaining kidney increases its function so that it assumes 70% of the workload, rather than the original 50%. If you're scheduled for bilateral nephrectomy or having your only kidney removed, the nurse will try to prepare you for lifestyle changes, notably the need for regular dialysis. If appropriate, the doctor may tell you a future kidney transplant may be necessary to restore normal function.
- You'll be informed of the need for postoperative deep breathing and coughing to prevent lung problems.

What happens during the surgery?

Once the kidney is exposed, the surgeon frees it from the surrounding fatty tissue, adhesions, and the ureter, and then removes the kidney and ties off the ureter. If necessary, the surgeon inserts a drain and closes the wound.

What are the possible complications?

Serious complications of nephrectomy are uncommon but include infection, hemorrhage, lung collapse, pneumonia, blood clots, and pulmonary complications.

What happens after the surgery?

- You'll have an indwelling urinary catheter in place after surgery to allow measurement of urine output, and a nasogastric tube to prevent abdominal pain, distention, and vomiting. You'll also have a dressing and, possibly, a drain at the incision site.
- The nurse will encourage coughing, deep breathing, and position changes. If you experience difficulty breathing, chest pain, and bloody sputum, the nurse will raise the head of your bed, administer oxygen, and notify the doctor.
- You'll receive fluids intravenously to ensure adequate hydration. Food and fluid restrictions will be in place until about the fourth day after surgery, when you'll resume oral feedings.
- To reduce the risk of circulatory problems, the nurse will encourage early and regular walking, apply antiembolism stockings, and en-

SELF-HELP

Recovering from kidney removal

When you've been discharged from the hospital, follow these important guidelines.

Know when to call your doctor
- Call the doctor immediately if you detect any significant decrease in urine output; this is a sign of kidney failure.
- Notify the doctor if fever, chills, blood in the urine, or flank pain occur. These signs and symptoms may indicate urinary tract infection, a common response to indwelling urinary catheter insertion.
- Also notify your doctor if you have weight loss, bone pain, altered mental status, and numbness in the extremities — signs that the cancer has spread to other areas of the body.

Other instructions
- Monitor how much you drink and how much you urinate. These measurements are used to help assess kidney function.
- Follow all of the doctor's guidelines on fluid intake and diet restrictions.
- Be aware that pain around the incision site and fatigue are common and may continue for several weeks after discharge.
- Avoid strenuous exercise or heavy lifting and refrain from sexual relations until the doctor lifts those restrictions (usually after at least 6 weeks).
- Remember to keep regular follow-up appointments to evaluate kidney function and to assess for possible complications.

courage leg exercises, such as calf-pumping and ankle circles. (See *Recovering from kidney removal.*)

KIDNEY TRANSPLANT

Ranked as the most commonly performed and most successful of all organ transplants, kidney transplantation is an attractive alternative to dialysis for many people with end-stage kidney disease. A successful transplant can allow the person to resume a normal lifestyle.

The major obstacle to a successful transplant is rejection of the donated organ by the recipient's body. Blood and tissue-typing tests are performed to determine the degree of compatibility between the recipient and donor. The most compatible donor is then selected to minimize the risk of rejection. Transplant success rates have improved in recent years and may be attributed to improved tissue typing, drugs that keep the recipient's body from rejecting the kidney, surgical techniques, and candidate selection. However, because donor kidneys are scarce, some people remain on waiting lists for months or years.

Why is this surgery done?

Kidney transplants exchange a diseased kidney for a healthy one in order to restore normal kidney function. This operation may be performed to treat end-stage kidney disease. Because of the inherent risks of surgery and the scarcity of donor organs, a careful evaluation of physiologic, psychological, and social factors is necessary. The results of this evaluation may be input into a complex rating system to determine transplant recipients.

When shouldn't this surgery be done?

Although there are few absolute guidelines for not performing a kidney transplant, they may include active cancer or another major organ or system disease such as liver failure. A history of substance abuse, severe psychiatric disorders, noncompliance with treatment, and a lack of support systems may also rule out a person as a transplant candidate.

What happens before the surgery?

- The transplant procedure will be explained to the person by the transplant team. They will discuss the benefits and risks of transplantation with the person and his or her family.
- The person will undergo a comprehensive pretransplant evaluation. It may include a thorough physical exam, a battery of lab tests, X-ray studies, an electrocardiogram, bowel preparation, and shaving of the operative area. Dialysis is usually necessary the day before surgery and may be needed for a few days after surgery if the transplanted kidney fails to function immediately.
- A consent form must be signed.

What happens during the surgery?

In this procedure, a surgeon implants a healthy kidney that has been surgically removed from a living relative or a cadaver donor. The organ's vessels are then connected to the appropriate blood vessels.

The donor ureter is connected to the bladder. The person's kidneys typically aren't removed unless they're structurally abnormal, infected, greatly enlarged, or are causing hypertension. They're left in place to ease management of dialysis and to reduce blood transfusion requirements in case of transplant rejection.

Understanding transplant rejection

Transplant rejection can occur immediately after surgery or may develop years later. But whenever it occurs, it demands prompt intervention.

Hyperacute rejection

Hyperacute rejection occurs several minutes to hours after transplantation as your circulating antibodies attack the donor kidney. The organ rapidly dies because of lack of blood supply to the area. If you experience hyperacute rejection, the nurse will prepare you for removal of the rejected kidney.

Acute rejection

This type of rejection may occur 1 week to 6 months after transplantation of a living donor kidney or 1 week to 2 years after transplantation of a cadaver kidney. Acute rejection is caused by an antigen-antibody reaction.

Acute rejection may be reversible with prompt treatment. Characteristic indicators of this condition include signs of infection (fever, rapid pulse, sluggishness, elevated white blood cell count), scanty or no urine output, high blood pressure, or a weight gain of more than 3 pounds (1.4 kilograms) in a day.

If you show signs of acute rejection, the nurse will reassure you that this complication is common and often reversible. You'll be prepared for dialysis.

Chronic rejection

This irreversible complication can start several months or years after transplantation. It's caused by long-term antibody destruction of the donor kidney. Typically, it's detected by serial lab studies.

If you're experiencing chronic rejection, you'll be informed that complete destruction of the donor kidney may not occur for several years. Next, you'll be prepared for a kidney scan, kidney biopsy (removal and analysis of tissue), and other tests as ordered. An increased dose of immunosuppressants will be administered and your dietary and fluid regimen adjusted; when necessary, you'll be prepared for dialysis or another transplant.

What are the possible complications?

Major complications include infection, increased incidence of cancer, and death. Rejection of the donor kidney is also a major complication. (See *Understanding transplant rejection.*)

What happens after the surgery?

- Pain relievers may be prescribed.
- With a living-donor kidney transplant, urine flow usually begins immediately after the ureter is connected to the bladder. After a cadaver kidney transplant, the person may be unable to urinate for 2 to 14 days; dialysis will be necessary during this period. The urine will be blood-tinged for several days before it gradually becomes clear.
- The person may gradually resume a normal diet, with restrictions as ordered. (See *Recovering from a kidney transplant,* page 322.)

SELF-HELP

Recovering from a kidney transplant

When you've been discharged from the hospital, follow these important guidelines.

Monitor yourself carefully

- Measure and record your fluid intake and urine output and weigh yourself on a daily basis. Take your temperature and blood pressure twice daily.
- Watch for and promptly report any signs and symptoms of transplant rejection, including tenderness or swelling over the graft site, fever exceeding 100° F (37.8° C), decreased urine output, weight gain, blood in the urine, general weakness, and elevated blood pressure.
- Report signs of infection promptly. Because you're at increased risk for infection, avoid exposure to crowds and persons with known or suspected infections for at least 3 months after surgery.

Resume your activities slowly

- You should engage in moderate exercise on a regular basis. For best results, begin exercising slowly and increase it gradually. Make sure to avoid excessive bending, heavy lifting, and contact sports.
- Avoid activities or positions that place pressure on the new kidney — for example, long car trips and lap-style seat belts.
- Refrain from sexual activity for at least 6 weeks after surgery.

Other instructions

- Take all prescribed medications as indicated.
- If you're a woman who's had a kidney transplant, you'll need to discuss family planning with your partner and health care provider because pregnancy poses an additional risk to a new kidney.
- Make sure to keep all regular follow-up visits; they're necessary to evaluate kidney function and the status of the transplant.
- Avoid strong sunlight. When outdoors, use a sunscreen because immunosuppressant therapy increases the risk of skin cancer.

URINARY DIVERSION SURGERY

A urinary diversion provides an alternative route for excretion of urine when disease prevents its normal flow through the bladder. A permanent urinary diversion should be performed when any condition requires that the entire bladder be removed. In conditions requiring temporary urine drainage or diversion, a catheter is usually inserted to divert the flow of urine. The catheter remains in place until the incision heals.

Several types of permanent urinary diversion surgery can be performed. Most require the person to wear a urine collection device and to care for the stoma (an opening created between a body cavity and the body's surface during surgery).

The two most common types of urinary diversion surgery are cutaneous ureterostomy and ileal conduit. Cutaneous ureterostomy offers several advantages. It's a shorter and easier-to-perform procedure than ileal conduit diversion and can be performed successfully on thick-walled ureters that are chronically dilated. It carries little risk of complications caused by intestinal absorption of urine contents.

Because ileal conduit diversion allows for creation of a much larger stoma than can be created from a ureter, an ileal conduit is usually easier to care for than a ureterostomy.

Continent urinary diversion procedures provide alternative methods of drainage that eliminate the need for external devices. Kock's pouch is a small-bowel reservoir for urine. In this diversion, the surgeon creates nipple valves to prevent reflux (backward flow) of urine. Intermittent catheterization is usually required to empty urine from the pouch. Alternative types of urinary diversion include the Indiana, Mainz, or UCLA pouches. For these procedures, the more muscular walls of the large bowel create the urine reservoir.

Why is this surgery done?

Most commonly performed in people who've had all or part of the bladder removed, urinary diversion provides an alternative route for excretion of urine when bladder dysfunction or removal doesn't allow normal drainage. This surgery may also be performed in people with congenital urinary tract defects; severe, unmanageable urinary tract infections that threaten kidney function; injury to the ureters, bladder, or urethra; obstructive cancer; or bladder dysfunction caused by lesions to the central nervous system or the nerves that directly supply the bladder.

What happens before the surgery?

- You'll be taught the proper technique for emptying a urine collection device and performing stoma care.
- Your health care team will explain the surgery to you and tell you that you'll have a nasogastric tube in place after surgery. This tube prevents abdominal pain, distention, and vomiting.
- You'll be told what to expect in terms of the appearance and location of the stoma, which varies depending on the type of surgery performed.
- You'll learn about the urine collection device you'll use after surgery. You'll be encouraged to handle the device to ease acceptance of it.
- If possible, the nurse will arrange for a visit by a well-adjusted ostomate (someone who's had similar surgery), who can provide a first-

hand account of the operation and offer some insight into the realities of caring for a stoma and a urine collection device.

- As appropriate, your family will be included in all aspects of preoperative teaching — especially if they'll be providing much of the routine care after discharge.
- Either you or a responsible family member will be required to sign a consent form.
- Your diet may be restricted. You may have to fast 8 hours before surgery and undergo a cleansing enema. If you're debilitated, other preparatory measures may include fluid replacement therapy and intravenous antibiotics to prevent infection.

What happens during the surgery?

You'll receive a general anesthetic, and the surgeon will choose the most appropriate type of urinary diversion.

In the simplest type, cutaneous ureterostomy, the surgeon dissects one or both ureters from the bladder and brings them out through the skin surface on the flank or the anterior abdominal wall to form one or two stomas.

In the ileal conduit procedure, the surgeon connects the ureters to a small portion of the ileum (part of the small intestine) that's excised (cut out) especially for the procedure and then creates a stoma from one end of the ileal segment.

In continent urinary diversion, the surgeon uses a portion of the small bowel to create both a reservoir for urine nipple valves, which prevent the reflux of urine. (See *Types of permanent urinary diversion*.)

What are the possible complications?

Because the intestinal lining is delicate, an ill-fitting urinary collection device can cause bleeding, especially with an ileal conduit.

The skin around the stoma may become reddened or abraded from too-frequent changing or improper placement of the device, poor skin care, or an allergic reaction to the device or adhesive. Continuous leakage around the urinary collection device can result from improper placement or poor skin elasticity.

What happens after the surgery?

- Your dressings are frequently checked and changed. (The surgeon will probably perform the first dressing change.)
- The nurse will provide you with emotional support throughout recovery and will also help you adjust to your altered body image and,

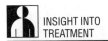
INSIGHT INTO
TREATMENT

Types of permanent urinary diversion

The types of permanent urinary diversion with stomas (surgically created openings between a body cavity and the body's surface) include ureterostomy, ileal conduit, and continent urinary diversion.

Ureterostomy

A stoma or stomas are formed when ureters are diverted to the abdominal wall or flank. There are five different types of ureterostomy.

Flank loop ureterostomy

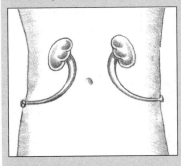

Ureters loop as they're brought to the skin surface.

Double-barrel ureterostomy

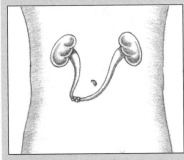

Both ureters are brought to the skin surface, forming a stoma.

Transureterostomy

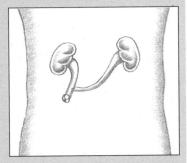

One ureter is surgically attached to the other, which is then brought to the skin surface to form a stoma.

Bilateral ureterostomy

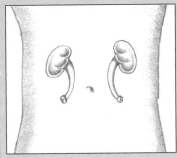

Both ureters are brought to the skin surface to form stomas.

(continued)

Types of permanent urinary diversion *(continued)*

Unilateral ureterostomy

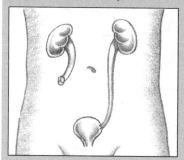

One ureter is brought to the skin surface to form a stoma.

Ileal conduit

A segment of the ileum (lower portion of the small intestine) is excised (cut out), and the two ends of the ileum that result from excision of the segment are stitched closed. Then the ureters are dissected from the bladder and surgically connected to the ileal segment. One end of the ileal segment is stitched closed; the opposite end is brought through the abdominal wall, thereby forming a stoma.

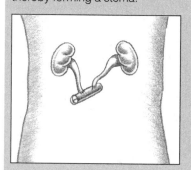

Continent urinary diversion

After total cystectomy (bladder removal), an 8-inch (20-centimeter) segment of the ileum is used to create the urine reservoir (Kock's pouch).

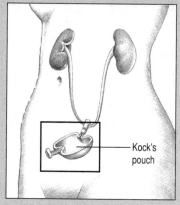

Kock's pouch

Kock's pouch

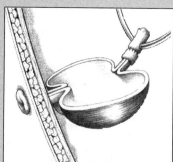

SELF-HELP

Recovering from urinary diversion

When you've been discharged from the hospital, follow these important guidelines.

Know what to expect

- You may be required to perform care of your stoma (a surgically created opening between a body cavity and the body's surface) and change your own pouches. If so, talk to your nurse about the best way to perform these self-care activities before you're discharged from the hospital.
- If you're discharged with an indwelling urinary catheter in place, make sure that you and a family member know how to care for it.
- Watch for and promptly report signs of complications, such as fever, chills, flank or abdominal pain, and pus or blood in the urine.

Keep follow-up appointments

Keep all scheduled follow-up appointments with the doctor and the enterostomal therapist so that they can evaluate your stoma care and make any necessary changes in equipment. For instance, stoma shrinkage, which usually occurs within 8 weeks after surgery, may require a change in pouch size to ensure a tight fit.

Resume normal activities

- If there are no complications, you should be able to return to work soon after discharge unless your work requires heavy lifting; in that case, you'll need medical approval before resuming work.
- You may safely engage in most sports, even such strenuous ones as skiing, skydiving, and scuba diving. However, you should avoid contact sports, such as football and wrestling.
- Many people who have undergone urinary diversion surgery are concerned that the stoma and pouch will interfere with their sexual pleasure. If you have some concerns, ask your nurse to refer you to a professional for sexual counseling.

Other instructions

- Although most women who've had this surgery can have safe pregnancies, it's a good idea to consult with your doctor before you plan to become pregnant.
- You may benefit from joining a support group. Ask a member of your health care team to refer you to the United Ostomy Association.

if applicable, to the stoma and urinary collection device. (See *Recovering from urinary diversion* for more details on how to care for yourself after this type of surgery.)

BLADDER SURGERY

A relatively quick and simple procedure, transurethral resection of the bladder involves insertion of a cystoscope (instrument for examining or surgically repairing the interior of the bladder and ureters) through the urethra and into the bladder to remove lesions. Tissue samples can then be collected for evaluation. (The procedure can also be performed using a Yag laser, if tissue's not being collected.)

When used to remove superficial tumors, this procedure may need to be performed as frequently as recurrences are identified, as long as these recurrences are not likely to spread. A typical schedule might involve treatment every 3 months for the first 2 years, every 6 months for the next 3 years, and annually thereafter.

Why is this procedure done?

Transurethral resection of the bladder is most commonly performed to treat small, superficial, low-grade bladder cancer and to obtain a biopsy (tissue sample for analysis) of suspicious lesions. It may also be used to remove benign papillomas (wartlike growths) in the bladder or remove abnormal fibrous tissue from the bladder neck. This procedure is also done to repair bleeding sites.

When shouldn't this procedure be done?

This procedure shouldn't be used to remove large tumors or to treat cancerous lesions that have spread to other sites.

What happens before the procedure?

The procedure will be explained to you. You'll be awake if a spinal anesthetic is used during the procedure. You should have little or no discomfort afterward, and posttreatment effects, such as blood in the urine and a burning sensation during urination, should subside quickly. Also, you'll be warned that you may have painful bladder spasms, but these can be relieved with antispasmodics.

What happens during the procedure?

After a general or a spinal anesthestic is administered, you'll be placed in the position typically used during a gynecologic exam. Then the doctor introduces a cystoscope into the urethra and passes it into the bladder in order to view the interior of the bladder. He or she then fills the bladder with a clear, irrigating solution, locates the lesion, and positions the cystoscope's cutting loop in place. The surgeon turns on the electric current, which runs through the loop, to cut or cauterize the lesion and finally removes the cystoscope. (See *Understanding transurethral resection of the bladder.*)

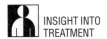

INSIGHT INTO
TREATMENT

Understanding transurethral resection of the bladder

In this procedure, the doctor inserts a cystoscope through the ure-thra into the bladder to remove small superficial lesions.

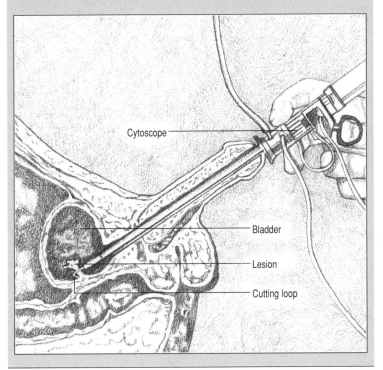

Cytoscope

Bladder

Lesion

Cutting loop

What are the possible complications?

Potential complications include blood in the urine, urine retention, bladder perforation, and urinary tract infection. The risk of compli-cations can be reduced by careful monitoring and meticulous care of the indwelling urinary catheter.

What happens after the procedure?

- Your doctor will prescribe antispasmodics for bladder spasm and pain relievers.
- You may get tests to further evaluate your condition. (See *Recovering from bladder surgery*, page 330.)

SELF-HELP

Recovering from bladder surgery

When you've been discharged from the hospital following transurethral resection of the bladder, keep in mind these important guidelines.

Know when to call the doctor
- You may notice that your urine contains a small amount of blood for several days after surgery. This is a normal occurrence and should not alarm you. However, persistent blood in the urine that lasts longer than a few days should be reported to the doctor.
- Report commonly occurring signs of a lower urinary tract infection (urinary frequency, urgency, and painful urination), as well as signs and symptoms of an upper urinary tract infection (fever, chills, or flank pain).

Modify your activities
To promote healing and reduce the risk of bleeding from increased intra-abdominal pressure, avoid sexual or other strenuous activity, don't lift anything heavier than 10 pounds (4.5 kilograms), and continue to take a stool softener or other laxative until the doctor approves a change.

Other points to remember
- Drink plenty of water (about ten 8-ounce glasses daily) and empty the bladder every 2 to 3 hours while gross hematuria (blood in the urine) persists. This will reduce the risk of clot formation, urethral obstruction, and urinary tract infection.
- Make sure that you respond promptly to the urge to urinate.
- Make sure to keep all appointments for follow-up examinations. They allow the surgeon to evaluate the need for repeat treatments.
- Early detection and removal of bladder tumors through transurethral resection of the bladder may prevent the need for bladder removal.

CYSTOSTOMY

Cystostomy is a type of urinary diversion. It involves insertion of a catheter through the skin of the region above the pubic area into the bladder, with connection of the device to a closed drainage system.

Why is this procedure done?
Typically, cystostomy provides temporary urinary diversion after certain gynecologic procedures, bladder surgery, or removal of the prostate and relieves urinary obstruction resulting from severe narrowing of the urethra or from pelvic injury. Rarely, it may be used to create a permanent urinary diversion to relieve urinary obstruction by an inoperable tumor or other lesions.

It's often useful in infants and young children, whose narrow urethras may hinder insertion of an indwelling urinary catheter.

What happens before the procedure?

- The procedure and postoperative care is explained to you or your family.
- You sign a consent form.

What happens during the procedure?

Cystostomy may be performed during other surgery while you're under general anesthesia. It may also be performed under local anesthesia as a bedside procedure. The procedure typically causes little or no discomfort and takes 5 to 10 minutes.

To perform a percutaneous cystostomy, the surgeon makes a stab wound in the area above the pubic bone, inserts a trocar (sharp surgical instrument used to remove fluid from cavities) and catheter, and advances them into the bladder until urine return is detected. Next, the surgeon stabilizes the catheter while the trocar is removed and then secures the catheter to the skin with sutures and tape. Percutaneous cystostomy requires a distended bladder and the absence of groin surgery or scarring of the operative site. If bladder distention is doubtful — for example, in an obese patient — it may be verified by ultrasonography.

To perform an open suprapubic cystostomy, the surgeon makes a short, 2- to 3-inch (5- to 7.6-centimeter) transverse incision two fingerbreadths above the pubic bone. He or she divides the membrane and separates the underlying muscles to expose the anterior bladder wall. Next, the surgeon introduces a Malecot catheter into the bladder and brings the catheter out to the skin surface through the stab incision, or, more commonly, through a stab wound above the incision. After closing the incision, he or she stitches the catheter in place and secures it with tape.

With either approach, the cystostomy tube is connected to a closed drainage system. After removal of the cystostomy tube, the doctor will place sterile dressings over the site. Rapid healing generally occurs, sealing over the insertion site. However, if a large-bore catheter is inserted, healing may be delayed.

What are the possible complications?

Cystostomy can lead to urine retention from catheter obstruction, evidenced by leaking around the catheter; bladder infection; blood in the urine; and skin breakdown.

Caring for yourself after cystostomy

When you've been discharged from the hospital, follow these important guidelines.

Know when to call your doctor
- Report an excessive amount of urine leakage around the catheter because it may indicate partial dislodgment, in which case you'll need to have the catheter replaced.
- Promptly notify the doctor of any signs of infection, such as discolored or foul-smelling discharge; impaired drainage; swelling, redness, or tenderness at the catheter insertion site; and decreased urine output.
- See your doctor or return to the hospital if the catheter becomes completely dislodged.

Other instructions
- Change the dressing as directed by your nurse.
- If the cystostomy tube is still in place, empty and reattach the collection bag as needed.
- Drink plenty of fluids.
- Keep all scheduled follow-up appointments because they allow for the early detection of complications.

What happens after the procedure?

You'll be encouraged to cough, do deep-breathing exercises, and get out of bed. (See *Caring for yourself after cystostomy.*)

MARSHALL-MARCHETTI-KRANTZ PROCEDURE

The Marshall-Marchetti-Krantz procedure, the most common surgery for stress incontinence in women, involves elevating the anterior vaginal wall to support the bladder and urethra. When stress incontinence in women doesn't respond to pubococcygeus muscle (Kegel) exercises or drugs, surgery may help restore urinary sphincter competence. This relatively simple surgery eliminates stress incontinence in most people, with minimal chance of recurrence.

A newer, less invasive procedure that elevates the urethra anteriorly is now being performed with similar results. This procedure uses a "needle-and-thread" method through the vagina and suprapubic area instead of a lower abdominal incision. The hospital stay is typically 24 to 72 hours, and the person is sent home with a suprapubic catheter to use if she's unable to urinate. It remains in place until the follow-up visit with the doctor.

Why is this surgery done?

The Marshall-Marchetti-Krantz procedure is recommended for stress incontinence when medical treatment and pubococcygeus muscle exercises fail.

What happens before the surgery?

- The procedure will be explained to you.
- You'll sign a consent form.
- You'll be advised that a catheter may be inserted during surgery.

What happens during the surgery?

With the person under general anesthesia, the surgeon makes an incision across the pubic region and frees the bladder neck, urethra, and anterior vaginal wall. He or she then suspends the urethra and bladder neck by suturing both sides of the anterior vaginal wall to the pubic bones and to the lower rectal membranes. Typically, the surgeon completes the procedure by inserting a drain and an indwelling urinary catheter or cystostomy tube (suprapubic catheter). He or she then closes the incision and applies a sterile dressing.

What are the possible complications?

This procedure carries the risk of urethral obstruction, with resultant urine retention, and infection caused by leakage of urine into the vagina. These complications are rare.

What happens after the surgery?

- The nurse will check the incisional drain and dressing every 4 hours for the first 24 hours.
- The amount and color of urine drainage from the indwelling urinary catheter or cystostomy tube will be monitored. Blood-tinged urine normally occurs for 24 to 48 hours after surgery.
- You may experience bladder spasms caused by the catheter or bladder manipulation during surgery. You'll be given medication to control this.
- If you show signs of urine retention, you may need intermittent catheterization. Intermittent catheterization isn't usually necessary after healing is complete and the swelling subsides.
- If you continue to experience difficulty urinating, the nurse will teach you how insert your own catheter. (See *Recovering from a Marshall-Marchetti-Krantz procedure.*)

PROSTATECTOMY

Prostatectomy is the partial or total surgical removal of the prostate gland. Depending on the person's disease, one of four approaches is used. Transurethral resection of the prostate, the most common approach, involves insertion of a resectoscope into the urethra. This approach is useful in the treatment of a benign growth with a moderately enlarged prostate and as a palliative measure in prostate cancer. It involves a short hospital stay and doesn't require a surgical incision.

Open surgical methods are used to treat a benign growth and prostate cancer if the prostate is too large for transurethral resection

 SELF-HELP

Recovering from a Marshall-Marchetti-Krantz procedure

When you've been discharged from the hospital, follow these important guidelines.

Know when to call your doctor
- Report signs of urinary tract infection, such as fever, chills, flank pain, and blood in the urine.
- Also report signs of wound infection, such as severe pain, redness, and swelling at the incision site.

Other instructions
- Get plenty of rest and avoid strenuous activity during the recovery period, when you'll feel weak, tired, and sore at the incision site.
- If you'll require intermittent catheterization after discharge, ask your nurse to provide you with written instructions on inserting your own catheter.
- Try to empty your bladder before each catheterization, and record the amount of urine in your catheter and the amount you urinated before catheterization. Note also the time.
- Keep follow-up appointments.

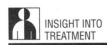
INSIGHT INTO
TREATMENT

Comparing types of prostatectomy

Depending on your disease, the surgeon may perform radical perineal, retropubic, suprapubic, or transurethral resection of the prostate.

Radical perineal prostatectomy
Advantages
- Allows direct visualization of the prostate gland
- Permits drainage by gravity
- Has low mortality and decreased incidence of shock

Disadvantages
- High incidence of impotence and incontinence
- Risk of damage to the rectum and external sphincter
- Restricted operative field

Retropubic prostatectomy
Advantages
- Allows direct visualization of the prostate gland
- Avoids bladder incision
- Requires short convalescence
- Carries small risk of impotence

Disadvantages
- Can't be used to treat associated bladder disorders
- Increased risk of hemorrhage

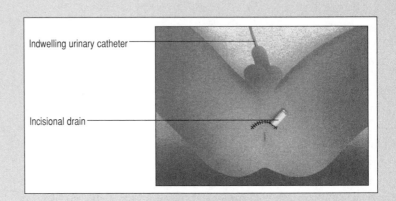

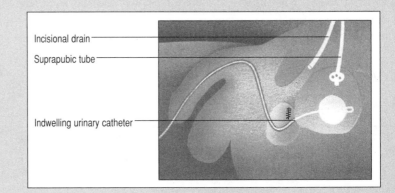

and when total removal of the prostate gland is necessary. (See *Comparing types of prostatectomy.*)

Why is this surgery done?
Prostatectomy should be performed when chronic prostatitis, benign prostatic growth, or prostate cancer fails to respond to drug therapy or other treatments. It also should be performed to remove diseased

Suprapubic prostatectomy

Advantages

- Allows exploration of wide area, such as adjacent lymph nodes
- Simple procedure

Disadvantages

- Requires bladder incision
- Hemorrhage control difficult
- Urine leakage common around suprapubic tube
- Prolonged and uncomfortable recovery

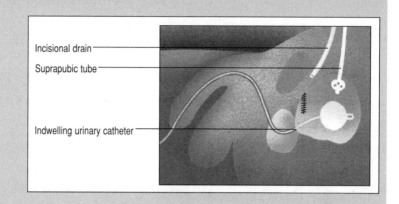

Incisional drain

Suprapubic tube

Indwelling urinary catheter

Transurethral resection of the prostate

Advantages

- Safer and less painful and invasive than other prostate procedures
- Doesn't require surgical incision
- Requires short hospital stay
- Carries small risk of impotence

Disadvantages

- Possible narrowing of the urethral passage and delayed bleeding
- Not a curative surgery for prostate cancer

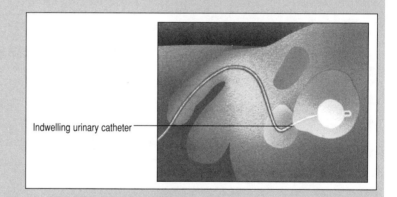

Indwelling urinary catheter

or obstructive prostate tissue and to restore urine flow through the urethra.

What happens before the surgery?

- You'll learn about the surgery and the expected course of recovery. Part of your preparation involves learning to overcome your fears and anxieties.

- Keep in mind that some types of prostatectomy may cause impotence. Typically, the doctor will discuss this possibility with you before surgery. If necessary, have your health care provider arrange for sexual counseling to help you cope with this. If you're scheduled for transurethral resection of the prostate, you should know that this procedure often causes retrograde (backward-flowing) ejaculation but no other impairment of sexual function.
- You'll get a cleansing enema and the nurse will shave the surgical site (unless you're scheduled for transurethral resection of the prostate).

What happens during the surgery?

The person receives a general or a spinal anesthetic and then, depending on the disease, the surgeon will choose one of several approaches. If the surgeon chooses the transurethral approach, he or she passes a resectoscope up the urethra to view the prostate. A heated wire loop or a cutting edge is passed through the resectoscope to cut away as much of the prostate as possible. Pieces of the prostate are washed out through the resectoscope, and the resectoscope is then withdrawn and replaced with an indwelling urinary catheter.

In other approaches, the surgeon makes an abdominal incision to expose the bladder and prostate and removes the prostate tissue. In radical perineal prostatectomy, the surgeon makes an incision near the sex organs to expose the prostatic tissue.

What are the possible complications?

Severe complications include hemorrhage, infection, and urine retention. Although temporary or permanent impotence is a rare occurrence after surgery, the radical perineal approach is associated with a high incidence of impotence and incontinence as well as the risk of damage to the rectum and anal sphincter. Transurethral prostatectomy may produce retrograde ejaculation.

What happens after the surgery?

- The nurse will frequently check the incision site for signs of infection and change dressings as necessary.
- The nurse will watch for and report fever, chills, and groin pain. These signs may indicate inflammation of the epididymides (small structures on the undersides of the testicles).
- You'll have an indwelling urinary catheter inserted for urine drainage. The catheter may remain in place for 2 to 5 days. It will be removed when the urine is clear, except after radical prostatectomy.

SELF-HELP

Recovering from a prostatectomy

When you've been discharged from the hospital, follow these important guidelines.

Know what to expect

- Some men who've undergone this operation experience transient urinary frequency and dribbling after the catheter is removed. Both of these conditions are temporary; you'll gradually regain control of your bladder.
- If you'll go home with the catheter in place, you or a caregiver will be responsible for keeping it clean.
- The nurse will teach you how to perform perineum-tightening (Kegel) exercises to speed the return of urinary control.

Report any problems

- It's normal for you to produce blood-tinged urine for the first few weeks after surgery. However, you should report bright red urine or persistent blood in your urine. You may see increased bleeding with increased activity.
- Watch for and immediately report any signs of infection, such as fever, chills, and flank pain.

Other instructions

- Avoid caffeine-containing beverages, if possible, because caffeine acts as a mild diuretic.
- Drink ten 8-ounce (236-milliliter) glasses of water a day, urinate at least every 2 hours, and notify the doctor promptly if you have trouble urinating.
- To decrease the risk of bleeding, avoid sexual intercourse, lifting any object heavier than 10 pounds (4.5 kilograms), performing strenuous exercise (short walks are usually permitted), and taking long car trips until the doctor gives permission (usually 6 weeks).
- Take prescribed medications, such as antibiotics, antispasmodics, and stool softeners. Stool softeners are ordered to reduce straining.

In that case, it can be in place for 3 to 4 weeks. Also, there may be a tube in your abdomen and, possibly, an incisional drain.

- The nurse will keep the collection container below the level of the bladder to promote drainage and keep the skin around the tube insertion site clean and dry.
- Commonly, antispasmodics are prescribed to control painful bladder spasms and pain relievers are given for discomfort from the incision.
- If you had a radical perineal prostatectomy, your doctor or a nurse will arrange for psychological and sexual counseling during recovery. (See *Recovering from a prostatectomy*.)

HYDROCELECTOMY

Hydrocelectomy is the surgical removal of a hydrocele (a collection of fluid in the tunica vaginalis [a membranous covering] of the testicle or along the spermatic cord). Hydrocelectomy is typically reserved for males over age 1; in infants, a hydrocele usually regresses spontaneously. Hydrocelectomies are usually performed on an outpatient basis.

Why is this surgery done?

Hydrocelectomy is necessary when needle aspiration fails to remove the fluid that has collected around the tunica vaginalis, when the hydrocele becomes large and uncomfortable, or when swelling caused by the collected fluid compresses testicular tissue, interfering with circulation to the testicles and causing loss of testicular function.

What happens before the surgery?

- The nurse will teach you about the procedure, explaining that there will be a drain in place after the surgery. This drain will prevent fluid buildup and help to prevent infection and promote healing.
- You'll be taught about the importance of wearing a scrotal support after the procedure. This support relieves swelling and pain and helps to keep the dressing in place.

What happens during the surgery?

After an anesthetic is administered, the surgeon makes a small incision in the scrotum through which the hydrocele is removed. The surgeon then uses electric sparks generated by a high-frequency current to destroy tissue of the involved vessels. The surgeon may then insert a small incisional drain before closing the opening.

Alternatively, the surgeon may plicate (fold) the hydrocele, permanently collapsing its walls and preventing refilling. No incisional drain is required after plication.

After the incision is closed, the surgeon applies a dressing and a scrotal support.

What are the possible complications?

Hydrocelectomy rarely causes complications if meticulous wound care is provided. Occasionally, infection, obvious bleeding from the incision or drainage site, and internal scrotal hemorrhage may occur.

SELF-HELP

Recovering from a hydrocelectomy

When you've been discharged from the hospital, follow these important guidelines.

Know what to expect
- If you're discharged on the day of surgery, you or a family caregiver will be responsible for changing the dressing using sterile technique. In addition, you'll be taught how much and what kind of drainage to expect and how to change the scrotal support. If you have any questions about what to do, clarify them with the nurse before discharge.
- Be aware that scrotal swelling may persist for up to a month after surgery but will gradually subside.
- You may shower but avoid taking baths until all wound drainage has ceased and healing is complete.

Report any problems
- Watch for and report signs of infection, including fever, chills, and worsening scrotal pain, tenderness, or swelling.
- Also notify the doctor of any obvious bleeding from the incision site or from the drain if one was inserted.

Other instructions
- Be sure that you understand when and how to take all prescribed medications.
- Avoid heavy lifting or straining for at least 6 weeks to reduce the risk of incisional hernia.
- Abstain from sexual activity as advised by your doctor (usually for 6 weeks).
- Keep all follow-up visits with the surgeon so that the healing of the wound can be regularly evaluated.

What happens after the surgery?

- You'll receive pain relievers. Most males experience moderate pain for the first 24 hours, but the pain should begin to rapidly decrease in severity.
- The scrotum will be kept elevated to minimize swelling and snugly supported to enhance comfort. The scrotal support will be changed when it becomes saturated with drainage.
- You'll receive anti-inflammatory drugs to reduce scrotal swelling. (See *Recovering from a hydrocelectomy.*)

ORCHIOPEXY

Orchiopexy is a surgical procedure that secures the proper position of a testicle in the scrotum. When successful, orchiopexy decreases the risk of sterility, testicular cancer, and testicular injury from abnormal positioning. If a testicle is missing or must be removed, a prosthesis (artificial body part) is inserted to achieve a normal appearance and foster the person's positive body image. Orchiopexy for correction of an undescended testicle is usually performed in children ages 1 to 6.

Why is this surgery done?

Orchiopexy is performed to treat an undescended testicle when other treatments, such as hormonal therapy, fail. It should be performed when the testicle is in a twisted position (testicular torsion) but remains viable.

What happens before the surgery?

The surgery will be explained to the person or, if the person is a child, to his parents.

What happens during the surgery?

Orchiopexy is performed under general anesthesia. If there's testicular torsion (twisting), the surgeon makes an incision in the scrotal skin and attempts to untwist and stabilize the spermatic cord. He or she may remove a hydrocele, if present, or perform an orchiectomy (removal of the whole testicle), if tissue death has occurred.

To treat an undescended testicle, the surgeon makes an incision in the groin or lower abdomen to expose the testicle and a small incision to open the scrotum. He or she then frees the testicle, lowers it into the scrotal sac, and secures it with stitches. If both testicles are undescended, this procedure is repeated for the other testicle.

In two-stage orchiopexy, an alternative procedure, the surgeon brings the testicle down into the scrotal sac and stitches it to the thigh; then, 2 to 3 months later, he or she embeds it in the scrotal sac. If the spermatic cord is too short to accommodate repositioning of the testicle, the surgeon may sever the spermatic cord before placing the testicle in the scrotal sac. After completing the procedure, the surgeon closes the incision and applies a dressing.

What are the possible complications?

Complications of this procedure are uncommon but include hemorrhage, infection, and painful urination.

What happens after the surgery?

- The nurse will provide ice packs or a scrotal support to relieve the discomfort. Pain relievers will be administered.

- Meticulous skin care will be given by the nurse. He or she will encourage good personal hygiene to prevent contamination of the operative site with stools or urine. (See *Recovering from orchiopexy*.)

CIRCUMCISION

Circumcision is the surgical removal of the foreskin from the glans penis. This procedure is commonly performed on infants; however, much controversy currently surrounds routine newborn circumcision. Its supporters say that circumcision helps reduce the risk of future penile cancer and of cervical cancer in female sexual partners and minimizes the risk of phimosis; they also believe that circumcision decreases the risk of urinary tract infections in men. However, in 1975, the American Academy of Pediatrics stated that there was no medical justification for routine circumcision. In 1989, however, the academy changed positions, stating that the procedure may have medical benefits as well as risks. Despite this controversy, circumcision remains the most commonly performed of all pediatric surgeries.

Why is this surgery done?
Circumcision may be performed on an adult to treat phimosis (abnormal tightening of the foreskin around the penis) or paraphimosis (inability to return the foreskin to its normal position after retraction). Most commonly, circumcision is performed on newborns 1 to 2 days after birth or later, if performed for religious or cultural reasons.

When shouldn't this surgery be done?
In newborns, circumcision shouldn't be performed on infants who have bleeding disorders or ambiguous genitalia. It also should not be performed on infants with hypospadias (urethral opening on the underside of the penis) because the foreskin will be needed for later surgical reconstruction. If the mother is infected with HIV, the doctor will delay circumcision until the newborn's HIV status is determined.

SELF-HELP

Recovering from orchiopexy

When you've been discharged from the hospital, follow these important guidelines.

Know when to call your doctor
- Promptly report increased scrotal pain, swelling, or other changes in the testicle.
- Because people with cryptorchidism are at increased risk for testicular cancer, perform regular testicular self-examinations to detect any lumps or unusual findings. These findings should be reported to your doctor.

Other instructions
- Gradually resume normal activities, beginning about 1 week after surgery, but avoid heavy lifting and other strenuous activities until the doctor advises otherwise.
- Wear a scrotal support to enhance comfort and control swelling for the first few weeks after surgery.
- Avoid sexual activity for about 6 weeks after surgery.

SELF-HELP

Circumcision care

After you're discharged from the hospital, follow these important guidelines.

Keep the wound clean
• Keep the wound clean and (if appropriate) change your wound dressing according to directions given by your doctor or nurse.
• Watch for and report any renewed bleeding or signs of infection, such as swelling at the incision site or drainage.
• Normally, a thin, yellow-white exudate will form over the site within 1 to 2 days after the procedure. Don't remove it because it protects the wound until healing occurs.

Resume normal activities
You can resume normal activities within 1 week and sexual activity as soon as healing is complete, usually after 1 to 2 weeks.

Other points to remember
• Your doctor may have prescribed a barbiturate sleeping medication, which suppresses rapid eye movements during sleep and thereby prevents normal nocturnal erections. This will eliminate tension on the suture line.
• Use pain relievers as prescribed to relieve discomfort.
• Even though the stitches will be absorbed and need not be removed, you should schedule a postoperative office visit with your doctor.

What happens before the surgery?

• The nurse will review the procedure with the person to be circumcised (or, if he's a newborn, with his parents) and will explain circumcision care. (See *Circumcision care*.)
• Before circumcision to relieve a foreskin disorder, the nurse will reassure the person that surgery will not interfere with urinary, sexual, or reproductive function.
• If the person to be circumcised is a newborn, the nurse will make sure that he hasn't been fed for at least 1 hour before surgery to reduce the risk of vomiting.

What happens during the surgery?

The doctor can choose from several different procedures. For a newborn, a plastic circumcision bell or a Gomco clamp may be used. If using a plastic circumcision bell, the doctor slides the device between the foreskin and head of the penis and then tightly ties a length of suture around the foreskin near the edge. After 5 to 8 days, the foreskin with the plastic bell attached will drop off, leaving a clean, well-healed line of excision.

If using a Gomco clamp, the doctor stretches the foreskin forward over the penis, applies the clamp on the edge of the penis, and then excises the foreskin and removes the clamp. After either procedure, sterile petroleum gauze is usually applied to the area.

If performing a sleeve resection, (the preferred method for an adult male) the doctor cuts and separates the inner and outer surfaces of the foreskin, then puts sutures in place to approximate the skin edges. Electrocoagulation may be used to control bleeding, if necessary, and a compression dressing may be applied. Alternatively, the doctor may use the clamp procedure for an adult as well.

An anesthetic is usually not administered to a newborn because of the risk of respiratory complications. However, some doctors now use a local anesthetic for a newborn to eliminate pain.

What are the possible complications?

Although circumcision is a relatively minor and safe operation, it can cause bleeding or, less commonly, infection and urethral damage. With application of the plastic circumcision bell, incomplete amputation of the foreskin may occur.

What happens after the surgery?

▪ The circumcised newborn will be left diaperless for 1 to 2 hours to check for bleeding and to reduce irritation.

▪ The nurse will bring your newborn to you for comfort as soon as possible after the procedure.

▪ At each diaper change, the nurse will apply antibiotic ointment, petroleum jelly, or petroleum gauze. The circumcised infant will be placed on his abdomen for at least 12 hours. He'll be diapered loosely to prevent irritation.

▪ The nurse will provide pain relievers for discomfort from the incision and will also apply a topical anesthetic ointment or spray, as needed, for an adult, who's more subject to pain from pressure exerted on the suture line by an erection.

SELF-HELP

Caring for a ureteral stent

When you've been discharged from the hospital, follow these important guidelines.

Keep the stent clean
• If you have a stent with external drainage, you must keep the stent entry site sterile and learn to change the dressing as necessary.
• Take showers rather than baths to reduce the likelihood of infecting the stent site.

Other instructions
• Monitor yourself for signs and symptoms of complications such as a fever and pus-filled drainage.
• Drink at least eight 8-ounce (240-milliliter) glasses of fluid daily to flush bacteria from the urinary tract.
• Discuss with your doctor when it's safe to resume sexual activity.
• Keep all follow-up appointments with the doctor. Stent replacements will be necessary.

URETERAL STENTS

A ureteral stent is a hollow tubular device designed for placement within the ureter (the tube that carries urine from the kidney to the bladder). The stent has side holes that allow urine to drain unimpeded from the kidney to the bladder. Typically made of soft, flexible silicone, it's inserted in a variety of ways.

Ideally, a ureteral stent provides a free, unobstructed flow of urine; remains in position; and causes few, if any, complications.

Why is this procedure done?
Ureteral stents may be used to maintain ureteral flow in people with ureteral obstruction caused by kidney stones, swelling, constriction, or tumors. Ureteral stents can also be used if significant injury to the mucous membrane occurs during procedures involving the urinary tract. After an operation, such as removal of a kidney stone, stents may be used to keep the ureter open. Stents may be inserted intraoperatively to identify the ureter and prevent ligation and are often used after shock-wave lithotripsy to ensure urine drainage and facilitate passage of kidney stone fragments. (See "Shock Wave Lithotripsy," pages 353 to 356.)

What happens before the procedure?
• The doctor or nurse will explain the procedure; show you, if possible, what the stent will look like; and describe the necessary postoperative care. (See *Caring for a ureteral stent.*)
• The nurse will involve the family and arrange for visits from a home health care nurse if you'll have a stent with external drainage.

What happens during the procedure?
You may be placed in a position typically assumed during a gynecologic exam. Cystoscopy is performed, and a guide wire is passed through the cystoscope and up the ureter. The stent is placed over the guide wire and advanced up the ureter under fluoroscopic guidance. When the correct position is confirmed by X-ray, the guide wire is removed; the stent will resume its original configuration and secure itself.

A stent may also be placed through an artificial opening into the kidney. If this is the option your surgeon chooses, you'll be placed either on your stomach or on your back for this procedure. A guide wire is passed through the nephrostomy and down the ureter. The stent is passed over this wire. The stent's position is checked before the guide wire is removed. Intraoperative placement during open surgery on a ureter may not require an X-ray to confirm the stent's position.

What are the possible complications?

Complications include inflammation or infection from a foreign body. Rarely, stents may become obstructed from clot formation or encrustation. Other complications include migration or dislodgment of the tube.

What happens after the procedure?

- The nurse will monitor your intake and output. Keep in mind that a decreased urine output and colicky pain with chills, nausea, and vomiting may indicate stent dislodgment or obstruction.
- The nurse will observe the surgical wound for leakage of urine, which may indicate stent dislodgment or obstruction.

DIALYSIS

HEMODIALYSIS

Hemodialysis removes wastes and other impurities from the blood of a person with kidney failure. This potentially lifesaving procedure removes blood from the body, circulates it through a dialyzer (purifying filter), and then returns the blood to the body. (See *Hemodialysis access sites,* pages 346 and 347.)

Why is this procedure done?

Hemodialysis extracts waste products from the blood and helps prevent uremia, a deadly condition caused by kidney failure.

Hemodialysis is one of the forms of dialysis that's performed in end-stage kidney disease. Hemodialysis may be performed in acute kidney failure and less commonly in acute poisoning, such as an overdose of barbiturates or pain relievers.

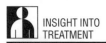

INSIGHT INTO
TREATMENT

Hemodialysis access sites

Hemodialysis requires blood vessel access. The site and type of access may vary, depending on the expected duration of dialysis, the surgeon's preference, and the person's condition.

Subclavian vein

The surgeon inserts an introducer needle into the subclavian vein, inserts a guide wire through the introducer needle, and removes the needle. Using the guide wire, he or she then threads a 5- to 12-inch (12.7- to 30.5-centimeter) plastic or Teflon catheter into the person's vein.

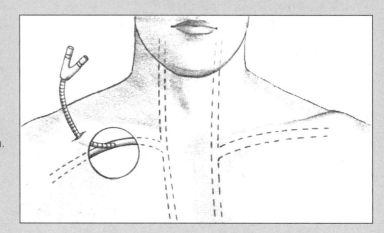

Femoral vein

The surgeon inserts an introducer needle into the left or right femoral vein in the leg. He or she then inserts a guide wire through the introducer needle and removes the needle. Using the guide wire, the surgeon then threads a 5- to 12-inch plastic or Teflon catheter with a Y-connector or two catheters into the vein. One opening is for removal of blood from the body; the other is for the return of blood to the body.

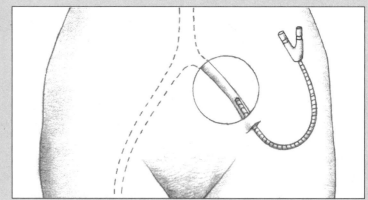

What happens before the procedure?

- The nurse will explain the purpose and duration of treatment, associated complications, and required aftercare.
- You'll lie on your back, with the blood vessel access site well supported.
- Required blood samples will be drawn.
- You'll be connected to a dialysis unit.

Fistula for the wrist or forearm

To create a fistula, the surgeon makes an incision into the person's wrist or lower forearm, then makes a small incision in the side of an artery and another in the side of a vein. He or she joins the edges of these incisions together to make a common opening about 1 to 3 inches (2.5 to 7.5 centimeters) long.

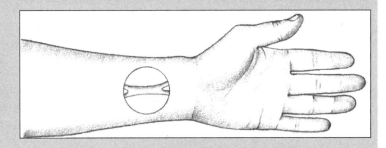

Shunt for the wrist or forearm

To create a shunt, the surgeon makes an incision in the person's wrist or lower forearm (or rarely an ankle), and then inserts a 6- to 10-inch (15- to 25-centimeter) transparent Silastic catheter into an artery and another into a vein. Finally, the surgeon tunnels the catheters out through stab wounds and joins them with a piece of Teflon tubing.

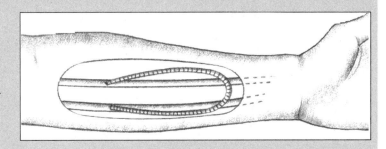

Graft for the arm or thigh

To create a graft, the surgeon makes an incision in the person's forearm, upper arm, or thigh. He or she then tunnels a natural or synthetic graft under the skin and stitches one end to an artery and the other end to a vein.

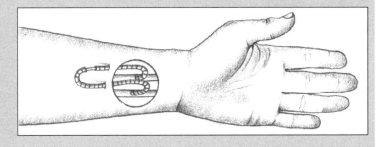

What happens during the procedure?

Specially prepared personnel usually perform this procedure in a hemodialysis unit. Special hemodialysis units are also available for home use.

A surgeon creates an access site in a blood vessel. The blood lines from the dialyzer are then connected to the access site. Blood samples are drawn for analysis. The hemodialysis unit is turned on and the

SELF-HELP

Caring for yourself while undergoing hemodialysis

Your chances of successfully completing a course of hemodialysis are better if you follow the steps outlined below.

Help prevent infection
- Keep the incision at the vascular access site clean and dry to prevent infection. Clean it with hydrogen peroxide solution daily until healing is complete and the stitches are removed (usually 10 to 14 days after surgery).
- Notify the doctor of any pain, swelling, redness, or drainage in the accessed arm.

Protect your arm
- Don't allow any treatments or procedures on the accessed arm, including blood pressure monitoring or needle punctures.
- Avoid putting excessive pressure on the arm; don't sleep on it or wear constricting clothing over it; and don't lift heavy objects or strain with it.
- Don't shower, bathe, or swim for several hours after dialysis.

- You may use the affected arm freely once the access site has healed. Exercise is beneficial because it increases blood flow, which stimulates vein enlargement.

Other instructions
- You'll need to learn to use the stethoscope correctly to detect the bruit (an unusual sound) and to feel the thrill (vibration). These will indicate good blood flow at the access site. Ask your nurse to demonstrate the appropriate techniques for you.
- If you'll be performing hemodialysis at home, familiarize yourself with all aspects of the procedure before leaving the hospital. Keep the phone number of the dialysis center handy, in case you need to call with any questions about the treatment.
- Keep an accurate record of your food and fluid intake, and comply with prescribed diet restrictions, such as limited protein, potassium, and salt intake; increased caloric intake; and decreased fluid intake.
- If you need additional information and support, contact the American Association of Kidney Patients or the National Kidney Foundation.

procedure usually continues for 3 to 6 hours. At the end of the procedure, additional blood samples are drawn, and you're disconnected from the dialysis unit.

For people with chronic kidney failure, dialysis is commonly prescribed for three times a week, 4 hours each treatment. This may vary in chronic kidney failure, depending on the person's condition and response to hemodialysis.

What are the possible complications?

Common complications of hemodialysis include a decrease in blood pressure, nausea and vomiting, muscle cramps, and disequilibrium syndrome (seizures, muscle twitching, and headache). Other complications include apprehension, restlessness, clammy skin, thready pulse, increased respirations, and decreased body temperature, difficulty breathing, chest pain, bluish discoloration of the skin, excessive external bleeding at the access site, and infection.

What happens after the procedure?

If you were treated in an outpatient dialysis center, the nurse will verify that your vital signs are stable and that your level of consciousness is adequate before discharge. (See *Caring for yourself while undergoing hemodialysis.*)

PERITONEAL DIALYSIS

In this procedure, a dialysis solution is put into the membrane of the abdomen to remove poisons from the body. Peritoneal dialysis may be performed manually, by an automatic or semiautomatic cycler machine, or as continuous ambulatory peritoneal dialysis (CAPD). As its name implies, CAPD allows the person to be out of bed and active during dialysis; it minimizes lifestyle disruption, as it doesn't require travel to a dialysis center.

Some people use CAPD in combination with an automatic cycler machine in a treatment called *continuous-cycling peritoneal dialysis.* In continuous-cycling peritoneal dialysis, the cycler performs dialysis at night while the person sleeps, and the person performs CAPD during the day.

Peritoneal dialysis offers several advantages over hemodialysis, such as ease of performance, high safety margin, portability, and availability. Disadvantages may include immobilization, low efficiency, protein loss, and metabolic complications.

Why is this procedure done?

Peritoneal dialysis should be performed for the person with chronic kidney failure who doesn't respond to other treatments or when a less rapid treatment is needed. It's performed for the person with severe defects in blood-clotting mechanisms, heart and blood vessel disease, and acute poisoning; it's also performed for those with extensive burns who can no longer sustain hemodialysis, and for those who have religious objections to hemodialysis.

When shouldn't this procedure be done?

Peritoneal dialysis shouldn't be performed for those people who've had abdominal surgery, adhesions, scarring, or infection. It's not advisable for anyone who would be unable to adequately perform the dialysis exchanges, either alone or with the help of a caregiver.

What happens before the procedure?

- If this will be your first time undergoing peritoneal dialysis, the nurse will explain the purpose of the treatment and what to expect during and after the procedure.
- Before insertion of the urinary catheter, the nurse will ask you to urinate to reduce the risk of bladder perforation and to increase comfort during catheter insertion. He or she will also perform straight catheterization if necessary.
- The nurse will put on a surgical mask and prepare the dialysis administration set. Any prescribed medication will be added to the dialyzing solution (dialysate) at this time. The drainage bag will be placed below you to facilitate drainage by gravity, and the outflow tubing will be connected to it.
- You'll be warned that you may feel cramping, shoulder aching, fullness in the abdomen or rectum, and aching in the penis, scrotum, or vagina during the dwell time (the time the dialysate remains in the peritoneal cavity). You'll be premedicated with pain relievers, if necessary, and positioned to promote comfort.

What happens during the procedure?

Peritoneal dialysis may be performed in the operating room or at the bedside, with a nurse assisting. The surgeon administers a local anesthetic in a small area of your abdomen below the navel, and makes a small incision, and inserts the catheter into the peritoneal cavity. The catheter is then secured in place and a dressing is applied.

In manual dialysis, you, the nurse, or a family member instills dialysate through the catheter inserted into the peritoneal cavity, allows it to dwell for a specified time, and then drains it from the peritoneal cavity. Typically, this process is repeated for 6 to 8 hours at a time, five or six times a week.

Peritoneal dialysis using a cycler machine requires sterile equipment and sterile connection technique. The programs are set up and the machine programmed to infuse the ordered volume of dialysate. The solution is allowed to dwell for the prescribed time and then is

SELF-HELP

Performing peritoneal dialysis at home

If you or a family member will perform continuous ambulatory peritoneal dialysis (CAPD) or continuous-cycling peritoneal dialysis (CCPD) at home, make sure you understand the procedures and can perform them safely.

Report any problems
- Watch for and report signs of infection and fluid imbalance. Make sure you know how to measure blood pressure, pulse, temperature, weight, and fluid intake and output to provide a record of response to treatment.
- Wear a bracelet or carry a card that identifies you as a peritoneal dialysis patient. Keep the phone number of the dialysis center on hand at all times in case of an emergency.

Other points to remember
- A dietitian will help you modify your diet to adjust for nutritional imbalances resulting from peritoneal dialysis.
- Keep follow-up appointments with your doctor and dialysis team to evaluate the success of treatment and detect any problems.
- A home health care nurse may visit to assess your adjustment to CAPD.
- You may benefit by meeting other people on peritoneal dialysis. Ask your health care team about meeting them.

allowed to flow out. The cycle of infuse, dwell, and outflow is repeated (usually every half hour) for 8 to 10 hours per session.

You can perform CAPD by filling a special plastic bag with dialysate and instilling the solution through a catheter into your peritoneal cavity. While the solution remains in the abdomen, you can roll up the empty bag, place it under your clothing, and go about your normal activities. After 6 to 8 hours of dwell time, the spent solution is drained into the bag. The full bag is removed and discarded. You may then attach a new bag of dialysate; repeat the process four times a day to ensure continuous dialysis 24 hours a day, 7 days a week. (See *Performing peritoneal dialysis at home.*)

What are the possible complications?

Peritoneal dialysis can cause severe complications. The most serious one, peritonitis, results from contamination of the peritoneal cavity by bacteria or fungi through the catheter or the insertion site. Other complications include catheter obstruction from protein debris, catheter lodgment against the abdominal wall, or kinking of the catheter; metabolic complications; low blood pressure; diminished blood volume from excessive plasma fluid removal; and respiratory distress from upward pressure of the dialysate on the diaphragm.

What happens after the procedure?

After dialysis is completed, the nurse will disconnect the equipment and change the dressings as needed every 24 hours. If you'll be performing peritoneal dialysis at home, your nurse will also instruct you in various self-care measures.

KIDNEY STONE TREATMENTS

KIDNEY STONE BASKETING

When kidney stones become lodged in a ureter (one of the two slender tubes that carry urine from the kidney to the bladder), removal with a basketing instrument is a treatment option. This procedure, called *basketing*, avoids major surgery and helps relieve pain, prevent infection, and restore the kidney function threatened by the stone's blockage of the ureter. The basketing instrument is inserted through a cystoscope or ureteroscope (instruments used to inspect the interior of the bladder and ureters) into the ureter to capture the stone and is then withdrawn to remove it. However, because of the risk of ureteral perforation, basketing is generally not performed for removal of an excessively large stone or one located above the lower one-third segment of the ureter.

Why is this procedure done?

This treatment should be performed when a stone is impacted in the ureter, the person has unmanageable pain, or if there is threatened kidney damage or suspected kidney or systemic infection.

What happens before the procedure?

You'll be prepared for tests to determine the location of the stones and your kidney function status. Such tests typically include abdominal X-rays.

What happens during the procedure?

You're placed in the lithotomy position (a position typically used in routine gynecologic exam) on an X-ray table, and a lower abdominal X-ray is taken to locate the obstructing stone. A general or spinal anesthetic is then administered as appropriate. After inserting a cystoscope or ureteroscope (which will also require the insertion of a guide wire) into the urethra, the surgeon passes the special loop or basket catheter through the cystoscope or ureteroscope and into the ureter where the stone is located.

After removing the stone, the surgeon typically inserts a ureteral catheter or stent to the level of the renal pelvis to drain urine into the bladder and, possibly, an indwelling urinary catheter to aid bladder drainage.

Depending on the location of the stone, the surgeon may first perform a percutaneous nephrostomy by creating an opening through the skin and inserting the cystoscope and the basketing instrument through this opening to remove the stone. This procedure is also performed to maintain kidney function and to drain infected urine until the stone can be removed. After the stone is removed, the percutaneous nephrostomy tube is left in place to ensure that the ureter is not blocked by blood clots or excessive accumulation of fluid. The stone is also examined and compared with the stone of the X-ray film to confirm that it has been totally removed.

What are the possible complications?

When performed properly, basketing should cause few complications. Potential complications include infection, bleeding, ureteral perforation, and ureteral tearing. Occasionally, the kidney stone basket becomes impacted, requiring surgical removal.

What happens after the procedure?

You'll be given pain relievers. (See *Avoiding recurrence of kidney stones.*)

SHOCK WAVE LITHOTRIPSY

Extracorporeal shock wave lithotripsy (ESWL) uses high-energy shock waves to break up kidney stones and allow their normal passage from the body. Depending on the type of equipment used, a person undergoing this treatment may be anesthetized and placed in a water tank. The affected kidney is positioned over an electric spark generator, which creates high-energy shock waves that shatter stones without damaging surrounding tissue. Afterward, the person is able to excrete the fine, gravel-like remains of the stones.

The newer types of equipment used for ESWL do not require submersion in water and may not require general anesthesia. Instead, a membrane coupling device can be directly applied to the skin over the affected kidney. Additional treatments may be necessary for large or multiple stones. ESWL is not as effective for cystine, uric acid, and some calcium oxalate stones.

Because ESWL is noninvasive, most people can be discharged the same evening or the next day and can resume normal activity after a few days. ESWL also minimizes the risk of many potentially serious complications, such as infection and hemorrhage, associated with invasive methods of stone removal.

Why is this procedure done?

This procedure may be performed as a preventive measure in a person with potentially obstructive kidney stones or as an emergency treatment for an acute obstruction; more often, a stent (retrograde or percutaneous) is inserted to ensure urine drainage and facilitate passage of kidney stones fragments. Kidney stones about 1 inch (2.5 centimeters) or smaller are ideal targets for ESWL. The larger the stone, the less likely is successful elimination of all stone fragments.

When shouldn't this procedure be done?

Depending on the circumstances, ESWL may not be performed during pregnancy or in the presence of a urinary tract obstruction distal to the stones, which would prevent passage of stone fragments. It may also not be performed in cases of unrelated infection, excessive obesity, a history of a bleeding or clotting disorder, kidney cancer, and stones that are attached to the kidney or ureter or located below the level of the iliac crest.

What happens before the procedure?

- A nurse will explain the procedure.
- If possible, the nurse will show you the equipment used during for the procedure before the first scheduled treatment.

What happens during the procedure?

At the beginning of the procedure, you'll receive some type of anesthetic because the shock waves can cause discomfort as they pass through the walls of your body. The type of anesthetic depends on the type of lithotriptor used. Some devices require general or epidural anesthesia; others, which pulverize stones effectively while delivering energy less painfully, can be used with local anesthesia alone. An intravenous line and catheter are inserted, and electrocardiograph electrodes are attached.

For lithotripsy in water, you're placed in a semireclining position on the machine's hydraulic stretcher and lowered into the water tank. In the tank, your position is adjusted so that the shock-wave generator focuses directly on the stones. Biplane fluoroscopy or ultrasonography can be used to enhance visualization of the stones and confirm their position. The generator's then activated to direct high-energy shock waves through the water at the kidney stones. To prevent disruption of your heartbeat, the shock waves are synchronized with your heart's R waves and fired during diastole. The number of waves fired during treatment depends on the size and composition of the stones but may range from 500 to 2,000 shocks. After the shocks are delivered, you're removed from the tub and the electrocardiograph electrodes are removed.

What are the possible complications?

Complications of ESWL, occurring in about 1% of those who have the procedure, include perirenal hemorrhage, urinary tract obstruction caused by stone fragments, severe pain, and urinary tract infection. Recent reports indicate that patients who have undergone ESWL have an increased incidence of high blood pressure, although the clinical significance of this response hasn't been determined.

What happens after the procedure?

- A nurse will monitor your vital signs every 4 hours for the first 24 hours after treatment, or until discharge if you're released within 24 hours, and will report any abnormal findings to the doctor.
- Your fluid intake and urinary output will be closely monitored.
- The nurse will tell you to maintain a fluid intake of at least 2 quarts (2 liters) of water a day to aid passage of stone fragments.
- The nurse will strain your urine for stone fragments and send them to the lab for analysis.

SELF-HELP

Aiding passage of kidney stone fragments

You can help ensure the effective elimination of kidney stone fragments and prevent them from recurring by taking the following precautions.

Watch for side effects

- There are a number of side effects of extracorporeal shock-wave therapy, including pain on the treated side as fragments pass, slight redness or bruising on the treated side, blood-tinged urine for several days after treatment, and mild gastrointestinal upset. Although these signs and symptoms may alarm you, they're normal.
- You should, however, report severe, persistent pain, persistent blood in the urine, an inability to urinate, fever and chills, or recurrent nausea and vomiting.

Resume normal activities

Because physical activity will promote the passage of kidney stone fragments, you're encouraged to resume normal activities, including exercise and work, as soon as you feel up to it (unless the doctor instructs otherwise).

Other instructions

- Drink 3 to 4 quarts (3 to 4 liters) of fluid each day for about 1 month after treatment. This will aid passage of kidney stone fragments and will help prevent formation of new stones.
- You'll be taught how to strain your urine for fragments. You'll be required to strain all urine for the 1st week after treatment, to save all fragments in the container provided, and to take the container along on your first follow-up doctor's appointment.
- Stick to the diet or drug regimen designed for you by your doctor.

■ The nurse will note the urine's color and test its pH, and notify the doctor of obvious or persistent bleeding. (See *Aiding passage of kidney stone fragments.*)

■ You'll be encouraged to move around as early as possible after treatment to aid passage of stone fragments.

■ To help remove any particles lodged in gravity-dependent kidney pockets, the nurse will instruct you to lie facedown with your head and shoulders over the edge of the bed for about 10 minutes and to perform this maneuver twice a day. You should drink fluids 40 to 45 minutes before starting this maneuver to enhance its effectiveness.

■ The nurse will monitor you for pain on the treated side and administer pain relievers if necessary. If you experience severe pain, which may indicate ureteral obstruction from new kidney stones, you should promptly report it to the doctor.

ULTRASONIC LITHOTRIPSY

In this lithotripsy technique, kidney stones are shattered by an ultrasonic probe inserted through a nephrostomy tube into the renal pelvis (expanded end of the ureter). Ultrahigh-frequency sound waves are generated to pulverize the kidney stones while continuous suctioning removes the fragments. Like extracorporeal shock-wave lithotripsy (ESWL), percutaneous ultrasonic lithotripsy (PUL) greatly reduces the person's recovery time as compared with open kidney surgery.

Why is this procedure done?

Lithotripsy techniques are used to remove kidney stones that cannot pass through the urinary tract spontaneously. This procedure is principally used in people with kidney stones larger than 1 inch (2.5 centimeters), including those in the upper ureter that cannot be manipulated back into the renal pelvis for ESWL. PUL may replace ESWL or may be performed after it to remove residual stone fragments. It's particularly useful for removing kidney stones that aren't treatable by ESWL.

When shouldn't this procedure be done?

This procedure shouldn't be performed for people with irreversible blood-clotting disorders or untreated urinary tract infections.

What happens before the procedure?

- The nurse will explain the procedure to you, including insertion of the nephrostomy tube and the lithotripsy technique.
- You'll be warned that you may experience discomfort from the nephrostomy tube but that the treatment should be otherwise painless.
- The day before the scheduled treatment, the nurse will prepare you for lower abdominal X-rays or other diagnostic tests to locate the kidney stones.
- All food and fluids will be withheld after midnight on the night before the procedure.

What happens during the procedure?

Because the shock waves can cause discomfort, you'll receive a general or an epidural anesthetic. The surgeon establishes a nephrostomy tract with a needle puncture performed under ultrasound guidance,

Passing kidney stones

If no complications develop, you may be discharged 2 to 4 days after lithotripsy. Even after you are discharged, you may continue to pass kidney stones. The following precautions will help you to deal with expected developments.

Know what to expect

- You should try to drink 3 to 4 quarts (or liters) of fluid each day for about a month after treatment to aid passage of any retained kidney stone fragments and to help prevent formation of new ones.
- You'll be taught to strain your urine for kidney stone fragments. Strain all urine for the first week after treatment, save all fragments in the container provided, and take the container along on your first medical follow-up visit.
- The nurse will review with you any prescribed changes in your diet or drug regimen to help prevent formation of new stones.

Other instructions

- Promptly report persistent bloody or cloudy and foul-smelling urine, an inability to urinate, fever and chills, or severe and unremitting flank pain. Also report redness, swelling, or pus-filled drainage from the tube insertion site.
- Avoid strenuous exercise, sexual activity, heavy lifting, or straining until your doctor instructs otherwise.
- Do take short walks because mild physical activity will help aid passage of any retained kidney stone fragments.
- If you're discharged with a drainage tube in place, make sure that you understand how to care for it before you leave the hospital.

threads an angiographic wire through the needle, and passes various-sized nephrostomy tubes over the wire to progressively dilate the tract. When the tract is sufficiently dilated, the surgeon inserts a nephroscope to visualize the kidney stone.

Next (or 1 or 2 days later, if PUL is being performed in two stages), the surgeon inserts a working tube that resembles a small cystoscope through the nephrostomy tract and into the kidney's urine collecting system and then passes an ultrasonic probe through the tube and positions it against the stones. When the probe is in position, the surgeon turns on the device, producing ultrahigh-frequency sound waves that shatter the stones into fragments. He or she then uses suction, irrigation, or a basketing instrument to remove the fragments. After treatment is complete, the surgeon withdraws the probe and the working tube and then reinserts the nephrostomy tube. The tube remains in place until it's confirmed that all stone fragments have been passed.

What are the possible complications?

Potential complications include postoperative bleeding, urinary tract infection, and leakage of irrigating fluid into surrounding tissue. PUL may also lead to kidney damage from insertion of the nephrostomy tube and ureteral obstruction from incomplete passage of stone fragments.

What happens after the procedure?

- It's normal for your urine to be slightly bloody for several days after PUL; however, obvious or persistent blood in your urine should be reported.
- To aid passage of retained fragments and hinder formation of new kidney stones, you'll be maintained on a high fluid intake — up to 4 quarts (about 4 liters) a day. For the same reason, you'll be encouraged to walk as soon as possible after the procedure.
- The doctor will determine if there are any retained fragments. This usually takes place 1 or 2 days after the procedure. If no fragments are revealed, the nephrostomy tube is clamped and removed the next day. You may be discharged with the tube in place if tests indicate existing stone fragments that have not been passed.
- Because the nephrostomy tract heals and closes within 24 hours after removal of the tube, you can return to work within days. Your nurse will make sure that you understand what to do to facilitate passage of shattered kidney stones. (See *Passing kidney stones.*)

BLADDER TREATMENTS

BLADDER TRAINING

Bladder training is a conservative approach to treatment of incontinence. Preferable to the use of drugs or surgery, bladder training uses behavior therapy techniques, such as pelvic muscle (Kegel) exercises to make the person more aware of the lower urinary tract and relaxation techniques to help the person control the urge to urinate. Successful bladder training requires a strongly motivated person with the ability to discern body sensations.

Biofeedback may be used to enhance bladder training and pelvic exercises. It uses sophisticated equipment that gives visual and auditory feedback to help people identify and use their bladder muscles more effectively.

Indwelling urinary catheters are a last resort in treating incontinence. They should be used only when incontinence cannot be managed medically, surgically, through behavior modification, or by periodic catheterization.

Why is this therapy done?

Bladder training should be performed for managing incontinence that results from neurologic disease or dysfunction of the bladder itself. Successful treatment results in establishing a regular schedule for urination, which allows the person to achieve urinary continence.

What happens before the therapy?

- The nurse explains the training program and ensures that you understand and are willing to cooperate.
- Just before the start of the program, the nurse takes a thorough medical history, which will include specific questions regarding your regular urination patterns.
- You'll be instructed to eat a high-fiber diet and to maintain an adequate fluid intake of about six to eight 8-ounce glasses (1,400 to 1,900 milliliters) per day but to limit fluid intake in the evening.

What happens during the therapy?

Bladder training is a joint effort between you and your caregivers. At the beginning of the bladder training program, you'll be instructed to perform muscle-strengthening exercises to increase the strength of the pelvic floor muscles. Next, you'll establish a urination record, which serves as the basis for the toileting schedule. The schedule indicates times when you should try to empty the bladder. In the early phase of bladder training, the interval between toileting is usually 1 ½ to 2 hours. Then, as you progress, the interval is gradually prolonged by 30 minutes until a goal (usually 4 hours) is reached. The established toileting schedule is maintained even if you have episodes of incontinence.

If you have an urge to urinate before the scheduled toileting time, you're encouraged to relax and perform pelvic muscle-strengthening exercises. Once the urge has passed, you then move slowly (to prevent incontinence) to the bathroom.

If you have difficulty starting a urine stream, you'll be instructed to either sit or stand with your thighs flexed and your feet and back supported. It's also helpful to massage the bladder or lean forward when sitting. These methods help initiate bladder emptying by increasing intra-abdominal pressure. (See *How to enhance bladder training*.)

What are the possible complications?

No complications are associated with bladder training.

CATHETERIZATION

Urinary catheterization is the insertion of a drainage device into the bladder using sterile technique. Catheterization may be intermittent or continuous. Intermittent catheterization drains urine that remains in the bladder after urination or when the person is unable to void naturally. Continous catheterization uses an indwelling urinary catheter to provide continuous drainage of urine.

Why is this procedure done?

Intermittent catheterization may be used postoperatively for people with urinary incontinence to remove residual urine or for people with other disorders that interfere with bladder emptying. The person may also perform this procedure at home if he or she has a chronic bladder disorder. (See *How to use a catheter*, pages 362 and 363.)

Continuous catheterization is indicated to relieve bladder distention caused by such conditions as urinary tract obstruction and neurogenic bladder (bladder dysfunction from lesions of the central nervous system). It also allows continuous urine drainage in people with a swollen urethral opening related to surgery, localized injury, or childbirth. What's more, continuous catheterization can provide accurate monitoring of urine output when normal urination is impaired. It also can be used to irrigate the bladder or instill medications.

 SELF-HELP

How to enhance bladder training

Take the following steps to increase your chances for success in bladder training:
- Arrange your living space so that you have easy access to the toilet when the urge to urinate occurs.
- Increase your intake of dietary fiber to promote regular urination and thus enhance the bladder training program.
- You and your caregiver should stick to the toileting schedule.

How to use a catheter

If you have impaired or absent bladder function, you may have to use the catheter to drain urine from your bladder.

Gathering the right supplies

To perform this technique, you'll need the following items: a rubber catheter, washcloth, soap and water, gloves, water-soluble lubricant, plastic storage bag. Optional equipment includes a drainage container, paper towels, and a catheterization record.

You should keep a supply of catheters at home and use each catheter only once before cleaning it. When all but the last one have been used, boil the catheters for 20 minutes in a pan of water, drain the water, and store the catheters in the pan or a freshly laundered towel. The catheters will become brittle with repeated use and should be checked often. A new supply should be ordered well in advance.

Getting started

Begin by trying to urinate into a toilet or, if you need to measure urine quantity, into a drainage container. You should then wash your hands thoroughly with soap and water, dry them, and put on the gloves.

Directions for women

Begin by separating the labia as widely as possible with the fingers of your nondominant hand to obtain a full view of the urethral opening. Then use your dominant hand to wash the perineal area thoroughly with a soapy washcloth, using downward strokes. The area is then rinsed with the washcloth in downward strokes.

Next, squeeze some lubricant onto the first 3 inches (7.6 centimeters) of the catheter. Then, holding the catheter like a pencil about ½ inch (1.3 centimeters) from its tip while keeping the vaginal folds separated, insert the lubricated catheter about 3 inches into the urethra. Pressing down with your abdominal muscles will help to empty your bladder, allowing urine to drain through the catheter and into the toilet or drainage container.

When the urine stops draining, slowly remove the catheter and then wash it with warm, soapy water, rinse it inside and out, and dry it with a paper towel.

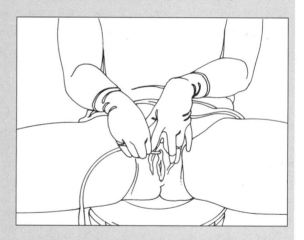

What happens before the procedure?

- The nurse will review the procedure with you.
- You'll be reassured that although catheterization may produce slight discomfort, it shouldn't be painful. If it's painful, let your nurse know so that the procedure can be stopped.

How to use a catheter *(continued)*

Directions for men

Thoroughly wash and rinse the end of your penis with soap and water, pulling back the foreskin if appropriate. Then keep the foreskin pulled back during the procedure.

Next, squeeze lubricant onto a paper towel and roll the first 7 to 10 inches (17.8 to 25 centimeters) of the catheter in the lubricant. This generous amount of lubricant will make the procedure more comfortable. Then use your nondominant hand to hold your penis at a right angle to your body.

Then, holding the catheter like a pencil in your dominant hand, slowly insert it 7 to 10 inches into the urethra until urine begins to flow. Advance the catheter about 1 inch (2.5 centimeters) farther, allowing all urine to drain into the toilet or drainage container. When the urine stops draining, remove the catheter slowly and, if necessary, pull the foreskin forward again. Then wash, rinse, and dry the catheter as described above.

The timing of catheterization is critical to prevent overdistention of the bladder, which can lead to infection. Catheterizations are usually done every 4 to 6 hours around the clock (or more often at first).

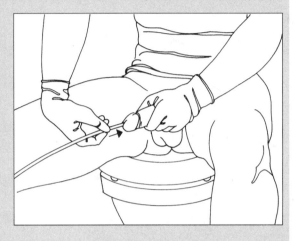

What happens during the procedure?

If you're female, you'll lie on your back, with your knees flexed and separated and your feet flat on the bed. If you're male, you also will lie on your back, but with your legs flat and extended.

Your genitalia and perineum (area between the genitalia and anus) are cleaned with soap and water or an antiseptic solution to avoid introducing bacteria into the bladder. Because this is a sterile procedure, the nurse will wear gloves throughout.

To accomplish intermittent catheterization, a nurse inserts a sterile straight catheter through the urethra into the bladder. This type of catheter is left in place only long enough to drain residual urine and is withdrawn when the urine flow stops.

If an indwelling urinary catheter will be used for continuous drainage of urine, a balloon at the proximal end of the catheter is inflated with sterile water to secure the catheter in place within the bladder. The catheter is connected to a collection bag that's positioned below the level of the bladder to enhance drainage and prevent urine from flowing back into the bladder, which can cause

SELF-HELP

How to avoid infection at the catheter site

Take the following precautions to help prevent infecting the catheterization site.

Secure the tubing
If you have an indwelling urinary catheter, you'll be taught how to secure the tubing and the leg bag. You may find it more comfortable to alternate legs every other day to prevent skin irritation. Always keep the leg bag or closed-system drainage bag lower than bladder level to make drainage easier. Always empty the bag when it's about half full, and apply a new bag according to the instructions given by your doctor or nurse.

Know when to call your doctor
- Notify your doctor immediately if you notice any urine leaking out around the catheter.

- Report any signs of urinary tract infection, such as fever, chills, flank or urinary tract pain, and cloudy or foul-smelling urine.

Other instructions
- If you're required to perform intermittent catheterization, make sure you familiarize yourself with the procedure before leaving the hospital.
- Drink at least 2 quarts of water daily, unless the doctor orders you to do otherwise.
- Minimize the risk of infection by cleaning the area around the catheter insertion site every day.
- Wash your hands thoroughly before and after handling the catheter and collection system.
- Take showers instead of tub baths while the catheter is in place.

infection. The catheter is then secured in position to prevent traction on the bladder and to maintain the normal direction of urine flow.

What are the possible complications?
People who have an indwelling urinary catheter are at risk for developing urinary tract infections or sustaining urethral injury.

What happens after the procedure?
- If you're female, the catheter will be strapped to your thigh to prevent tension in the urogenital area. If you're male, the nurse will secure the catheter to the thigh or lower abdomen.
- Expect a small amount of mucus drainage at the catheter insertion site from irritation of the urethral wall, but notify the doctor or nurse of excessive, bloody, or pus-filled drainage.
- You'll be encouraged to keep an adequate fluid intake (up to 3 quarts [liters] per day, if necessary) to maintain continuous urine flow through the catheter and decrease the risk of infection and clot formation. (See *How to avoid infection at the catheter site*.)

8

TREATING OBSTETRIC & GYNECOLOGIC DISORDERS

DRUG THERAPIES

PROGESTINS

The progestins are progesterone, one of the naturally occurring female hormones, and its synthetic derivatives. Studies have shown that adding progestins to supplemental estrogens (in postmenopausal women, for example) may reduce some of the toxic effects of estrogens alone. Progestins are also used for contraception.

Progestins can restore the body's steroid hormone balance. In menstrual disorders caused by hormonal imbalance, they can induce a normal menstrual cycle. These drugs can also be given to stop uterine bleeding or to treat endometriosis or premenstrual syndrome. Some forms may be used as an oral contraceptive; medroxyprogesterone injections are used as a long-term (3-month) contraceptive.

What are progestins used for?
- To prevent pregnancy
- To restore the body's normal hormonal balance
- To supplement the effects of prescribed estrogens

What are some commonly used progestins?
- hydroxyprogesterone, known by the brand names Duralutin, Hy/Gesterone, and Pro-Span
- medroxyprogesterone, known by the brand name Depo-Provera
- megestrol, known by the brand name Megace
- norethindrone, known by the brand names Aygestin and Norlutate
- norgestrel, known by the brand name Ovrette
- progesterone

What are the possible side effects?
- Mental changes, depression
- Breakthrough bleeding, spotting, changes in menstrual flow, changes in cervical secretions, breast changes (including tenderness)
- Swelling of the hands or feet, weight change
- Allergic rash with or without itching, acne
- Jaundice (yellow skin)
- Blood-clotting abnormalities

What are the guidelines for taking progestins?

- If you're taking the drug as a contraceptive, take it at the same time each day. If you miss a dose, take it as soon as you remember and take the next pill according to your regular schedule. Use an alternative method of contraception (such as contraceptive foam, with your partner wearing a condom) whenever you miss a dose. If you miss two doses, take only one of the missed doses; resume the regular schedule and use an alternative method of contraception until your next menstrual period.
- Tell your doctor if you have diabetes, seizures, migraines, heart or kidney disease, asthma, or mental illness. Also tell the doctor if you have a history of cancer or if you have thrombophlebitis or other blood-clotting disorder.
- Immediately report a severe or sudden headache, loss of coordination, slurred speech, visual changes, and severe depression or irritability. Also report pain in your chest, groin, or legs, and any shortness of breath, especially if it's unrelated to exertion.
- Report changes in menstrual flow.
- Take the drug after meals to reduce stomach upset.
- If you smoke, try to quit. Smoking increases the risk of thromboembolic disorders.
- Perform monthly breast self-examinations.

What else you should know

- Progestins can harm a developing fetus. Be sure to tell the doctor immediately if you suspect you're pregnant.
- Tell other health care providers that you're taking progestins. See your gynecologist every 6 to 12 months for a pelvic and breast examination and a Pap test.
- If you're diabetic, monitor your urine glucose level closely and report any abnormalities.

Progestins can harm a developing fetus. Be sure to tell the doctor immediately if you suspect you're pregnant.

ESTROGENS

Estrogens are naturally occurring female hormones that participate in the complex cycle of ovulation and menstruation. Studies have also shown that estrogens play an important role in maintaining a healthy heart and bones. Decreasing estrogen levels during menopause cause many uncomfortable symptoms.

Estrogen supplements have become more common as medical researchers uncover the benefits of estrogen therapy. They're given orally, by injection, by insertion into the vagina, or by application to the skin.

What are estrogens used for?
- To restore normal hormonal balance
- To treat certain forms of estrogen-sensitive cancers
- To relieve symptoms of estrogen deficiency

What are some commonly used estrogens?
- chlorotrianisene, known by the brand name TACE
- dienestrol, known by the brand name Ortho dienestrol cream
- diethylstilbestrol, known by the brand name Stilphostrol
- esterified estrogens, known by the brand names Estratab and Menest
- estradiol, known by the brand names depGynogen, Depogen, Estrace, and Estraderm
- estrone, known by the brand names Gynogen, Kestrin Aqueous, and Theelin Aqueous
- estropipate, known by the brand name Ogen
- quinestrol, known by the brand name Estrovis

What are the possible side effects?
- Breakthrough bleeding, spotting, changes in menstrual flow, dysmenorrhea, premenstrual-like syndrome, amenorrhea during and after treatment, an increase in the size of uterine fibromas, vaginal fungal infections
- Digestive problems
- Skin reactions
- Visual problems
- Mood changes, insomnia

What are the guidelines for taking estrogens?
- Be sure to tell your doctor if you have a history of thrombophlebitis, thromboembolic disorders, or other blood-clotting problems. Also tell the doctor if you have a history of high blood pressure, gallbladder disease, blood diseases, migraines, seizure disorders, diabetes, heart failure, liver or kidney disorders, or a family history of breast, ovarian, or cervical cancer.

- Review the package insert and, if you have any questions, ask your doctor or pharmacist. Estrogens are considered safe to take if you have regular, thorough physical exams. Perform monthly breast self-examinations and report any changes immediately.
- Seek emergency treatment immediately if you experience sudden or severe headache; sudden loss of coordination or change in vision; pains in the chest, groin, or leg (especially the calf); shortness of breath; sudden slurring of speech; or weakness or numbness in an arm or a leg.
- Report swollen ankles or feet, changes in vaginal bleeding, breast lumps or discharge, abdominal or flank pain, rash, yellow skin or eyes, or dark urine.
- Take the drug with food if nausea develops during the first few weeks of therapy. Nausea disappears with continued therapy.
- Take a missed dose as soon as you remember, unless it's time for the next dose. Never double the dose.
- Stop taking the drug and check with the doctor if you suspect that you're pregnant. Continued estrogen therapy during pregnancy may cause birth defects in the fetus.
- If you're using the transdermal form of estradiol, apply the patch to a clean section of your abdomen (not to the breasts or to any areas where the patch may be rubbed loose). Apply the patch twice weekly and wait at least a week before applying a patch to the same area.

What else you should know

- If you're receiving cyclic therapy for postmenopausal symptoms, withdrawal bleeding may occur during the week you are off the drug. Spotting is a common side effect of estrogen therapy and is a sign that the body is responding to the drug just as it once did to its own estrogen supply. You can't get pregnant while on estrogen therapy because you haven't ovulated.
- If you smoke, try to stop. Smoking during estrogen therapy increases the risk of serious cardiovascular effects, especially if you're over age 35.
- Schedule an annual pelvic and breast examination and a Pap smear with your gynecologist.
- Have an annual eye examination because estrogens can worsen your vision.

Smoking during estrogen therapy increases the risk of serious cardiovascular effects, especially if you're over age 35.

FERTILITY DRUGS

Fertility drugs are used to stimulate the ovaries to release an egg in order to be fertilized by sperm. These drugs only work in women who have at least one functioning ovary.

Eggs develop in ovarian follicles. When the follicles mature, the eggs are released and travel down the fallopian tube into the uterus. The fertilized egg becomes implanted in the wall of the uterus, and pregnancy occurs. Typically, ovulation occurs 4 to 10 days after the last day of treatment.

What are fertility drugs used for?

These drugs are used to achieve pregnancy.

What are some commonly used fertility drugs?

- clomiphene, known by the brand name Clomid
- gonadorelin acetate, known by the brand name Lutrepulse
- human chorionic gonadotropin (HCG), known by the brand names A.P.L., Follutein, Pregnyl, and Profasi HP
- menotropins, known by the brand name Pergonal

What are the possible side effects?

- Enlarged or overstimulated ovaries, ovarian cysts, fibroid enlargement, premenstrual syndrome
- Allergic reactions
- Depression, insomnia, dizziness or light-headedness, nervousness, restlessness
- Blurred vision
- Hot flashes

What are the guidelines for taking fertility drugs?

- The use of fertility drugs may lead to multiple births. The incidence varies from 5% with Clomid to 20% with HCG.
- Tell your doctor if you have a history of thrombophlebitis, asthma, seizure disorders, or heart disease.
- Immediately call your doctor if you have bloating or abdominal pain. Also immediately report hives, wheezing, or difficulty breathing.
- During therapy, you'll need regular pelvic exams, blood tests, and ultrasound scans.

- The use of fertility drugs may cause visual difficulties, dizziness, or light-headedness. Avoid driving until you know how you respond to the drug.
- Take a missed dose as soon as you remember. If you don't remember until the time of your next dose, double the dose. Call the doctor if you miss more than one dose.
- Have sexual intercourse every day or every other day during your fertile period.
- Take your basal body temperature and chart it on a graph. Consider using a test kit for predicting ovulation.
- Bring a first-voided morning urine specimen for testing at each follow-up visit.

What else you should know
- Clomid is usually the first drug used. If it fails to induce ovulation after three trials, menotropins and HCG may be given. Menotropins must be used with HCG to stimulate ovulation, which should occur within 18 hours after administration. HCG may also be used 7 to 10 days after Clomid.
- Women with primary hypothalamic amenorrhea may receive Lutrepulse. This drug is administered every 90 minutes for 21 days with a special portable intravenous pump.

OXYTOCICS

These drugs mimic the effects of the hormone oxytocin, which stimulates the uterus to contract. The hormone also promotes milk production in the breasts. When used during a normal childbirth, oxytocics can promote the natural pattern of rhythmic uterine contractions and speed the movement of the baby through the birth canal. These drugs are often used when the natural labor doesn't progress in a timely fashion. Following delivery, oxytocics can enhance the delivery of the placenta and minimize postpartum bleeding.

Following delivery, oxytocics can enhance the delivery of the placenta and minimize postpartum bleeding.

What are oxytocics used for?
- To assist in a normal vaginal delivery
- To decrease bleeding after delivery
- To stimulate lactation

What are some commonly used oxytocics?

- ergonovine, known by the brand name Ergotrate
- methylergonovine, known by the brand name Methergine
- oxytocin, known by the brand names Pitocin and Syntocinon

What are the possible side effects?

- Fluid overload, high or low blood pressure, severe bleeding after delivery
- Abnormal heartbeats (in the mother or baby)
- Blood-clotting problems
- Nausea and vomiting
- Pelvic bruising
- Uterine hyperstimulation or rupture
- Allergic reactions (in the mother or baby)

What are the guidelines for taking oxytocics after delivery?

- Ergotrate and Methergine will be given to you after delivery. Tell the doctor or nurse if you experience a headache, palpitations, dizziness, or any other unusual reactions.
- Contact the doctor immediately if you have any abnormal vaginal bleeding.
- If you are using Syntocinon nasal spray to promote lactation, clear your nasal passages before administering the solution.

TOCOLYTICS

Drugs that relax uterine muscles to suppress premature labor are called *tocolytics.* Currently, only the drug ritodrine has the Food and Drug Administration's approval for inhibiting preterm labor; however, clinicians often use and prefer another drug, terbutaline. Studies have repeatedly shown that both drugs have advantages and disadvantages, but both appear to be safe and effective.

Tocolytics usually are given intravenously during hospitalization until uterine contractions stop. After discharge from the hospital, a woman may continue with oral doses until the delivery of a mature infant is ensured. Alternatively, some doctors prescribe a 5-day treatment course, which avoids prolonged maternal and fetal exposure to the drug. Infusion may be repeated if premature labor recurs.

What are tocolytics used for?

These drugs are used to halt premature labor and to allow a pregnancy to continue.

What are some commonly used tocolytics?

- ritodrine, known by the brand name Yutopar
- terbutaline, known by the brand name Brethine

What are the possible side effects?

- Changes in blood pressure, palpitations, rapid heart rate
- Nausea, vomiting, skin rash
- Nervousness, headache, tremors
- Elevated blood sugar

What are the guidelines for taking tocolytics?

- If you feel palpitations, chest pain, difficulty breathing, or tightness in the chest, notify the doctor immediately. Check your pulse rate before taking the drug. If your pulse rate exceeds 130 beats per minute, skip the dose and notify the doctor promptly. Immediately report any contractions, lower back pain, cramping, or increased vaginal discharge.
- Expect doctors and nurses to closely monitor you and your baby during intravenous therapy. The drug should have minimal effects on your baby.
- Tell the doctor if you experience headache, nervousness, tremors, restlessness, nausea, or vomiting; such reactions probably signal the need to reduce the drug's dosage. Notify the doctor if your urine output decreases or if you gain more than 5 pounds (2.3 kilograms) in a week.
- Take your temperature every day and report a fever, which may be a sign of infection.
- Take oral doses of the drug with food to avoid an upset stomach, and take the last dose several hours before bedtime to avoid insomnia.

What else you should know

- Maintain bed rest as much as possible. Don't prepare your breasts for breast-feeding until about 2 weeks before your due date because this can stimulate uterine contractions.
- Keep follow-up appointments so that the doctor can monitor your progress with lab tests and fetal monitoring.

SURGERIES

MASTECTOMY

Mastectomy is the surgical removal of all or part of one or both breasts. Primarily performed to remove cancerous breast tissue and any affected lymph nodes, mastectomy is commonly combined with radiation therapy and chemotherapy. In the past, radical mastectomy was the treatment of choice for breast cancer. Today, different types of mastectomy can be performed depending on the size of the tumor and whether or not the cancer has spread to other parts of the body.

A *partial (segmental) excision* should be performed for a small tumor in a breast's periphery. This approach leaves a cosmetically satisfying breast but may fail to remove all malignant tissue or to detect the cancer's spread to axillary lymph nodes, which are located in the armpit. A *subcutaneous mastectomy* may be used to treat a tumor in the center of the breast that hasn't spread.

Simple mastectomy may be performed if a tumor is confined to breast tissue. It's also used to relieve pain in advanced breast cancer and as treatment for extensive noncancerous breast disease.

A *modified radical mastectomy*, the standard surgery for the early stages of breast cancer, removes small, localized tumors. It causes less disfigurement and disability than radical mastectomy.

A *radical mastectomy* should be performed to treat large tumors that affect the underlying tissues and axillary lymph nodes. Later, breast reconstruction may be performed using muscle from the back.

Why is the surgery done?
Mastectomy should be performed for operable breast cancer and any cancerous cells that may have spread to the surrounding tissues. It's also performed to treat various other breast disorders such as fibrocystic disease.

What happens before the surgery?
- The doctor explains the procedure and all treatment options to you.
- The nurse will provide you with information about the types of breast prostheses available, if appropriate.
- You must sign a consent form.

Primarily performed to remove cancerous breast tissue and any affected lymph nodes, mastectomy is commonly combined with radiation therapy and chemotherapy.

What happens during the surgery?

For all types of mastectomy, you'll receive a general anesthetic. (See *Types of breast surgery*, pages 376 and 377.) In a *partial mastectomy*, the surgeon removes the entire tumor along with at least 1 inch (2.5 centimeters) of the surrounding healthy tissue. In a *subcutaneous mastectomy*, the surgeon removes all breast tissue but preserves the overlying skin and nipple and may also insert a prosthesis (artificial body part). In a *simple mastectomy*, the surgeon removes the entire breast and may apply a skin graft if necessary. Axillary lymph nodes closest to the breast may be removed.

To perform a *modified radical mastectomy*, the surgeon will use one of several techniques to remove the entire breast. All axillary lymph nodes are also removed while the large pectoralis muscle is left intact. The surgeon may or may not remove the small pectoralis muscle. If a woman has small, localized lesions, the surgeon may perform breast reconstruction immediately or a few days or months later.

In a *radical mastectomy*, the surgeon removes the entire breast, the axillary lymph nodes, the underlying muscles, and adjacent tissues. During the operation, he or she covers skin flaps and exposed tissue with moist packs for protection and, before closure, irrigates the chest wall and armpit area.

In an *extended radical mastectomy*, the surgeon removes the breast, underlying muscles, axillary contents, and the upper internal mammary lymph node chain.

After closing the mastectomy site, the surgeon may make a stab wound and insert a catheter. The catheter removes blood that may collect under the skin flaps, preventing healing and predisposing you to infection. Less commonly, large pressure dressings are applied rather than insertion of a catheter. If a graft was needed to close the wound, a pressure dressing will be placed over the donor site.

A new technique, *laser mastectomy*, doesn't involve overnight hospitalization and is currently gaining attention. To be considered for this procedure, a woman must have been diagnosed with breast cancer and must have one or more supportive family members living with her. If a woman undergoes this procedure, she'll be sedated beforehand and then given a general anesthetic. The breast is removed using a laser. Drains are inserted and local anesthetics are injected into the wound before closing the incision to reduce postoperative pain.

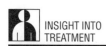

Types of breast surgery

The type of procedure the surgeon chooses depends on the size and location of the tumor and the degree of cancer spread.

Partial (segmental) excision
In this procedure, the surgeon removes the lump, approximately 1 inch (2 to 3 centimeters) of healthy tissue surrounding it, and the membranes over the chest muscles directly behind the lump. The axillary lymph nodes (in the armpit) also may be removed. Some breast tissue remains. Radiation therapy may follow surgery.

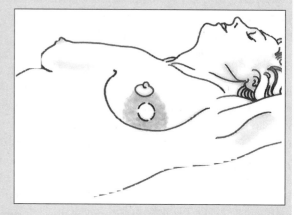

Subcutaneous mastectomy
In this procedure, the surgeon removes breast tissue while retaining breast skin. The tissue is examined for invasive cancer. If cancer is found, more extensive surgery is scheduled. If staging was performed during an earlier biopsy (removal and analysis of tissue), the subcutaneous mastectomy and breast implant insertion may take place at the same time.

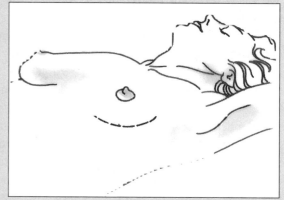

Simple (total) mastectomy
In this procedure, the surgeon removes the breast tissue and the axillary (underarm) lymph nodes closest to the breast. Radiation therapy typically follows.

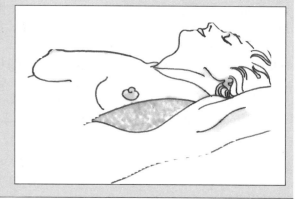

Types of breast surgery *(continued)*

Modified radical mastectomy
In this procedure, the surgeon removes the breast, axillary lymph nodes, and chest muscle but preserves the pectoralis major muscle. It's the most common surgery for breast cancer.

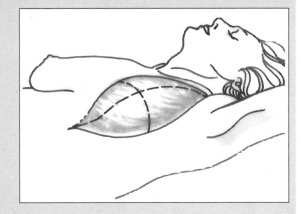

Radical mastectomy
In this procedure, the surgeon removes the breast, all the axillary lymph nodes, chest muscle, pectoralis major and pectoralis minor muscles, and surrounding fat, tissue, and skin.

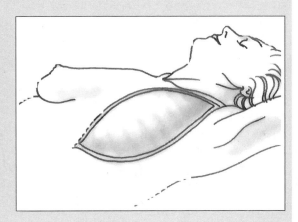

What are the possible complications?
After any type of mastectomy, infection and delayed healing are possible complications. However, the major complication of radical mastectomy is swelling of the lymph vessels, which typically occurs soon after surgery and persists for years. Removal of the lymph nodes that drain the axilla may interfere with lymphatic drainage of the arm on the affected side.

What happens after the surgery?
▪ After the operation, your arm on the affected side will be elevated on a pillow to enhance circulation and prevent swelling. (See *Recovering from a mastectomy,* page 378.)

SELF-HELP

Recovering from a mastectomy

After you have been discharged from the hospital, follow these important guidelines.

Take care of yourself
- Make sure to wash cuts and scrapes on the affected side promptly and contact the doctor immediately if you notice itching, swelling, or hardening of tissue.
- Use the arm on the affected side as much as possible. Avoid keeping it in a lowered position for a long period.
- Perform daily range-of-motion exercises with both arms to maintain symmetry in size and to prevent additional deformities.
- You may find that you're more easily fatigued than you were before the surgery. Rest frequently during the day for the first few weeks after discharge.

Continue to examine yourself
Even though you've lost one breast to cancer, you should continue to give yourself monthly breast self-examinations of the remaining breast and the mastectomy site. You might want to verify that you're performing the technique correctly by having the nurse observe you performing the breast self-examination.

Consider a prosthesis
If necessary, discuss the possibility of a permanent prosthesis with your health care provider. This can be fitted 3 to 4 weeks after surgery. Prostheses (artificial body parts) are available in a wide range of styles, skin tones, and weights from lingerie shops, medical supply stores, and department stores.

Other points to remember
- Make sure that you don't allow any other health care providers to take blood pressure readings, give injections, or perform venipunctures on the affected arm. It's a good idea to wear a medical identification bracelet that states these restrictions.
- Keep all scheduled postoperative appointments.
- Many women feel self-conscious after a mastectomy and tend to dress so as not to draw attention to themselves. However, you may find that dressing the way you used to before the mastectomy boosts your self-confidence.

- The nurse will teach you arm exercises to prevent muscle shortening and contracture of the shoulder joint and to make lymph drainage easier. Arm exercises can usually begin on the first day after surgery, and other exercises can be added each day depending on the procedure and your needs.
- Because mastectomy causes emotional distress, the nurse will need to teach you to conserve your energy and to recognize the early signs of fatigue. You'll be encouraged to view the operative site, describe its appearance, and express your feelings about it. The nurse will be there to offer support when you look at the wound for the first time.
- Your nurse will contact the American Cancer Society's "Reach to Recovery" rehabilitation program to arrange for a volunteer who's had a mastectomy to talk with you.

- After 2 to 3 days, you'll be fitted for a temporary breast pad. Soft and lightweight, the pad may be inserted into a bra without stays or underwires.

DILATATION AND CURETTAGE OR EVACUATION

A dilatation and curettage (D&C) involves widening the cervical canal with a dilator and scraping the uterus with a spoon-shaped instrument called a *curette*. A dilatation and evacuation (D&E) involves widening the cervical canal with a dilator and then removing the fetus or fetal tissue with a curette or a curette with suction attached.

Why is this procedure done?

A D&C is performed to remove tissue after an incomplete abortion, to diagnose and control abnormal uterine bleeding, to explore the uterus, and to obtain tissue samples for study.

A D&E can also be used to remove tissue after an incomplete abortion in the late first trimester or early second trimester. It may also be done to effect an abortion, usually up to 12 weeks of gestation but occasionally up to 16 weeks. The procedure may be done as late as 20 weeks but is associated with increased risks. (See *Recovering from a D&C or D&E*.)

What happens before the procedure?

- The doctor or nurse will explain the procedure to you and answer your questions.
- You'll be instructed to have nothing to eat or drink after midnight before the procedure.
- You must sign a consent form.

What happens during the procedure?

The doctor performs these procedures in the operating room, short procedure unit, clinic, or specially equipped office. After administration of an anesthetic, the doctor will perform a pelvic examination, expand the cervix with an instrument called a *dilator*, and then remove the superficial layer of the endometrium (uterine lining) with a

SELF-HELP

Recovering from a D&C or D&E

When you've been discharged from the hospital, follow these important guidelines.

Know when to call the doctor
- Report any signs of infection, such as fever, chills, and bloody discharge.
- Take pain relievers to control discomfort, but report any unrelenting sharp pain to your doctor.
- Expect spotting and discharge for a week or longer after the procedure. This is normal. However, report any bright red blood to your doctor immediately.

Other instructions
- Be sure to keep your scheduled follow-up appointments with your doctor so that your progress can be evaluated.
- If you need birth control counseling, be sure to ask the nurse for an appropriate referral.
- Resume activity as tolerated, but don't use tampons, douch, or engage in vigorous exercise or sexual intercourse for 10 days after the procedure.

curette. He or she may also perform a biopsy (removal and analysis of tissue), if necessary.

If a D&C is used to treat an incomplete abortion, the doctor also removes the remaining products of conception.

In an elective abortion, the surgeon may use a synthetic dilator or wedges that are inserted the evening before surgery. The surgeon then uses a curette to remove the fetus or fetal tissue.

What are the possible complications?

Potential complications of a D&C include uterine perforation, hemorrhage, and infection. Second-trimester D&E may cause cervical injury and may affect future pregnancies; it can lead to miscarriage, cervical incompetence, or premature birth.

What happens after the procedure?

- You'll have a pad in place to absorb vaginal discharge.
- You'll be given pain relievers for cramps and pelvic and lower back pain.
- You'll be instructed to report any continuous, sharp pain that doesn't diminish with pain relievers; this symptom indicates perforation of the uterus.
- You'll be groggy and won't be able to drive.

HYSTERECTOMY

A hysterectomy is the removal of the uterus. It can be performed using a vaginal or an abdominal approach, but the latter approach gives the doctor a better view of the pelvic organs and a larger operating field.

Hysterectomy may be classified as subtotal, total, panhysterectomy, or radical. A *subtotal hysterectomy*, which is performed rarely, is the removal of all of the uterus except the cervix. In *total hysterectomy*, the surgeon removes all of the uterus, including the cervix. In *panhysterectomy*, which requires the abdominal approach, the surgeon removes all of the uterus (hysterectomy) as well as the ovaries and the fallopian tubes (bilateral salpingo-oophorectomy). *Radical hysterectomy* is the removal of the uterus, ovaries, fallopian tubes, adjoining ligaments and lymph nodes, the upper one-third of the vagina, and surrounding tissues.

Why is the surgery done?

Hysterectomy (and sometimes removal of surrounding tissue) should be performed for treating malignant and nonmalignant growths of the uterus, cervix, and surrounding tissue; control of uterine bleeding and hemorrhage; irreparable uterine rupture or perforation; life-threatening pelvic infection; treatment of endometriosis when conservative treatment has failed; and correction of problems involving pelvic floor relaxation.

What happens before the surgery?

- The nurse will reinforce the surgeon's explanation of the procedure and make sure that you've signed a consent form.
- If necessary, the nurse will review with you the preparation that may be required: a douche, enema, shower with an antibacterial soap, and shaving the site.
- You'll be taught about postoperative techniques such as turning, coughing, and deep breathing; performing range-of-motion exercises; and early walking.

What happens during the surgery?

A hysterectomy is usually performed while you're under general anesthesia. Using an abdominal approach, the surgeon makes a vertical incision from the navel to the pubic region or a horizontal incision in the lower abdomen and removes the uterus and necessary accompanying structures. Then the surgeon closes the abdomen and applies an abdominal dressing and a pad to absorb any discharge.

The vaginal approach doesn't require an external incision. Instead, the surgeon makes an incision above and around the cervix, removes the uterus, and then stitches the opening closed and applies a pad. This approach is not used in panhysterectomy or radical hysterectomy.

What are the possible complications?

Possible complications of hysterectomy include wound infection, urine retention, abdominal distention, inflammation and clotting of blood vessels, pneumonia, hemorrhage, ureteral injury, and bowel injury. Abdominal hysterectomy may also be complicated by wound rupture, obstruction of the pulmonary artery, and intestinal paralysis. Psychological complications may include depression, loss of sexual desire, and a perceived loss of femininity.

SELF-HELP

Recovering from a hysterectomy

When you've been discharged from the hospital, follow these important guidelines.

Take it easy
- Avoid driving, heavy lifting, or heavy housework for at least 1 month (longer, if your doctor recommends). Also avoid vigorous exercise, including jogging, aerobics, dancing, and active sports, for the same amount of time.
- Moderate exercise such as walking is helpful. You should increase the distance you walk a little each day.
- Avoid sex, douching, and the use of tampons as prescribed by your doctor — usually for 3 to 6 weeks.

Other instructions
- Call your doctor right away if you have any complications: fever, increased bleeding, and difficulty with urination or bowel movements.
- Eat foods high in protein, vitamin C, and iron to aid healing.
- You may feel depressed or irritable temporarily because of abrupt hormonal fluctuations. The change in your mood may make it difficult for your family members to know how to respond to you. It may help them to know that your reactions are normal; knowing this may enable them to respond calmly and supportively to your needs.

What happens after the surgery?

- Immediately after surgery, you'll probably have to lie on your back but will be asked to turn from side to side. On the day after surgery, you'll be encouraged to walk to promote adequate circulation.
- You'll have a catheter inserted to prevent urine retention.
- You should expect some abdominal cramps and moderate drainage from the incision site that will require a perineal pad.
- The nurse will encourage you to cough, deep breathe, and turn frequently — at least every 2 hours — and to listen to your breath sounds to note any respiratory complications.
- You'll be given medications to relieve pain and may be offered a heating pad to relieve abdominal pain.
- You'll perform leg exercises to maintain adequate circulation. (See *Recovering from a hysterectomy.*)

Laparoscopy and Laparotomy

A laparoscopy is the examination of the upper abdominal cavity and reproductive organs using an endoscope (an instrument that allows the surgeon to observe the inside of a hollow organ). A laparotomy is any surgical incision into the abdominal cavity.

After a laparoscopy, the person may go home the next day; after a laparotomy, the hospital stay will be the same as for any other abdominal surgery.

Why is the procedure done?

A laparoscopy lets the doctor visualize the organs in the pelvis and upper abdominal cavity for diagnosis or further surgery. Laparoscopic procedures may include tubal ligations, removal of ovarian cysts, salpingectomy (removal of the fallopian tubes), oophorectomy (removal of the ovaries), cholecystectomy (removal of the gallbladder), and appendectomy, among others. They may also be used in staging cancer, some liver biopsies and, possibly, removal of an ectopic pregnancy.

Laparoscopy may also help detect abnormalities such as cysts, adhesions, fibroids, and infection; identify the cause of pelvic pain by diagnosing endometriosis, ectopic pregnancy, or pelvic inflammatory disease; and evaluate pelvic masses or the fallopian tubes of infertile patients.

Laparotomy may be performed to treat gynecologic conditions unsuited for treatment by laparoscopy — for example, to remove ovarian cysts that may rupture or to remove growths that are too large for removal by laparoscopy.

When shouldn't the procedure be done?

Laparoscopy should be avoided in a person with a blocked intestine, abdominal cancer, acute abdominal tuberculosis, or ruptured ectopic pregnancy with massive bleeding.

What happens before the procedure?

- The nurse or doctor will describe the laparoscopic procedure and answer any questions you may have.

Recovering from a laparoscopy or a laparotomy

After you have been discharged from the hospital, follow these important guidelines.

Report any problems

After a laparoscopy, it's important to report bright red vaginal bleeding; a fever of 100.4° F (38° C) or higher; severe abdominal pain; redness, puffiness, or drainage from the incision; or any nausea, vomiting, or diarrhea.

Other instructions

• Wait until the day after a laparoscopy to bathe or remove the bandage.
• Eat lightly after a laparoscopy because there may be residual abdominal gas.
• After a laparoscopy, wait 2 days before you resume your normal activities.
• Avoid strenuous work and sports for 1 week or as recommended by the doctor.
• Keep all follow-up medical appointments.
• After a laparotomy, follow the prescribed activity restrictions.

• You must fast 6 to 8 hours before the procedure because a general anesthetic will most likely be administered.
• If you're a smoker, you mustn't smoke for about 12 hours before the procedure.

What happens during the procedure?

A regional or a general anesthetic is administered for a laparoscopy. The surgeon makes a small incision slightly below the navel and introduces a trocar (a surgical instrument used for removing fluids) and a catheter into the incision. The trocar is then removed, and carbon dioxide gas is pumped into the abdominal cavity to distend the area to be visualized. If additional instruments are needed, they may be inserted through another incision made below the initial one or they may be passed through the laparoscope. The laparoscope allows passage of surgical instruments such as lasers. When the surgeon has completed the specific procedure, the carbon dioxide gas is removed; the incision is stitched with absorbable suture; and a dressing is applied.

A laparotomy is performed under general anesthesia. The surgeon makes an abdominal incision and explores the entire abdomen for disease. Any diseased organ is removed or repaired, the incision is closed, and a dressing is applied.

What are the possible complications?

Possible complications of laparoscopy include excessive bleeding, abdominal cramps, and shoulder pain. These effects may result from infection of the abdomen with carbon dioxide.

What happens after the procedure?

• You'll have some minor vaginal bleeding.
• If you've had a laparoscopy, you may have abdominal cramps or shoulder pain. You'll be given pain relievers. Feelings of bloating or abdominal fullness will subside as the gas in the abdomen is absorbed into the bloodstream, exchanged in the lungs, and exhaled.
• You may be discharged the same day if you had a laparoscopy. (See *Recovering from a laparoscopy or a laparotomy.*)

CERVICAL CONIZATION

Also called a *cone biopsy*, cervical conization is the surgical removal of a cone-shaped portion of the uterine cervix for diagnostic and therapeutic purposes. Before development of colposcopic evaluation, conization was the method of choice for evaluating abnormal Pap tests. It's currently done less often. (See *Performing cervical conization.*)

Why is the procedure done?
Cervical conization is usually performed to remove a precancerous portion of the endocervix (inside the cervical canal) when there's an abnormality.

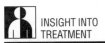
INSIGHT INTO
TREATMENT

Performing cervical conization

These illustrations indicate the area that is removed during conization.

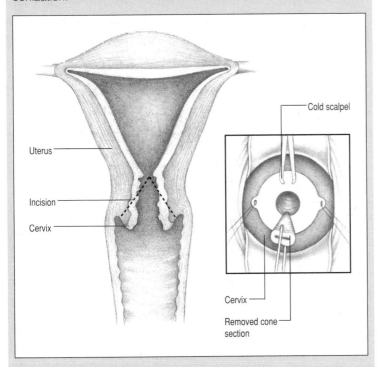

Recovering from cervical conization

When you've been discharged from the hospital, follow these important guidelines.

Get follow-up care
- Make sure that you return for a follow-up examination in 2 to 4 weeks.
- Keep in mind the importance of lifelong follow-up care. Current recommendations are for Pap tests every 6 to 12 months.

Other instructions
- Remember that it's very important for you to take all prescribed prophylactic antibiotics to prevent infection. (Doxycycline for 5 to 7 days may be ordered.)
- Immediately report any signs or symptoms of infection or excessive bleeding.
- Be aware that menstrual bleeding may be heavier, with a brownish premenstrual discharge.
- Avoid sexual intercourse and the use of douches until after the postoperative visit.

Conization is also performed when colposcopic examination can't rule out cancer and when there is evidence of severe dysplasia (abnormal cell growth) and cancer, especially if multiple lesions are present. (Laser carbon dioxide therapy may be used for lesser lesions, to retain optimum fertility, or for conditions such as chronic cervicitis, condylomata, and moderate dysplasia.)

What happens before the procedure?
Because conization is performed on an outpatient basis, a nurse will teach you before the procedure about home care, possible complications, and follow-up care.

What happens during the procedure?
The procedure is performed in the outpatient department, and you receive a general anesthetic. The surgeon uses a scalpel or a laser to make a circular cut around the external opening of the cervix to remove a cone-shaped piece of tissue. A laser is believed to cause less bleeding at the operative site. The surgeon then sutures the site.

What are the possible complications?
Potential complications include cervical perforation, heavy bleeding, infection, infertility, cervical stenosis, decreased cervical mucus, and premature labor in future pregnancies due to weakening of the cervix.

What happens after the procedure?
- Your vital signs are monitored.
- Check your sanitary pad, monitoring the amount and color of all vaginal discharge. (See *Recovering from cervical conization.*)

CERVICAL SUTURING

Also called *cerclage*, cervical suturing uses a purse-string suture to reinforce an incompetent cervix in order to maintain pregnancy. Typically performed between the 14th and 18th week of pregnancy, after the major risk of spontaneous abortion has passed, cervical suturing

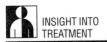

INSIGHT INTO
TREATMENT

Understanding cervical suturing

In a patient with an incompetent cervix, the cervical canal partially dilates, allowing the membranes to prolapse. To help correct this defect and allow a pregnancy to continue, the doctor may perform cervical cerclage. In this procedure, he or she places Mersilene, a nonabsorbable suture, around the cervix beneath the mucous membrane to constrict the opening as shown here.

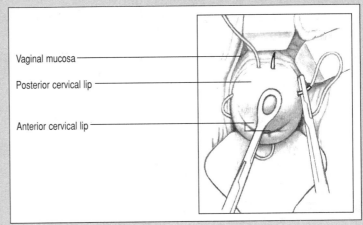

As shown in this cross section, the suture works much like the string in a drawstring bag. The key to this procedure's success is placing the suture high enough on the cervix so that it remains in place.

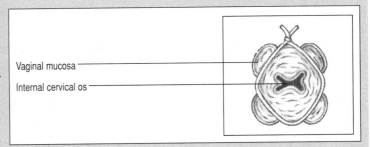

should be performed for women with a history of premature delivery caused by an incompetent cervix.

Two cervical suturing procedures are commonly used. The modified Shirodkar technique involves threading and tying a Mersilene band around the internal cervical os, which provides the opening into the uterus. Cervical cerclage, or the McDonald procedure, places a nonabsorbable suture around the cervix. Both techniques are successful in maintaining pregnancy for about 90% of the women who have it done. (See *Understanding cervical suturing*.)

Why is the procedure done?
Cerclage keeps the internal cervical os closed until the pregnancy has reached term, preventing premature labor and delivery. It should be done when an incompetent cervix is confirmed. Some predisposing

SELF-HELP

Recovering from cervical suturing

When you've been discharged from the hospital, follow these important guidelines.

Know when to call the doctor

- Immediately report uterine contractions, amniotic membrane rupture, vaginal bleeding, fever, or pain.
- Normally, there will be some spotting from the cervical incision for several days after the procedure. This is nothing to worry about. However, you should immediately report any bright red blood or excessive bleeding to the doctor.

Other instructions

- Change the perineal pad as needed or at least every 8 hours. Don't be alarmed if you find tiny pieces of suture on the pad. These come from the absorbable suture used to close the incision — not from the suture holding the cervix closed.
- Don't have sexual intercourse until you've had your postoperative checkup. Your doctor may put you on pelvic rest (no sexual intercourse, tampons, or douching) and bed rest for the remainder of the pregnancy.

factors of cervical incompetence are previous second-trimester elective abortion, previous difficult delivery, or injury to the cervix.

When shouldn't the procedure be done?

Cervical suturing should not be done if the woman has vaginal bleeding or uterine cramps.

What happens before the procedure?

- The doctor or nurse will briefly explain the procedure to you.
- After fetal viability has been established, you'll receive a spinal or a general anesthetic.

What happens during the procedure?

If the modified Shirodkar technique is used, the surgeon will pull back the vaginal walls with an instrument and elevate the vaginal mucosa (mucous membrane). After making an incision, the surgeon will weave a narrow nonabsorbable suture around the internal cervical os of the uterus, tighten the suture to close the os, restore the vaginal mucosa to its original position, and suture it in place, usually with an absorbable suture.

The sutures are allowed to remain in place until the pregnancy has reached full term, at which time they are removed and labor is allowed to begin spontaneously.

What are the possible complications?

Cervical suturing can cause complications such as preterm labor, hemorrhage, blood infection, or rupture of the amniotic membranes. Occasionally, scarring and narrowing of the os occur as a result of suturing and render the cervix incapable of dilating after the suture is removed. When this happens, a cesarean delivery is necessary.

What happens after the procedure?

You'll need to rest in bed for the first 24 hours. Your activity level will be increased afterward as appropriate. (See *Recovering from cervical suturing.*)

CESAREAN SECTION

Cesarean section is an operation in which the fetus is delivered by surgical incisions in the abdominal wall and uterus. It becomes necessary when vaginal delivery is unsafe for the mother or fetus.

Several approaches may be used. The procedure of choice, lower segment cesarean delivery, involves a vertical or horizontal abdominal incision as well as an incision in the lower uterine segment. This characteristically leads to less blood loss for the woman and a stronger uterine scar than the classic procedure, which involves vertical incisions in both the abdomen and uterus.

Cesarean sections are done in about 25% of all pregnancies.

Why is the surgery done?

Most cesarean sections are performed to manage or prevent complications that make vaginal delivery impossible or hazardous for the mother or fetus. For instance, cesarean delivery is commonly performed when the woman's pelvis is too small to allow passage of the fetal head. It may also be performed in a number of other conditions, including pregnancy-induced high blood pressure, maternal diabetes, fetal distress, breech presentation, previous uterine surgery, and an ineffective labor pattern caused by uterine dysfunction.

What happens before the surgery?

- The doctor or nurse will explain the procedure to you and tell you what to expect after the birth.
- You'll have an urinary catheter inserted to prevent bladder damage during surgery.
- You'll be required to sign a consent form.
- If your partner is allowed in the operating room, he'll be required to scrub or dress according to hospital policy.

What happens during the surgery?

You'll receive a general or a regional (spinal or epidural) anesthetic. Shaving and cleaning the incision site may be performed in the operating room immediately before the operation.

The surgeon makes an incision in the abdomen, draws back the bladder with a retractor, and makes an incision in the uterus. He or she then removes the retractor and delivers the baby. Next, the sur-

SELF-HELP

Recovering from a cesarean section

When you've been discharged from the hospital, follow these important guidelines.

Know when to call the doctor
- Immediately report hemorrhage, chest or leg pain, shortness of breath, separation of the edges of the incision, and signs of infection (fever, difficult urination, or flank pain).
- Check with your doctor before resuming an exercise program. Your doctor will probably allow you to engage in walking and isometric exercises, but you should avoid strenuous exercises until after your postpartum checkup.

Other instructions
- Be sure to keep your follow-up appointment (usually in 4 weeks) so that your doctor can evaluate your progress.
- Express your concerns to the doctor about which contraceptive measures to use and when you can resume sexual intercourse.

geon suctions the baby's nose and mouth with a bulb syringe to clear the breathing passages and then completes the delivery. After clamping and cutting the umbilical cord, the surgeon transfers the infant to the newborn care team.

Next, the surgeon administers the drug Pitocin to contract the uterus. This helps reduce blood loss and promotes delivery of the placenta. Then the surgeon closes the incision. Finally, the uterus is massaged to promote contraction and thus prevent heavy bleeding.

What are the possible complications?

Complications for the woman may include anesthesia reactions, infection, hemorrhage, ruptured wound, and injury to pelvic or abdominal organs. Fetal complications may include oxygen insufficiency, respiratory distress, and prematurity.

What happens after surgery?

- The nurse will feel the uterus to determine uterine relaxation.
- If you received a spinal or an epidural anesthetic, you'll experience tingling when sensation returns. If you received a spinal anesthetic, you may have a headache. Measures to prevent such headache include drinking adequate fluids and lying flat in bed for 8 hours after the operation.
- If appropriate, every attempt will be made to provide for early contact between you and your infant. (See *Recovering from a cesarean section.*)

REMOVAL OF OVARIES AND FALLOPIAN TUBES

The surgical removal of one or both ovaries is called an *oophorectomy*. The removal of one or both fallopian tubes is called a *salpingectomy*. When the procedures are done together, they may be referred to as a *salpingo-oophorectomy*.

The removal of both ovaries eliminates much of the woman's production of estrogen and progesterone, and her loss of estrogen may result in a variety of symptoms. For young women especially, this procedure must be considered carefully beforehand because of the loss of estrogen's benefits.

Why are the surgeries done?

Oophorectomy should be performed to treat ovarian cysts, ovarian cancer, an estrogen-dependent tumor, or an ectopic pregnancy. Both ovaries may be removed during a hysterectomy if uterine disease has spread to them.

Salpingectomy may be performed to treat infection of the fallopian tubes, severe pelvic inflammatory disease, endometriosis, or an ectopic pregnancy, or to provide permanent contraception.

Salpingectomy almost always accompanies routine hysterectomy because the fallopian tubes offer no benefit if the woman will never again be pregnant. Many experts debate whether one or both ovaries should also be removed routinely. The removal of only one ovary ensures that the woman will continue to have the benefit of estrogen production. If both ovaries are removed, the woman will probably require estrogen replacement therapy, which carries risks of its own.

What happens before the surgeries?

- If both of your ovaries are to be removed, discuss your feelings related to the loss of reproductive abilities with your doctor.
- The nurse may instruct you to douche with Betadine solution before the operation, if ordered, to clean the vagina and to prevent infection.
- You'll have an urinary catheter inserted. It will be in place for 24 hours after surgery.

What happens during the surgeries?

While you're under general anesthesia, the surgeon will make an incision and locate and remove one or both ovaries or fallopian tubes. If a hysterectomy is to be performed, the uterus will also be removed. If the ovary is being removed because of cancer, the surgeon will also perform a biopsy (removal and analysis of tissue) on adjacent lymph nodes.

What are the possible complications?

Complications are rare but include hemorrhage, infection, a collapsed lung, obstruction of the pulmonary artery, psychological problems resulting from changes in self-concept, and physical (menopausal) changes resulting from loss of estrogen. Menopausal symptoms are usually delayed for several days or weeks after surgery unless both ovaries were removed.

Recovering from gynecologic surgery

When you've been discharged from the hospital following surgery to remove your ovaries or fallopian tubes, follow these important guidelines.

Talk to your doctor

- Take your medications. However, if you have any doubts about estrogen replacement therapy, discuss your concerns about its risks and benefits with your doctor.
- Immediately report any abnormal bleeding, pain, fever, or problems with urination.
- If the uterus was also removed, you'll no longer get your monthly menstrual period.

Keep follow-up appointments

- It's important that you return for a follow-up pelvic examination 6 to 8 weeks after surgery to check healing of the internal incisions.
- Even if you've had a hysterectomy, you'll still need to have annual Pap tests to screen for cervical cancer.

What happens after the surgeries?

- The nurse will have you cough and breathe deeply every hour to prevent lung problems.
- You'll be encouraged to walk as soon and as frequently as possible to prevent inflammation of veins and lung collapse.
- Medication will be administered to control pain, and estrogen replacement may be prescribed (usually once you've begun to walk again). (See *Recovering from gynecologic surgery.*)

OTHER TREATMENTS

Infertility therapies

Medically speaking, infertility is the inability to conceive and carry a pregnancy to viability after 1 year of regular intercourse without contraception. Almost one-fifth of all couples in North America have difficulty conceiving. The causes of infertility are varied. Female causes account for about 40% of all cases, male causes account for about 40%, and interactive or unexplained causes account for 20%.

Once the cause of the infertility is known, treatment can be initiated. Several types of treatment are available, depending on the diagnosis. Drug therapy and surgery are commonly used to restore normal reproductive function. Other treatments include artificial insemination, in vitro fertilization, gamete intrafallopian transfer, and zygote intrafallopian transfer. (See also "Fertility Drugs," pages 370 to 371.) Couples have an 18% to 25% chance of conception through in vitro fertilization and gamete intrafallopian transfer, respectively, in reputable programs. The zygote transfer, abbreviated ZIFT, is the newest option and has a success rate of approximately 40% among certain couples. (See *Coping with infertility.*)

Why are the treatments done?

Infertility therapies are undertaken to have biological children.

When are the treatments done?

In women, infertility therapies may be performed to counteract a cervical problem such as a cervical environment hostile to sperm.

They may also be done if a woman has cervical incompetence or a uterine problem, such as a bicornuate uterus or uterine tumors. What's more, they may be done if a woman has a fallopian tube problem such as adhesions from endometriosis, or an ovarian problem such as absence of ovulation.

In men, infertility therapies may be done to treat insufficient sperm production, inadequate motility of the sperm, blockage of the sperm within the reproductive system, and problems in ejaculation. In a joint problem, the therapies may address sexual dysfunction or female antibody reaction to healthy sperm. Unexplained infertility, however, is possible.

What happens during the treatments?

Treatments vary depending on the cause of infertility, and even when the cause is unknown, various therapeutic approaches might be tried. Therapy might consist of changing habits. For instance, treatment of a low sperm count might consist of eliminating factors that reduce sperm production, such as tight-fitting underwear or use of hot tubs or saunas. The workup may indicate the need for sexual counseling. Surgery might be warranted if, for example, the male has a varicocele. Advances in tubal microsurgery have offered treatment of various tubal problems. Medications, such as drugs used to induce ovulation, may be needed.

Sophisticated techniques may now be able to help infertile couples more than ever before, but there are significant physical, emotional, and financial costs.

Artificial insemination

Artificial insemination is the instillation of seminal fluid into the vaginal canal, cervix, or directly into the uterus (in cases where the cervical mucus isn't conducive to the sperm's survival). The partner's sperm or donor sperm (in cases of male infertility) may be used.

In vitro fertilization

In vitro fertilization may be performed when infertility is due to fallopian tube problems. This procedure bypasses the fallopian tubes by harvesting mature eggs from the ovary, fertilizing them in a test tube, and then implanting the fertilized eggs in the woman's uterus.

Gamete intrafallopian transfer

In this technique, the eggs are retrieved from the ovary and implanted into the fallopian tube, along with sperm. The goal is for fertilization to occur naturally.

SELF-HELP

Coping with infertility

Infertility is often an emotionally wrenching experience for couples. Here are some tips to help you get through it.

Seek professional help
- If you remain infertile, seek out professional counseling to help you decide on other options, which may include adoption, choosing to remain childless, or using a surrogate mother (if not legally prohibited).
- Seek counseling if you're having difficulty communicating your feelings or express uncontrollable anger or grief.
- Make sure that your doctor provides you with telephone numbers of support groups, such as Resolve, a national organization for infertile couples and individuals.

Other instructions
- If you're involved in lengthy fertility programs, try to get on with other aspects of your lives.
- Make sure that you return for follow-up appointments as necessary.

Zygote intrafallopian transfer

In this new technique, the eggs are harvested from the ovary and fertilized in a test tube. The fertilized egg is then placed directly into the fallopian tube, the natural site for conception.

What are the possible complications?

Infertility therapies cause few physical complications but produce considerable emotional stress. There may be complications associated with drug therapy or secondary to surgery. Reputable sperm banks test donors for antibodies to HIV to avoid spreading AIDS. Sperm banks also use frozen semen to ward off the problem.

DOUCHING

Douching is the instillation of fluid with or without medication into the vagina. Commonly used solutions include sterile water, normal saline solution, and antiseptic solutions such as povidone-iodine. Various disposable douches are commercially available for the treatment of vaginal inflammation. When performed after surgery, douching requires aseptic technique.

Douching for treatment of infection or infertility is usually done by the woman in her own home.

Why is the treatment done?

Douching is commonly used to treat gynecologic disorders, such as vaginal infection and inflammation. It's also used before and after operations, either to instill medication or sterilize the vagina. For example, vaginal douching with a povidone-iodine and water solution is frequently performed before a hysterectomy to prevent the transmission of infectious organisms from the vagina into the operating field.

Solutions that contain vinegar or sodium bicarbonate and water, which alter the protective pH balance and thereby create a compatible environment for sperm, are commonly used in the treatment of infertility. Many women douche with commercial solutions for personal hygiene after intercourse or at the end of the menstrual cycle to remove blood and tissue.

When shouldn't the treatment be done?

Women who are pregnant or who have untreated sexually transmitted diseases shouldn't douche because it may cause an air embolism and death. It also shouldn't be done for 4 to 6 weeks after miscarriage or childbirth because it may increase the risk of infection.

Frequent douching (more than twice a month) isn't recommended unless prescribed because it can irritate the vaginal lining and increase the risk of infection by disrupting the vagina's normal protective mechanism. Self-prescribed treatment for vaginal irritation or infections is strongly discouraged by most health care providers.

What happens before the treatment?

- The nurse will explain the procedure to you and provide privacy.
- You'll be instructed to empty your bladder.
- You should wash your hands before administering the douche.

What happens during the treatment?

Preoperative douching is usually performed by the nurse and given while you're in bed on a bedpan to ensure maximum cleaning. You may also douche in the bathtub or while sitting on the toilet.

One tablespoon of povidone-iodine solution is mixed with approximately 1,000 milliliters (about 1 quart) of warm tap water. Water temperature should be between 100° and 110° F (37.7° and 38.3° C).

Douching for the purpose of altering pH for infertility is usually done by you in the privacy of your own home and should be performed about 30 minutes before sexual intercourse. Vinegar and water solutions are prepared with 1 tablespoon of white vinegar in about 16 ounces (500 milliliters) of warm tap water; sodium bicarbonate douches require 1 tablespoon of baking soda in 1 quart of warm tap water.

You should empty your bladder before the procedure. After mixing the douche solution, the irrigating receptacle is hung at a level just above your hips to allow the solution to flow freely and gently. The nozzle is lubricated and gently inserted about 2 inches (5 centimeters) into the vagina in a downward and backward direction to prevent injury to the vaginal lining. Then, the solution is allowed to flow until the container is empty. The nozzle can be gently rotated during the instillation. If you're using a prefilled container, the nozzle is usually prelubricated. The nozzle is inserted in the same way; then

SELF-HELP

How to douche

To avoid the discomfort and complications of improperly administered douches, take the following precautions:
- Follow the nurse's written instructions for performing the procedure at home. If you're not sure you understand the given instructions, ask the nurse to clarify them for you.
- Report vaginal discharge, itching, odor, or irritation to your health care provider immediately.
- Don't douche frequently unless you're instructed to do so by your doctor. If you do, you may upset your vaginal pH and increase your susceptibility to infection.

the container is gently squeezed to instill the premeasured solution. The nurse will monitor you for signs of any irritation caused by the douching.

What are the possible complications?
Complications are rare, but routine, frequent douching may lead to vaginal dryness, irritation and, possibly, infection.

What happens after the treatment?
You'll be encouraged to lie down for 1 hour after the povidone-iodine douche to obtain maximum therapeutic benefit. (See *How to douche*.)

9

*T*REATING SEXUAL DISORDERS

PROSTHETIC AIDS

PENILE PROSTHESES

A penile prosthesis is a pair of semirigid rods or inflatable cylinders surgically implanted in the penis. This device is commonly used when other treatments for impotence prove ineffective.

Of the two types of penile prostheses, the semirigid device costs less, is easier to implant, and is less likely to require additional surgery to correct mechanical problems. This device is especially beneficial for a man with limited hand or finger function because its use doesn't demand manual dexterity. Its major disadvantage is continuous semierection, which may embarrass the man. (More flexible models have been developed that can be bent into less conspicuous positions.) Some couples also complain that the semirigid prosthesis produces an erection that isn't sexually satisfying because penile girth doesn't increase.

The inflatable prosthesis more closely mimics a normal erection. The person controls erection by squeezing a pump in the scrotum that releases fluid from a reservoir into the implanted cylinders. He then presses the release valve to return fluid to the reservoir and thus lose the erection.

Why is this procedure done?

Penile prostheses are implanted to correct problems with achieving an erection. They're used for men whose impotence results from diabetes, arteriosclerosis, surgical removal of the prostate gland, spinal cord injury, or prolonged use of alcohol or drugs such as antihypertensives. Men whose impotence results from a psychological problem—including sexual performance anxiety, low self-esteem, and past failure at sustaining an erection—are usually referred for sexual counseling. Use of penile prostheses in these men is controversial.

What happens before the procedure?

You shower the evening before and the morning of the surgery, using a special infection-fighting soap. A nurse shaves you in the operating room to reduce the risk of infection.

What happens during the procedure?

Usually the prosthesis is implanted in the operating room under general or spinal anesthesia. The semirigid device may also be implanted on an outpatient basis under local anesthesia.

To implant a semirigid prosthesis, the surgeon makes channels in the spongy penis tissue. The prosthetic rods are inserted into the channels, and the incisions are closed.

To implant an inflatable prosthesis, the surgeon follows the same steps to position the cylinders, then makes an abdominal and a perineal incision and places a reservoir, filled with a small amount of fluid, in the groin. Next, the surgeon places a pump in the lateral portion of the scrotum and connects the cylinders, reservoir, and pump with tubing. Then the surgeon squeezes the pump to test the function of the prosthesis.

What are the possible complications?

An implanted prosthesis may cause infection, erosion of the penis, and persistent pain, which may require removal of the implant. (See *Caring for yourself after implantation of a penile prosthesis.*)

Both types of prostheses place the person at risk for infection, but the incidence is low (about 1% to 4%). The inflatable prosthesis may also leak fluid, or the tubing connecting the pump reservoir and cylinders may become kinked.

What happens after the procedure?

- Ice packs will be applied to your penis for 24 hours after surgery. Your doctor may prescribe pain relievers.
- Your doctor will warn you not to inflate the implant until he or she says it's safe to do so.

SEX THERAPY

SEMANS' TECHNIQUE

This technique helps treat premature ejaculation. In this technique, the partner manually stimulates the penis, halting just before ejaculation so that a man becomes more aware of his sexual response. Also

---

SELF-HELP

Caring for yourself after implantation of a penile prosthesis

After you're discharged from the hospital, follow these important guidelines.

Take special precautions

- Pull the scrotal pump downward to ensure proper alignment.
- Wash the incision site daily with an antibacterial soap. Watch for signs of infection and report them immediately to your doctor.
- Keep all follow-up appointments to ensure that the incision is healing properly.

Other points to remember

- Be aware that scrotal swelling and discoloration may last up to 3 weeks.
- Be aware that your partner may experience discomfort or pain when you're permitted to resume sexual activity — usually about 6 weeks after surgery. This may result from an inability to have intercourse for a prolonged period before surgery. She should use a water-soluble jelly, such as K-Y Jelly, to minimize or avoid discomfort.

SELF-HELP

Using Semans' technique

When you begin to practice what you were taught, follow these important guidelines:
- Be sure to set aside time to satisfy your partner's sexual needs.
- Go to counseling sessions where you and your partner can discuss your progress in using Semans' technique.
- Be aware that honest communication between you and your partner is important.

called the start-stop technique, it was developed by Dr. Semans in 1956. Typically, Semans' technique is combined with nongenital and genital touching exercises between a man and his partner to increase communication and reduce sexual anxiety.

Why is this therapy done?
- To treat premature ejaculation
- To help a man gradually regain control over ejaculation through start-stop stimulation

What happens during the therapy?
Semans' technique is taught by a sex therapist, doctor, or psychologist. The partner begins by stimulating the man's penis with her hands until he feels the urge to ejaculate. She then stops the stimulation and waits until his urge to ejaculate passes before she begins stimulating his penis again. This stimulation is repeated four times, each time stopping short of ejaculation. Next, the partner stimulates the man's penis one more time, allowing him to ejaculate. The couple should avoid progressing to intercourse until this controlled manual stimulation has been mastered. (See *Using Semans' technique.*)

What are the possible complications?
There are no reported complications associated with this procedure. However, sexual dysfunction can cause feelings of anger, guilt, rejection, avoidance, and insecurity. Therapy to help enhance communication is important.

SQUEEZE TECHNIQUE

Developed by the sex therapists Masters and Johnson, the squeeze technique is the treatment of choice for premature ejaculation. In this technique, the sex partner briefly squeezes the man's penis just behind the head of the penis when the man feels the urge to ejaculate. This delays ejaculation and helps the man gradually gain control over it.

Why is this therapy done?
The squeeze technique prevents premature ejaculation.

What happens during the therapy?

This technique is taught by a psychologist, doctor, or sex therapist. The partner manually stimulates the man's penis. He lets her know when he feels the urge to ejaculate. She then positions her fingers around the penis and squeezes firmly for 3 to 4 seconds. This will cause slight flaccidity and forestall ejaculation. (See *Using the squeeze technique*.)

What are the possible complications?

The squeeze technique may cause temporary impotence, but this is uncommon.

SENSATE FOCUS THERAPY

Sensate focus therapy involves nongenital and genital touching exercises between the person and his or her partner to increase communication and reduce sexual anxiety. Helpful in treating various sexual disorders, sensate focus therapy encourages a couple to relax and express intimacy. This therapy can be one of several methods employed by the therapist to help couples experiencing sexual dysfunction. Initially, vaginal penetration is prohibited during these exercises to encourage each partner to focus on sensual feelings without being burdened by preset goals or performance anxiety. As a result, many couples discover or renew a deep sense of intimacy.

Why is this therapy done?

Sensate focus therapy decreases sexual anxiety by increasing a couple's awareness of touch and sexual intimacy. It's recommended for people who suffer from various sexual dysfunctions, especially when personal and emotional difficulties interfere with sexual expression.

What happens during the therapy?

Sensate focus therapy is taught by a sex therapist, doctor, or psychologist. The couple are told that they may feel uncomfortable or embarrassed when they first practice sensate focus exercises but that, with time, they'll overcome these inhibitions. It's important for each partner to let the other know what feels good and what doesn't.

 SELF-HELP

Using the squeeze technique

When you begin to practice what you were taught, follow these important guidelines.

Follow the proper technique
- After your partner squeezes your penis, have her wait 15 to 30 seconds before resuming penile stimulation. Each time you near ejaculation, have your partner do the squeeze technique until you can control ejaculation on your own.
- Once you achieve control, progress to inserting your penis into your partner's vagina, but avoid thrusting. As you develop control, attempt thrusting, gradually increasing speed. Have your partner use the squeeze technique as necessary to delay ejaculation to the optimal time.

Communicate openly
- You and your partner should express your feelings throughout this activity.
- Be aware that timing and hand placement are the keys to success.
- Be sure to set aside time to satisfy your partner's sexual needs.
- Attend follow-up counseling sessions with your partner to discuss your progress in using this technique.

Using sensate focus therapy

When you begin to practice what you were taught, follow these important guidelines.

Minimize distractions
- A relaxed atmosphere, with no distractions, is important. Focus on giving pleasure to your partner.
- When you both feel sufficiently at ease to progress to intercourse, you may begin intromission (insertion of the penis) without thrusting. But check with your therapist before taking this step and the next: intromission with thrusting.

Try to enhance sensations
- Use moisturizing creams and lotions to enhance sensation. Start touching with the hands, then blowing, sucking, and stroking with objects such as a feather.

- Encourage your partner to concentrate on the pleasurable sensations of being touched.
- Don't rush sensate focus exercises. Repeat each exercise until you feel completely at ease before moving on to the next one. Each couple progresses at their own pace.

Other instructions
- Communicate with each other throughout the exercise. Both of you should be assertive and take responsibility for your sexual pleasure by frankly discussing what you find enjoyable and what you find unpleasant.
- Identify feelings of guilt, anxiety, fear, and frustration. These feelings need to be dealt with through therapy in addition to sensate focus exercises.

The couple remove all their clothes. One partner touches and explores the other's body, except for the genitals and breasts. Then the partners reverse roles so that each one gives and receives pleasurable sensations. Once both partners are comfortable performing this exercise, touching progresses to include the genitals and breasts. However, the couple should avoid intercourse until they're fully at ease. (See *Using sensate focus therapy.*)

What are the possible complications?
Feelings of anger, guilt, frustration, avoidance, rejection, and insecurity can result from or lead to sexual dysfunction. Interpersonal problems may surface during therapy.

TREATING HORMONAL DISORDERS

DRUG THERAPIES

INSULIN

Insulin is a circulating blood hormone that allows glucose, a naturally occurring sugar, to enter the body's cells. Insulin is released by the pancreas after a meal.

Glucose provides a source of readily available energy for cells to live. Without insulin, glucose can't enter cells and it accumulates in the blood (elevated blood sugar levels are a classic sign of diabetes). When levels rise sufficiently, glucose enters the urine, where it attracts excess water from the blood and causes an increase in urine volume. Early symptoms of diabetes often include excessive urination and excessive thirst.

Insulin is the treatment of choice for Type I (insulin-dependent) diabetes. People with this disease need additional insulin because their pancreas is no longer producing this hormone. Insulin may also be used to treat Type II (non-insulin–dependent) diabetes under certain circumstances, such as when an affected person has an acute infection or too much physical or emotional stress.

Semisynthetic and recombinant DNA human insulins and "purified" insulins are recommended for people who've never received insulin, those with Type II diabetes who need insulin during stress or illness, those with pregnancy-induced diabetes, and nondiabetic people receiving total parenteral nutrition.

What is insulin used for?
Insulin is used to control diabetes mellitus.

What are some commonly used insulin preparations?
See *Comparing insulin preparations.*

What are the possible side effects?
- Excessively low blood sugar levels
- Rash, breakdown of fat under the skin in the area of injections

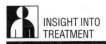

Comparing insulin preparations

Insulin comes in many types and purities, with various times of onset, peak effects, and durations of effects. The doctor may prescribe any of the insulins listed below or a mixture of several.

PREPARATION	INITIAL EFFECT (hours)	PEAK EFFECT (hours)	DURATION OF EFFECT (hours)
Rapid-acting insulins			
Insulin injection (regular, crystalline zinc)			
Regular Iletin I	½ to 1	2 to 4	6 to 8
Regular insulin	½	2½ to 5	8
Pork Regular Iletin II	½ to 1	2 to 4	6 to 8
Regular (concentrated) Iletin II	½	1 to 5	24
Velosulin	½	1 to 3	8
Purified Pork insulin	½	2½ to 5	8
Humulin R	½ to 1	2 to 4	6 to 8
Humulin BR	½ to 1	2 to 4	6 to 8
Novolin R	½	2½ to 5	8
Prompt insulin zinc suspension (semilente)			
Semilente insulin	1½	5 to 10	16
Semilente Purified Pork Prompt	1½	5 to 10	16
Intermediate-acting insulins			
Isophane insulin suspension (NPH)			
NPH Iletin I	2	6 to 12	18 to 26
NPH insulin	1½	4 to 12	24
Pork NPH Iletin II	2	6 to 12	18 to 26
NPH Purified Pork Isophane Insulin	1½	4 to 12	24
Insulatard NPH	1½	4 to 12	24
Humulin N	1 to 2	6 to 12	18 to 24
Novolin N	1½	4 to 12	24

(continued)

Comparing insulin preparations *(continued)*

PREPARATION	INITIAL EFFECT (hours)	PEAK EFFECT (hours)	DURATION OF EFFECT (hours)
Intermediate-acting insulins *(continued)*			
Isophane (NPH) 70%, regular insulin 30%			
Humulin 50/50	½	2 to 12	18 to 24
Mixtard 70/30	½	4 to 8	24
Mixtard Human	½	4 to 8	24
Humulin 70/30	½	2 to 12	24
Novolin 70/30	½	4 to 8	24
Insulin zinc suspension (lente)			
Lente Iletin I	2 to 4	6 to 12	18 to 26
Lente insulin	2½	7 to 15	24
Pork Lente Iletin II	2 to 4	6 to 12	18 to 26
Lente Purified Pork insulin	2½	7 to 15	22
Humulin L	1 to 3	6 to 12	18 to 21
Novolin L	2½	7 to 15	22
Long-acting insulins			
Protamine zinc insulin suspension			
Protamine Zinc & Iletin I	4 to 8	14 to 24	28 to 36
Beef Protamine Zinc & Iletin II	4 to 8	14 to 24	28 to 36
Pork Protamine Zinc & Iletin II	4 to 8	14 to 24	28 to 36
Extended insulin zinc suspension (ultralente)			
Ultralente insulin	4	10 to 30	36
Humulin U Ultralente	4	10 to 30	36

What are the guidelines for taking insulin?

- Insulin preparations vary as to how long their effects last. (See *Comparing insulin preparations,* pages 405 and 406, for details.) These preparations may also be prescribed in a mixed regimen, in which two or three types of insulin with different durations of action are combined to improve control over blood sugar levels.

- If insulins must be mixed, follow the doctor's directions for their proportions. After mixing NPH or Lente insulin in the same syringe with regular insulin, be sure to administer the mixture immediately. Letting the drug sit in the syringe for 10 minutes or more may change the characteristics of the insulin mixture. (See *How to inject insulin under the skin,* pages 408 and 409.)

- Closely monitor your blood and urine sugar levels as shown by your doctor. Studies have shown that people who maintain good blood sugar control have fewer long-term complications from their diabetes.
- Insulin is only part of the treatment. Diet and regular exercise also contribute to good blood sugar control. Consult your doctor if your caloric intake or activity level changes or if you become ill because such conditions may change insulin requirements.
- Rotate injections within a site on your abdomen, thighs, or upper arms. Full use of an injection site can allow for indefinite use of that area. Also, rotate between sites and don't use the same site more than once every 2 months. To help you remember where you've given yourself the injections, use a site rotation chart.
- Store insulin in a cool, dry place but never freeze it. (Refrigeration isn't necessary, but it may be convenient.)
- Wear a medical identification bracelet and carrying ample supplies of insulin and syringes with you on trips. Also carry a fast-acting carbohydrate, such as hard candy or fruit juice, in case of a low blood-sugar episode.

What else you should know

- Standard insulins, made primarily from beef or pork pancreas, are being replaced by semisynthetic and synthetic human insulins. These newer insulins reduce the risk of allergic reactions.
- Be sure to tell the doctor about all of the other medications you are taking, including nonprescription drugs. Don't take any other medicine without first checking with your doctor.
- Insulin is available across the United States without a prescription (except for concentrated U-500 insulin, which is used only in insulin-resistant diabetics). However, insulin syringes are often available only with a prescription. Check with your doctor or pharmacist to see what the regulations are in your area.
- Insulin treats diabetes but doesn't cure it. Lifelong medical follow-up is necessary, and you should never stop taking insulin because of the risk of a life-threatening coma from excessively high blood sugar levels.

(Text continues on page 410.)

SELF-HELP

How to inject insulin under the skin

To inject insulin under the skin, wash your hands thoroughly and re-move your prescribed insulin from the refrigerator if it's stored there. Then follow these steps.

Warm and mix the insulin by roll-ing the vial between your palms.
Caution: Never shake the vial. Check the expiration date; then read the label to make sure that the medication is the correct strength and type. Use an alco-hol sponge to clean the rubber stopper of the vial.

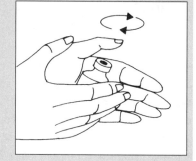

Before drawing up the insulin, in-ject an equal amount of air into the vial. That way, you won't cre-ate a vacuum in the vial, and it will be easier to withdraw your in-sulin.

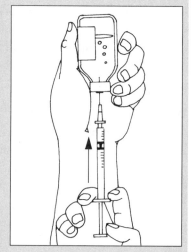

If air bubbles appear in the sy-ringe after you fill it with insulin, tap the syringe lightly to remove them. Draw up more insulin if necessary.

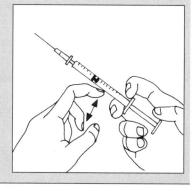

How to inject insulin under the skin *(continued)*

Select an appropriate site. (Refer to the guide your nurse gave you, showing how to rotate your injection sites correctly. To help you remember which site to use, write it on a calendar.) Pull the skin taut; then clean it with an alcohol sponge or a cotton ball soaked in alcohol, using a circular motion.

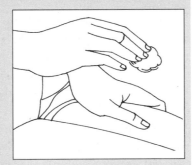

Using your thumb and forefinger, pinch the skin at the injection site. Then quickly plunge the needle up to its hub into the fat fold at a 90-degree angle. As you hold the syringe with one hand, pull back on the plunger slightly with your other hand to check for blood backflow. If blood appears in the syringe, discard everything and start again. If no blood appears, inject the insulin slowly.

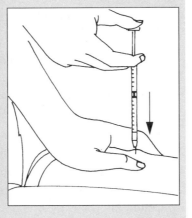

Place the alcohol sponge or cotton ball over the injection site; then press down on it lightly as you withdraw the needle. Snap the needle off the syringe, and dispose of the needle and syringe properly.

   Important: When you travel, keep a bottle of insulin and a syringe with you at all times. The insulin doesn't need to be refrigerated as long as you keep it away from heat.

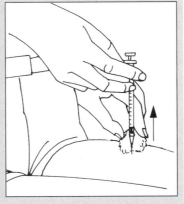

SULFONYLUREAS

Diabetes is generally classified into two types: Type I, which necessitates insulin injections, and Type II, which doesn't necessitate insulin injections.

Type II diabetes, often called *adult-onset diabetes,* occurs when the body's cells become resistant to the effects of insulin. This type of diabetes occurs despite normal levels of circulating insulin.

Sulfonylureas are given orally for Type II diabetes. They're ineffective in treating Type I (insulin-dependent) diabetes. Sulfonylureas make tissue more sensitive to the effects of insulin and may aid insulin synthesis and release by the pancreas.

What are sulfonylureas used for?

Sulfonylureas normalize blood sugar levels by increasing the production of insulin and enhancing its action.

What are some commonly used sulfonylureas?

- acetohexamide, known by the brand names Dimelor and Dymelor
- chlorpropamide, known by the brand names Apo-Chlorpropamide, Diabinese, and Novo-Propamide
- glipizide, known by the brand names Glucotrol and Gulcotrol XL
- glyburide, known by the brand names Apo-Glyburide, DiaBeta, Micronase, and Novo-Glyburide
- tolazamide, known by the brand names Tolamide and Tolinase
- tolbutamide, known by the brand names Apo-Tolbutamide, Mobenol, Orinase, and Tol-Tab

What are the possible side effects?

- Allergy
- Itching, rash
- Facial flushing
- Heartburn, nausea, vomiting, abdominal pain, diarrhea

What are the guidelines for taking sulfonylureas?

- Make sure that your doctor knows about all of the other medications you're taking, including nonprescription medicines. Don't take any other drugs without checking with your doctor.

- Take this drug 30 minutes before a meal to increase its effectiveness. Dividing the daily dosage improves gastrointestinal tolerance. Check with your doctor before altering the prescribed dosage.
- If you're switching from insulin therapy to an oral sulfonylurea, check your urine glucose and ketone levels at least three times daily before meals.
- Elderly, debilitated, or malnourished persons may have an increased response to sulfonylureas. Promptly report any side effects to your doctor.
- If you're taking Diabinese or Orinase, avoid alcohol. Even small amounts of alcohol can cause discomfort with facial flushing, light-headedness, a pounding headache, nausea, vomiting, palpitations, and shortness of breath. These symptoms can last for up to an hour.
- You'll need continued follow-up care. Don't discontinue this medication without your doctor's approval. Take your medication at the same time each day to help stabilize blood sugar levels. Take a missed dose as soon as you remember, unless it's almost time for the next dose; never take a double dose.
- Test your blood or urine glucose levels. If your blood sugar level remains uncontrolled after several months of therapy or if it becomes uncontrolled after initial successful control by sulfonylureas, you may require insulin therapy. You may need insulin during an acute infection or traumatic injury or if surgery is required.
- Wear a medical identification bracelet containing information about your condition and the prescribed drug.
- Know the signs and symptoms of low blood sugar. If they occur, immediately notify your doctor and ingest a quick-acting sugar, such as hard candy, orange juice, or table sugar.
- Sulfonylurea therapy represents only part of your diabetes care plan. The drug may be effective only temporarily or even ineffective if you fail to follow the prescribed diet and exercise program.

Sulfonylurea therapy represents only part of your diabetes care plan. The drug may be effective only temporarily or even ineffective if you fail to follow the prescribed diet and exercise program.

THYROID HORMONES

Thyroid hormone replacements were first used to treat hypothyroidism (an underactive thyroid gland) in the 1890s. These extracts of animal thyroid hormone, such as desiccated thyroid and thyroglobulin, are still used today, although most doctors prefer to use synthetic levothyroxine (T_4).

There are actually two active thyroid hormones — thyroxine (also called levothyroxine or T_4) and triiodothyronine (also called liothyronine or T_3). However, body tissue converts T_4 to T_3, so most doctors prefer only to supplement T_4 in persons with hypothyroidism. Some persons, however, benefit from direct supplement with T_3 and T_4 (commercially available as a drug called Thyrolar), or they may get T_3 supplements alone.

What are thyroid hormones used for?

Thyroid hormone replacements restore hormonal and metabolic balance in a person with deficient endogenous thyroid hormone levels.

What are some commonly used thyroid hormones?

- levothyroxine, also known as T_4, L-thyroxine, or by the brand names Levoid, Levothroid, or Synthroid
- liothyronine, also known as T_3, or by the brand names Cyronine or Cytomel
- liotrix, also known by the brand names Euthroid and Thyrolar

What are the possible side effects?

- Hyperthyroidism, or an overactive thyroid gland (nervousness, insomnia, tremors, rapid heart rate, nausea, and headache)
- Weight loss
- Menstrual irregularities
- Sweating
- Heat intolerance, fever

What are the guidelines for taking thyroid hormones?

- Tell your doctor about all drug and food allergies. If you're allergic to aspirin, you may also be allergic to tartrazine dye, which may present in Euthroid and Synthroid. Also, some persons with lactose intolerance may not tolerate Synthroid.
- Tell your doctor about all other medications that you're taking. Don't take any other drugs — including nonprescription drugs — without first checking with your doctor.
- Expect the doctor to closely monitor blood levels of thyroid hormones, especially at the beginning of therapy. Be sure to report for all follow-up appointments.
- Adhere to your medication schedule. Take the drug at the same time each day to maintain constant hormone levels and to reduce the risk of forgetting a dose. Take a missed dose as soon as possible unless

it's almost time for the next dose; never take a double dose. Call the doctor if you miss two or more doses.

- Report symptoms of hypothyroidism (a sluggish, lethargic feeling) or hyperthyroidism (anxiousness, sweating, palpitations) immediately because such symptoms indicate a need for dosage adjustment.

What else you should know

You should understand that thyroid hormone replacement doesn't cure your disease; it only relieves the symptoms. The drug must be taken continuously, although it may take a few weeks for your symptoms to subside.

> *You should understand that thyroid hormone replacement doesn't cure your disease; it only relieves the symptoms.*

THYROID HORMONE ANTAGONISTS

Persons who suffer from hyperthyroidism (an overactive thyroid gland) often experience bouts of excessive thyroid activity. This excessive thyroid activity is often accompanied by uncomfortable symptoms, including palpitations, sweating, nervousness, weight loss, and insomnia.

The thyroid hormone antagonists don't permanently affect the thyroid gland, but they inhibit hormone production until spontaneous remission of hyperthyroidism occurs. They are often administered before thyroid surgery because they decrease the number of blood vessels in the thyroid gland, making it easier for the surgeon to remove the gland with less blood loss.

What are thyroid hormone antagonists used for?

- To provide temporarily normal thyroid hormone levels in a person with hyperthyroidism
- To reduce thyroid hormone levels before surgery

What are some commonly used thyroid hormone antagonists?

- methimazole, known by the brand name Tapazole
- potassium iodide, known by the brand name Pima, and also called SSKI (for saturated solution of potassium iodide) and Lugol's solution (for strong iodine solution)
- propylthiouracil, or PTU, known by the brand name Propyl-Thyracil (in Canada)

What are the possible side effects?

- Fever, chills, sore throat
- Weakness
- Hepatitis
- Blood disorders
- Backache, joint pain
- Swelling of the ankles or feet
- Severe skin eruptions
- With excessive doses: cold intolerance; dry, puffy skin; headache; sleepiness; muscle aches; and unusual weight gain

What are the guidelines for taking thyroid hormone antagonists?

- If you're taking Pima, dilute the solution in juice or milk to counteract its metallic taste. Sip it through a straw to avoid discoloring your teeth. Take this solution after meals to prevent stomach irritation.
- If you're taking Pima for a prolonged period, tell the doctor if you experience a brassy taste or burning sensation in the mouth, skin eruptions, eye infections, fever, swelling, or irritability.
- Be sure to report for all follow-up exams. Several lab tests may be required in order to monitor for the effectiveness of therapy and to detect the early signs of drug toxicity.
- If you're taking this drug in preparation for surgery, be sure to take the drug exactly as prescribed. If taking it for hyperthyroidism, maintain the medication schedule to prevent recurrence. You may not notice improvement for several weeks until the stores of thyroid hormones are depleted from the thyroid gland. Symptoms related to increased thyroid activity may disappear rapidly. If not, other drugs may be prescribed. However, other symptoms, such as weight loss, muscle problems, and problems related to a high calcium blood level, will take longer to resolve.
- Report skin eruptions immediately. Also, promptly report a sore throat, fever, or mouth sores, especially during the 4th to 8th week of therapy.
- Don't stop taking the prescribed drug without medical approval; abrupt withdrawal may worsen the disease.
- Take your medication at the same time each day to enhance its effectiveness and to help you remember to take the drug. Take a missed dose as soon as possible; however, if it's almost time for the next dose, take both doses together. If you miss two doses, call your doctor for specific instructions.

- Don't take any nonprescription drugs (especially decongestants and cough medications, which may contain iodine) without your doctor's approval. Limit your daily intake of iodine.
- Advise all of your doctors and dentists of your medication regimen before any invasive procedures.

What else you should know

Thyroid hormone antagonists are the primary treatment for persons with transient hyperthyroidism (from Graves' disease, goiter, or thyroiditis), for those who refuse radioactive iodine treatment, and for those for whom surgery isn't an option.

SURGERIES

REMOVAL OF PITUITARY GLAND OR TUMOR

Microsurgical methods have dramatically reversed the high death rate once associated with removal of the pituitary gland or a pituitary tumor. As a result, hypophysectomy (surgical removal of the pituitary gland) and adenectomy (surgical removal of a pituitary tumor) are the treatments of choice for many pituitary tumors.

The most commonly used surgical method is transsphenoidal hypophysectomy in which the pituitary gland is reached through the sinuses. This approach uses powerful microscopes and improved radiologic techniques. It allows removal of microadenomas and causes fewer complications. Another approach, which goes through the skull, carries a high risk of death. This rarely used approach is performed only if the tumor is too large for or inaccessible by the transsphenoidal approach.

Why are these procedures done?

Hypophysectomy and adenectomy are the treatments of choice for pituitary tumors, which can cause acromegaly, gigantism, and Cushing's disease. They are done:
- to remove pituitary tissue that's secreting excessive levels of pituitary hormones or that's causing pressure on adjacent structures (hypophysectomy)
- to remove a pituitary tumor (adenectomy).

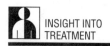

INSIGHT INTO
TREATMENT

Transsphenoidal hypophysectomy

When removing a pituitary tumor, the neurosurgeon will perform a transsphenoidal hypophysectomy. For this procedure, the person is placed in a semi-sitting position and given a general anesthetic. The surgeon makes an incision under the upper lip in order to reach the sella turcica (area around the pituitary gland) through the sphenoidal sinus. The surgeon can then remove the tumor.

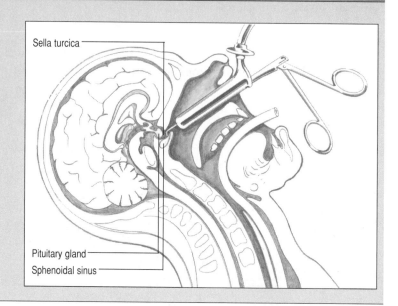

Sella turcica

Pituitary gland
Sphenoidal sinus

When shouldn't these procedures be done?

Hypophysectomy and adenectomy should not be performed if sinus or nasal infection is present or if the person has an anatomic defect that prevents access to the pituitary gland.

What happens before the procedures?

- You'll be told to expect headaches and discomfort after surgery. The presence of nasal packing for 2 to 3 days after the surgery will require breathing through your mouth. The doctor will tell you to expect a mustache dressing under your nose and, possibly, a urinary catheter.
- Diagnostic tests and exams will be completed.
- You'll sign a consent form.

What happens during the procedures?

Transsphenoidal hypophysectomy is performed with you in a semi-sitting position and under general anesthesia. (See *Transsphenoidal hypophysectomy.*)

What are the possible complications?

Brief diabetes insipidus frequently occurs after the operation. Other complications may include infection, spinal fluid leakage, hemorrhage, and visual defects. Total removal of the pituitary gland causes a hormonal deficiency that requires monitoring and hormonal replacement therapy.

Most people will receive a steroid such as hydrocortisone during surgery even if they did not have a previous hormonal deficiency because removal of all or part of the pituitary gland causes hormonal deficiency.

What happens after the procedures?

- You'll be on bed rest for 24 hours after surgery, then encouraged to walk. The head of the bed is elevated to avoid placing tension or pressure on the suture line. You'll be told not to brush your teeth, sneeze, cough, blow your nose, or bend over for several days.
- The nurse administers mild analgesics for headache caused by loss of spinal fluid during surgery or for paranasal pain. Typically, paranasal pain subsides when catheters and packing are removed — usually 24 to 48 hours after surgery.
- You must report postnasal drip, which may indicate a spinal fluid leak. (See *Recovering from pituitary gland surgery.*)

REMOVAL OF THE PARATHYROID GLANDS

Called a *parathyroidectomy* by doctors, this surgery removes one or more of the four parathyroid glands, which are located in the neck at the back of the thyroid gland. It's performed to treat parathyroid cancer or primary hyperparathyroidism.

The parathyroid glands release parathyroid hormone, which contributes to calcium metabolism. In primary hyperparathyroidism and most parathyroid cancers, the glands secrete too much parathyroid hormone, causing high levels of calcium in the blood and, often, low levels of another mineral, phosphorus.

The number of glands removed depends on the person's underlying condition. For example, if the person has a single tumor, removal of the affected gland corrects the problem. However, if more than

SELF-HELP

Recovering from pituitary gland surgery

After you've been discharged from the hospital, follow these important guidelines.

Take special precautions
- Don't brush your teeth for 2 weeks, to avoid injuring the incision. Instead, use a mouthwash and dental floss.
- Avoid bending over or blowing your nose.

Other instructions
- If you experience excessive thirst or urination, notify your doctor immediately. You may need to limit your fluid intake or take prescribed medications.
- You may need hormonal replacement therapy as a result of decreased pituitary secretion of thyroid-stimulating hormone. If you need such therapy, be sure to wear a medical identification bracelet.

one gland is enlarged, subtotal parathyroidectomy (removal of the three largest glands and part of the fourth gland) can correct the hyperparathyroidism. The surgeon usually tries to leave some glandular tissue so that adequate levels of calcium are maintained.

Why is this procedure done?

Parathyroidectomy is performed to remove diseased parathyroid tissue, decreasing levels of parathyroid hormone and calcium. Parathyroidectomy treats primary hyperparathyroidism. Total parathyroidectomy and removal of all abnormal adjacent tissue are necessary in parathyroid cancer. The surgeon may also perform a partial thyroidectomy if the abnormal tissue or tumor is hard to locate or if a problem in the thyroid gland is suspected.

People who undergo total parathyroidectomy may require treatment for hypoparathyroidism.

What happens before the procedure?

- The doctor will tell you that a partial thyroidectomy or a second surgery may be necessary if the surgeon can't find the diseased parathyroid tissue or all of the glands that are affected.
- You'll need to restrict the amount of calcium in your diet.
- You'll need to drink plenty of fluids to dilute the excess calcium in your blood.

What happens during the procedure?

While you're under general anesthesia, the surgeon makes a slit in the neck and exposes the thyroid gland. He or she then locates the four parathyroid glands, examines them for enlargement, and removes the affected ones. The surgery may be extended to the thyroid gland, or further studies may be needed and a second surgery performed if the doctor is unable to locate the abnormal tissue or all the parathyroid glands. Some surgeons may insert a drain or a closed wound drainage device before closing the incision and applying a bandage.

What are the possible complications?

Complications are rare but include hemorrhage, damage to the recurrent laryngeal nerves, respiratory problems, and hypoparathyroidism.

What happens after the procedure?

- You'll sit up after surgery to promote venous return from the head and neck and to decrease oozing from the incision.
- The nurse will administer mild analgesics to relieve pain.
- You must report numbness and tingling of the fingers, toes, and around the mouth (early signs of decreased calcium levels in the blood) as well as muscle cramps. (See *Recovering from parathyroidectomy.*)

REMOVAL OF THE THYROID GLAND

Called a *thyroidectomy* by doctors, this surgery removes part or all of the thyroid gland. A total thyroidectomy eliminates the possibility of recurrent hyperthyroidism but requires lifelong thyroid hormone replacement therapy. A partial thyroidectomy removes up to 80% of the gland; the remaining 20% supplies enough thyroid hormone for normal function.

Why is this procedure done?

Thyroidectomy is the treatment of choice for thyroid cancer, goiter, and hyperthyroidism that doesn't respond to medication and when radiation therapy can't be performed. It's done:

- to remove overactive thyroid tissue and thereby lower thyroid hormone levels
- to remove enlarged thyroid tissue and relieve breathing difficulty
- to remove thyroid cancer.

What happens before the procedure?

- You must follow a prescribed regimen of antithyroid drugs and iodine preparations.
- You must maintain an adequate caloric intake: About 4,000 to 5,000 calories daily may be necessary to regain and maintain weight lost due to the effects of excess thyroid hormone.
- You must avoid caffeine and other stimulants, which would cause additional nervousness and anxiety. Tranquilizers may be administered to promote rest.

 SELF-HELP

Recovering from parathyroidectomy

After you've been discharged from the hospital, follow these important guidelines.

Take special precautions

- Keep your incision site clean and dry. It will need to be checked at follow-up appointments.
- Avoid taking nonprescription drugs without your doctor's approval. Also avoid magnesium-containing laxatives and antacids, mineral oil, and vitamins A and D; these may affect calcium absorption or blood levels.

Other instructions

- If you've had a total parathyroidectomy, follow a high-calcium diet and take calcium and other medications as prescribed.
- Be aware that you'll need to undergo periodic checks of the level of calcium in your blood to help evaluate the outcome of surgery.

SELF-HELP

Recovering from thyroidectomy

After you've been discharged from the hospital, follow these important guidelines.

Promote healing
- Keep the incision site clean and dry.
- Use a mild body lotion to soften the healing scar and improve its appearance.
- Get adequate rest and nutrition to promote healing and regain or maintain weight.

Other instructions
- Support your head with a pillow and put your hands together behind your neck as you rise to prevent strain on the neck muscles.
- Take your prescribed thyroid hormone replacement. Recognize and report symptoms of hypothyroidism, hyperthyroidism, and infection.
- If parathyroid damage occurred during surgery, you'll need to take calcium supplements.
- Keep follow-up appointments to monitor serum thyroid hormone levels.
- Wear loosely buttoned collars, high-necked blouses, or scarves to hide the incision until it has healed.

What happens during the procedure?

After receiving a general anesthetic, you lie on your back, with sandbags or an air pillow under your shoulders and your neck hyperextended. The surgeon makes an incision ⅜ to ¾ inches (.75 to 2 centimeters) above the clavicle and exposes and removes the thyroid. Drains are inserted, and the wound is closed with clips or staples before a bandage is applied.

What are the possible complications?

Complications are rare after a thyroidectomy if you've been prepared with thyroid hormone antagonists before surgery. Potential complications include thyroid storm; hemorrhage; parathyroid damage, resulting in decreased levels of calcium in the blood or tetany; and laryngeal nerve damage, causing hoarseness or a permanent voice change.

What happens after the procedure?

- Immediately after surgery you'll have bandages and drains in place. You may experience some hoarseness, a sore throat, or temporary difficulty speaking.
- Your mouth and trachea may be suctioned. Steam inhalation may be used to promote expectoration of secretions.
- Your head is elevated to promote venous return from the head and neck, facilitate drainage, and decrease swelling.
- An ice collar is applied to your neck to promote comfort and decrease swelling. (See *Recovering from thyroidectomy*.)

REMOVAL OF THE PANCREAS

Called a *pancreatectomy* by doctors, this surgery removes all or part of the pancreas. It may involve removal of various parts of the organ, drainage procedures, and bypasses, depending on the person's condition, the extent of disease, and how poorly the pancreas is functioning. Usually the type of procedure is determined only after the surgeon explores the abdomen.

Why is this procedure done?

Pancreatectomy is used when more conservative techniques for treating pancreatic diseases have failed. It's done to relieve pain in persons with pancreatic cancer and chronic pancreatitis related to alcohol abuse. It's also used to treat insulin-producing tumors. It's done:

- to remove diseased pancreatic tissue
- to preserve functioning pancreatic tissue through adequate drainage and the prevention of the spread of cancer
- to relieve pain when the pancreas no longer functions.

What happens before the procedure?

- Diagnostic tests are performed.
- If you smoke, you're told to stop smoking before surgery.

What happens during the procedure?

While you're under general anesthesia, the surgeon makes an abdominal incision. The surgeon then selects the type of procedure based on evaluation of the pancreas, liver, gallbladder, and common bile duct. If the disease is localized, he or she may remove a portion of the pancreas and the surrounding organs. If the surgeon detects either metastatic disease in the liver or lymph nodes or tumor invasion of the aorta or superior mesenteric artery, he or she may bypass the obstruction to relieve your pain.

What are the possible complications?

Major complications of pancreatectomy include hemorrhage (during and after surgery), fistulas, abscesses (common with distal pancreatectomy), common bile duct obstruction, and pseudocysts. Partial pancreatectomy sometimes causes insulin dependence; total pancreatectomy always causes lifelong insulin dependence. (See *Recovering from pancreatectomy.*)

What happens after the procedure?

- You'll usually spend the first 48 hours in the intensive care unit.
- Oxygen may be administered, and deep-breathing techniques and coughing will be encouraged.
- If no complications develop, your gastrointestinal function will return in 24 to 48 hours. Then you may begin taking oral fluids.

 SELF-HELP

Recovering from pancreatectomy

After you've been discharged from the hospital, follow these important guidelines.

Take special precautions

- Carefully clean and bandage your wound each day.
- Report any signs of wound infection promptly.

Other instructions

- Test your urine for glucose and ketones and monitor your blood sugar levels.
- After a total pancreatectomy, you and a responsible family member must learn how to administer insulin.
- Because you may have problems with food absorption, you will need to follow special dietary instructions. Eventually, you may need pancreatic enzyme replacement therapy.
- If you have chronic pancreatitis, get regular medical follow-up and avoid alcohol consumption.

REMOVAL OF THE ADRENAL GLANDS

Called an *adrenalectomy* by doctors, this surgery removes all or part of one or both adrenal glands. It may be performed when an adrenal tumor overproduces any of the adrenal hormones.

Why is this procedure done?

Adrenalectomy is the treatment of choice for adrenal hyperfunction caused by adrenal hyperplasia or an adrenal adenoma. The prognosis is good when adrenalectomy is used to treat a benign adrenal adenoma. The prognosis is less favorable for adrenal cancer. The procedure can also be used to treat a pheochromocytoma (a catecholamine-secreting tumor of the adrenal medulla) in one or both adrenal glands, and it has also been used occasionally to treat some breast or prostate cancers. It's done:

- to remove adrenal tissue, reducing adrenal hormone hypersecretion
- to remove a malignant tumor from one or both adrenal glands.

What happens before the procedure?

- If the goal of surgery is to remove a pheochromocytoma, a rare cancer that causes the body to release too much of two hormones, the doctor may prescribe medication 1 to 2 weeks before surgery.
- If you have adrenal hyperfunction, the nurse will give you glucocorticoids on the morning of surgery to prevent adrenal insufficiency during surgery.

What happens during the procedure?

The surgeon explores the adrenal glands, looking for a tumor. If one's found, the surgeon either removes it or removes the involved adrenal gland.

What are the possible complications?

Hemorrhage, shock, low or high blood pressure, and decreased sodium levels in the blood can complicate recovery from surgery. However, better use of medications such as Dibenzyline, or Demser and Inderal before surgery has dramatically decreased the risk of complications.

SELF-HELP

Recovering from adrenalectomy

After you've been discharged from the hospital, follow these important guidelines.

Take your medicine
- Take your medication as directed. If you've had a unilateral adrenalectomy, be aware that medications may be discontinued in a few months when your remaining adrenal gland resumes functioning. If you've had a bilateral adrenalectomy, you'll need lifelong medication.
- Because the adrenal gland also regulates sodium and potassium, you'll need hormone replacement therapy, commonly with fludrocortisone acetate (Florinef).

Be alert for problems
- Learn to recognize symptoms of adrenal insufficiency, which can progress to adrenal crisis if not treated. Promptly report such symptoms as weight gain, acne, headaches, fatigue, and increased urinary frequency to the doctor. Take cortisone as prescribed with meals or antacids to reduce stomach irritation.

- Because sudden withdrawal of cortisone can trigger adrenal crisis, get continued medical follow-up to ensure appropriate adjustment of the cortisone dosage during stress or illness.
- If you've had adrenal hyperfunction, expect your physical symptoms to reverse over the next few months. However, these improvements don't mean you can discontinue cortisone medications.

Other instructions
- If your surgical wound isn't completely healed, keep the incision clean, and avoid wearing clothing that may irritate it. Follow your doctor's instructions regarding use of ointments or dressings.
- Report fever or increased drainage, inflammation, or pain at the incision site.
- Wear a medical identification bracelet or carry a card to ensure adequate care in an emergency.

What happens after the procedure?

After adrenalectomy, the nurse administers pain medication and replacement steroids. Glucocorticoids from the adrenal cortex are essential to life and must be replaced to prevent adrenal crisis. (See *Recovering from adrenalectomy.*)

DIET THERAPY

DIABETIC DIET

Diet is the cornerstone of diabetes treatment. A diabetic diet requires the development of an individual meal plan that allows the person to maintain a normal lifestyle while keeping blood sugar and weight at appropriate levels.

The person with Type I (insulin-dependent) diabetes can't produce insulin. So, he or she must administer insulin, schedule meals and snacks to offset peak insulin action, and follow a prescribed diet to avoid low and high blood sugar levels. The person also needs to follow an exchange system to balance dietary protein, carbohydrate, and fat. (See *Following a diabetic diet.*)

The person with Type II (non-insulin–dependent) diabetes produces some insulin but also has insulin resistance (the inability of the cells in the body to effectively use the insulin). Insulin resistance worsens if the person is overweight, so diet therapy in Type II diabetes focuses on weight loss to reduce insulin resistance; a balance of dietary protein, carbohydrate, and fat; and avoidance of both low and high blood sugar levels.

Why is this diet prescribed?

A diabetic diet provides the diabetic with a meal plan tailored to that individual's nutritional requirements, weight goals, lifestyle needs, and activity level.

What happens when the diet is prescribed?

- Your doctor commonly prescribes a caloric level, which is adjusted as necessary to maintain stable weight.
- A thorough dietary history is taken by the nurse or dietitian. What you eat and when you eat are taken into account.
- A dietitian or nurse develops a meal plan for you, often using an exchange list. These exchange lists have been developed by the American Diabetes Association and American Dietetic Association to meet the needs of diabetics. The lists are based on the principles of good nutrition, and they divide foods into equivalent groups (exchanges) according to calories and nutritional content. In the diabet-

SELF-HELP

Following a diabetic diet

As you begin your diet, follow these important guidelines.

Keep track of what you eat

- Because your prescribed diet is based on your individual needs, you must keep track of all the foods you eat. If you use the food exchange system, you may need to categorize foods. No foods are exempt — even so-called dietetic foods.
- Keep a food diary so you can see how and where your current eating habits deviate from your prescribed diet. Your food diary can be used to make necessary diet adjustments. Plan meals a few days in advance so you have the needed ingredients on hand. Avoid inappropriate substitutions.

Eat the right foods at the right times

- Eat foods that contain unrefined carbohydrates and are high in fiber. Daily intake of 25 to 30 grams of fiber delays gastric emptying and slows carbohydrate absorption, which can lower your blood sugar level and reduce insulin requirements.
- If you are insulin-dependent or taking oral antidiabetic agents, be sure to eat on a regular, consistent schedule, even during an illness, to balance insulin therapy. Lack of food, vomiting, diarrhea, or too much exercise can cause a low blood sugar level.
- If you're able to eat regular meals during an illness, you should also increase your fluid intake to three times your typical daily intake, or 12 ounces per hour for the average adult. If you're vomiting, try to drink liquids containing sugar and electrolytes (regular soda, fruit juices, fluid electrolyte replacement — such as Gatorade — or ice pops containing 15 grams of carbohydrate) every 30 minutes.

Use alcohol with caution

- If you drink alcohol regularly, you must follow certain restrictions to avoid complications. For instance, drinking alcohol without eating food can cause your blood sugar level to drop. The American Diabetes Association recommends limiting alcohol consumption to two exchanges of an alcoholic beverage once or twice a week. One alcohol exchange is ½ ounce of whiskey, 4 ounces of wine, or 12 ounces of beer.
- If you take insulin, you can use alcohol exchanges in addition to the usual meal plan. If you don't need to take insulin, substitute alcohol for fat exchanges; one alcohol exchange is equal to two fat exchanges.

Other instructions

- Continue to take prescribed insulin and oral antidiabetic agents during stress or illness unless told to stop by your doctor. Notify your doctor of any illness because illness and stress can cause your blood sugar level to rise.
- Carry a form of simple carbohydrate, such as hard candy or a fruit juice, to prevent low blood sugar levels when away from home or if a meal may be delayed.
- Make sure you and your family learn to recognize the symptoms of low and high blood sugar levels.
- Consider joining a local support group for diabetics. For information, contact the American Diabetes Association.

ic diet, carbohydrates contribute 50% to 60% of the total daily calories; proteins contribute 12% to 20%; and fat contributes no more than 30%.

For the person taking insulin, a bedtime snack may be necessary to prevent low blood sugar during sleep. The scheduled times for other snacks depend on the person's activity level, mealtimes, and the type of insulin or oral antidiabetic agents used.

What are the possible complications?

Low or high blood sugar levels are the primary complications of a diabetic diet. Either may occur if you don't follow the diet, if you change your activity level or lifestyle, or if your drug dosage is altered without corresponding diet changes.

11

TREATING BLOOD & IMMUNITY DISORDERS

DRUG THERAPIES

GOLD COMPOUNDS

Gold compounds slow the degenerative course of arthritis and may even induce remission. Three gold compounds are used for treating arthritis: aurothioglucose and gold sodium thiomalate, which are given by injection, and auranofin, which is taken orally. All three drugs are equally effective, but auranofin appears to be the least toxic.

Treatment with gold salts can only prevent additional damage to bone and cartilage; it doesn't repair existing damage. Therefore, gold therapy is most beneficial in the early stages of disease before irreversible joint damage has occurred. The beneficial effects develop slowly.

What are gold compounds used for?

The gold compounds reduce inflammation in rheumatoid arthritis.

What are some commonly used gold compounds?

- auranofin, known by the brand name Ridaura
- aurothioglucose, known by the brand name Solganal
- gold sodium thiomalate, known by the brand name Myochrysine

What are the possible side effects?

- Severe allergy
- Pain in the joints
- Inflammation of the mouth, lips, and mucous membranes
- Metallic taste
- Dermatitis, excessive sensitivity to sunlight
- Upset stomach, diarrhea
- Unusual bleeding or bruising

What are the guidelines for taking gold compounds?

- Expect the doctor to closely monitor your blood and urine during treatment. These studies are needed to ensure early detection of the drug's possible toxic effects. Be sure to report for all follow-up studies.
- Tell the doctor about all other drugs you are currently taking, including nonprescription ones. Don't take any other drugs without checking with the doctor first.

- Be alert for toxic effects, which may occur at any time during therapy or even several months after its discontinuation. Call your doctor immediately if you experience itching, shortness of breath, a metallic taste, coughing, unusual bleeding or bruising, nausea, vomiting, diarrhea, or abdominal pain.
- Joint pain may get worse for 1 to 2 days after an injection, but this usually stops after the first few injections.
- The benefits of gold therapy may not be apparent for 6 weeks or longer. Record the date that you first notice any relief from stiffness and pain or improvement of joint function.
- Gold compounds may lead to mouth ulcers and a sore throat. To help prevent these problems, brush your teeth and use a mouthwash after every meal.
- Tell your doctor if you have a history of blood diseases, diabetes, circulation problems, colitis, kidney or liver disease, skin rashes, or allergy to the drug.
- Avoid excessive exposure to sunlight, which can worsen skin reactions. Use a sunscreen and wear protective clothing if you're going to have prolonged exposure to the sun. Don't sunbathe or use a tanning bed.

Gold compounds may lead to mouth ulcers and a sore throat. To help prevent these problems, brush your teeth and use a mouthwash after every meal.

IMMUNOSUPPRESSANTS

The idea of using drugs to suppress the body's immune response was first considered nearly 100 years ago, but the actual development and use of such drugs is recent, coinciding with the development of organ transplants. In combination with steroid drugs, immunosuppressants have been used to prevent and treat organ transplant rejection. They have also been used experimentally to treat many immune diseases.

Azathioprine treats severe rheumatoid arthritis that doesn't respond to other treatments; it's also used for kidney transplants. Cyclosporine helps prevent rejection in various organ or bone marrow transplants. When used with steroid drugs, cyclosporine reduces inflammation in rheumatoid arthritis. Levamisole helps to treat colon cancer after surgery. Muromonab-CD3 and lymphocyte immune globulin help to prevent kidney rejection after transplant.

What are immunosuppressants used for?
Immunosuppressants are used to block immune responses.

What are some commonly used immunosuppressants?

- azathioprine, known by the brand name Imuran
- cyclosporine, known by the brand name Sandimmune
- levamisole, known by the brand name Ergamisol
- lymphocyte immune globulin, known by the brand name Atgam
- muromonab-CD3, known by the brand name Orthoclone OKT3

What are the possible side effects?

Azathioprine

- Nausea, vomiting, diarrhea, and mouth ulcerations
- Blood disorders

Cyclosporine

- Kidney damage
- Elevated blood potassium or sugar levels
- High blood pressure
- Tremor
- Tooth or gum problems
- Excessive hair growth
- Nausea, vomiting, diarrhea, abdominal distention
- Sinus disorder
- Breast enlargement
- Hearing loss, ringing in the ears
- Muscle pain, swelling of the hands, feet, or ankles

Levamisole

- Blood disorders
- Skin disorders
- Increased susceptibility to infections
- Nausea, vomiting, diarrhea

Lymphocyte immune globulin

- Fever
- Flulike illness
- Chest pain
- Nausea, vomiting, diarrhea
- Severe allergic reactions

Muromonab-CD3

- Pain in the joints
- Fever
- Tremor

- Flulike illness
- Severe allergic reactions

What are the guidelines for taking immunosuppressants?

- Expect the doctor to order a lot of blood and urine tests to detect early signs of drug toxicity. It's important that you report for all follow-up exams.
- Watch for signs of infection, such as fever, sore throat, chills, and malaise. Report these symptoms to the doctor immediately.
- Watch for bruises, blood in the urine, easy bleeding of the gums, or black, tarry stools. Report these to the doctor immediately. Be sure to use a soft toothbrush, and switch to an electric razor if possible.
- It's important that you follow the prescribed medication schedule. If you're taking cyclosporine and you miss a dose, take the drug as soon as possible, unless it's almost time for the next dose (in which case you should simply continue the regular schedule). If you're taking azathioprine several times a day, take a missed dose as soon as possible. If it's time for the next dose, take two doses. If you miss two consecutive doses of either of these drugs, notify the doctor immediately.
- Take steps to avoid infection: avoid crowds and people suffering from colds, flu, and other contagious illnesses; don't get vaccinated, especially with live-virus vaccines such as polio vaccines; avoid contact with anyone who's recently received a live-virus vaccine; and wash your hands before handling food.
- Be sure to tell your doctor about all of your allergies. Some immunosuppressants are derived from horse or mouse products and can cause severe reactions in certain sensitive people.
- Be sure to tell your doctor about all of the other medications you are taking, including nonprescription medicines. Avoid aspirin and aspirin-containing compounds.
- The prescribed drug may cause loss of hair; it may also cause you to lose your appetite or may produce nausea and vomiting. If gastrointestinal effects occur, take the drug with meals. If they persist, the doctor may prescribe an antiemetic.
- Symptoms of refractory arthritis may not improve for up to 12 weeks.
- If you're taking cyclosporine, report symptoms of high blood pressure, such as frequent headaches or dizziness. Watch for signs of liver damage, such as clay-colored stools, itching, or yellowing of the skin or eyes. If such signs occur, call the doctor immediately.

Be sure to tell your doctor about all of your allergies. Some immunosuppressants are derived from horse or mouse products and can cause severe reactions in certain sensitive people.

What else you should know

Tell your doctor if you've recently had chickenpox or shingles (herpes zoster) because these diseases increase your risk of developing a severe generalized infection. Also tell the doctor if you've recently had any vaccines; you shouldn't be vaccinated while taking these drugs without first checking with your doctor. And tell the doctor if you've ever had kidney or liver disease.

TRANSFUSIONS

BLOOD TRANSFUSION

A transfusion adds blood to the body. Depending on why it's done, a transfusion may involve whole blood or one or more of its components: packed red blood cells, platelets, fresh frozen plasma, cryoprecipitate, or granulocytes. (Cryoprecipitate contains the stable clotting factors. Granulocytes are the blood cells that help fight bacterial infection.)

Why is this procedure done?
- To replace blood lost from heavy bleeding
- To help treat anemia and other blood disorders

What happens before the procedure?
- A blood sample is taken to determine your blood type.
- If you have a history of blood transfusion reactions, the nurse will give you medications.
- Your vital signs are checked just before the transfusion starts.

What happens during the procedure?
Depending on the severity of your condition, transfusions are performed in the hospital or in an outpatient setting. The blood is delivered into your veins through special tubing. Commonly, saline solution is used to keep the vein open if the transfusion must be stopped or delayed.

What are the possible complications?

Blood transfusions carry the risk of serious complications, including an acute hemolytic reaction (in which red blood cells are destroyed) or an allergic reaction. Reactions can occur during, immediately after, or up to 10 days after a blood transfusion but most often occur immediately after the transfusion begins or within an hour after it's completed.

Another serious complication is the transmission of infectious diseases, such as hepatitis C, cytomegalovirus, and AIDS. Because of current techniques for testing donor blood for these diseases, such transmission is uncommon. However, because of these risks, many people elect to donate their own blood so that it can be used subsequently — for example, during a planned surgery.

Certain complications — such as hypothermia and bleeding tendencies — typically result from multiple or massive transfusions.

What happens after the procedure?

If the transfusion was given on an outpatient basis, you'll be observed for at least 2 hours before discharge. (See *Recovering from a blood transfusion.*)

*F*ACTOR REPLACEMENT

Factor replacement is the transfusion of blood clotting factors. Various blood products are used, depending on the disorder being treated.

Why is this procedure done?

Factor replacement corrects clotting factor deficiencies and thereby stops or prevents serious bleeding.

What happens before the procedure?

The nurse inserts an intravenous line and explains the procedure to you.

What happens during the procedure?

Factor replacement products are administered intravenously.

 SELF-HELP

Recovering from a blood transfusion

After you're discharged from the hospital, follow these important guidelines.

Avoid aspirin

If you're receiving platelets, don't use aspirin. It interferes with platelet function. Use Tylenol or another product that contains acetaminophen for pain relief or fever.

Watch for delayed reaction

You and your caregiver must learn the symptoms of a delayed transfusion reaction and of hepatitis: fever, headache, loss of appetite, nausea, vomiting, and abdominal pain. These symptoms most often occur 3 to 10 days after the transfusion and must be reported to your doctor immediately.

SELF-HELP

Receiving factor replacement at home

More and more people are receiving factor replacement at home, either by giving it to themselves or by having a family member perform the procedure. In fact, children as young as age 9 have been taught how to do it.

If you'll be continuing factor replacement therapy at home, a nurse will show you and your family the correct venipuncture and infusion techniques before you leave the hospital. Once you've been discharged, remember these important guidelines.

Stay prepared
Keep factor replacement and infusion equipment available, and begin treatment immediately if you or a family member experiences a bleeding episode.

Report side effects
- Become familiar with and immediately report symptoms of allergic reactions and fluid overload. For example, allergic reactions to factor replacement may cause hives, wheezing, red skin, or painless swelling of the face, neck, lips, throat, hands, feet, or genitals. Ask your doctor which other symptoms to watch for.
- Watch for symptoms of hepatitis, which may appear 3 weeks to 6 months after treatment with blood components. Symptoms include yellowish skin, appetite loss, upset stomach, clay-colored stools, and dark urine.

What are the possible complications?

A transfusion reaction can result from a single or massive transfusion of blood or blood products.

Reactions generally occur during or within 96 hours of the transfusion. Infections, such as those caused by HIV, hepatitis virus, or cytomegalovirus, may also be transmitted during a transfusion and can go undetected for weeks, months, and even years. Prothrombin complex carries a special risk of transmitting hepatitis because it's collected from large pools of donors.

What happens after the procedure?

The nurse monitors you for signs of bleeding and a transfusion reaction. (See *Receiving factor replacement at home*.)

EXCHANGE TRANSFUSION

An exchange transfusion is the replacement of a person's blood with an equal amount of donor blood. The treatment may be used for newborns and certain individuals with sickle cell anemia.

Why is this procedure done?
- To reduce high bilirubin levels in newborns
- To remove sensitized red blood cells and replace them with healthy donor cells
- To correct the anemia resulting from Rh incompatibility
- To correct severe anemia or break a cycle of frequently recurrent crisis in sickle cell anemia

What happens before the procedure?
The parents must sign a consent form. (See *Questions parents ask about an exchange transfusion*, page 436.)

What happens during the procedure?
The doctor inserts a catheter into the infant's umbilical vein (although a central venous catheter can be used) and threads it into the inferior vena cava, a large vein that returns blood from the outer parts of the body to the right chamber of the heart. The procedure usually takes 1 to 2 hours. Depending on the baby's weight, a specified amount of blood is withdrawn within 15 to 20 seconds and the same volume of donor blood is infused over 60 to 90 seconds.

After the procedure, the doctor may remove the umbilical catheter unless further transfusions are anticipated. In that case, the doctor will flush the catheter with saline solution and leave it in place.

What are the possible complications?
Exchange transfusions carry many risks. A condition known as *necrotizing enterocolitis* (intestinal inflammation marked by death of intestinal cells) may result from compromised bowel circulation or a misplaced or clogged catheter. Low blood sugar may result from increased insulin production in response to the sugar level of the donor blood. Cardiac arrest may result from heart overload.

Low calcium levels in the blood may develop from calcium depletion by sodium citrate in the donor's blood. With massive transfusions, high

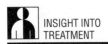

Questions parents ask about an exchange transfusion

Exchange transfusion is the treatment of choice for conditions sometimes seen in newborns called *erythro-blastosis fetalis* and *neonatal sepsis*. These are some common questions parents ask.

Is it safe?
Specially trained doctors will perform the procedure, and trained nurses will assist and constantly monitor your baby's progress. As a result, fewer than 1% of children develop complications. Erythroblastosis fetalis, however, poses a great risk to your child; if untreated, it causes nerve damage and mental retardation.

How will my baby survive if you take out all of his blood?
Only a small amount—about a tablespoon— is removed at any one time, and it's replaced immedi-

ately with an equal quantity of donor blood. This process is repeated until about 85% of the blood has been replaced.

Will my baby get AIDS from the transfusion?
Blood donors are carefully screened and all blood is tested for AIDS before it's used. Since the development of the blood test for AIDS, the risk of acquiring AIDS from a transfusion is extremely low.

If the father's blood type is compatible, he may donate a unit of blood for his child. Similarly, other relatives or friends may be encouraged to donate blood because the baby will need several units.

---

blood potassium levels may result from the breakdown of red blood cells. Bleeding and infection at the catheter site may also occur.

What happens after the procedure?
- The nurse observes the infant for signs of complications.
- If the umbilical catheter is removed, the nurse bandages the area and observes it for bleeding and infection.
- Once the infant is discharged from the hospital, the parents must remember to keep all follow-up appointments with the doctor.
- The parents should call the doctor immediately if the baby develops fever, malaise, or a yellowish skin discoloration.

*B*ONE MARROW TRANSPLANT

In this procedure, fresh or stored healthy bone marrow is used to replace diseased bone marrow. It aims to allow the recipient to resume normal production of blood cells. Whether or not bone marrow transplantation is attempted depends on the recipient's underlying disease, age, health status, and the availability of a compatible donor.

There are several types of bone marrow transplants. In an *autologous transplant,* the person's own bone marrow is procured and frozen. After the person receives chemotherapy or radiation therapy, the bone marrow is returned to him or her. An autologous transplant may not be an option for people with diseased bone marrow.

A *syngeneic transplant* uses the bone marrow of an identical twin. When possible, it's the ideal option because the bone marrow of the twin is identical, yet free of disease.

An *allogeneic transplant* uses marrow from a compatible donor. Donors for this type of transplant are usually siblings but may also be unrelated to the person. Tissue typing is done to determine the compatibility of the recipient and donor. It tests for a specific set of antigen markers. If both the donor and the recipient have the same antigen markers, their bone marrow is considered compatible. Other antigens exist but aren't detectable at this time. Therefore, the tissue of the recipient and donor may not be perfectly matched, even though the bone marrow is considered compatible. For this reason, the recipient requires medication to suppress the immune system after the transplant.

Why is this procedure done?

The procedure replaces the bone marrow of people whose marrow has been suppressed by chemotherapy, radiation therapy, or immunosuppressant therapy.

Bone marrow transplantation is the treatment of choice for aplastic anemia and severe combined immunodeficiency disease. It's also used to treat leukemia and lymphoma. In addition, bone marrow transplantation is being explored as a treatment for other blood diseases such as multiple myeloma.

What happens before the procedure?

The person is placed in reverse isolation to protect him or her from infection.

To prepare a person for a bone marrow transplant, high doses of chemotherapy and sometimes total body irradiation are given. This is done in an attempt to destroy diseased bone marrow and hidden cancer cells and to empty the marrow spaces to make room for healthy marrow. In a person receiving an allogeneic bone marrow

---

Bone marrow procurement

The timing of bone marrow procurement depends on the type of transplant to be done.

When is the marrow obtained?
Bone marrow for an autologous bone marrow transplant is usually obtained at least 2 weeks before the day of transplantation. But it can be obtained much sooner and preserved for long periods, even years. If necessary, the person's bone marrow may undergo a process that removes or destroys cancer cells before it is frozen until the day of transplantation.

Bone marrow from syngeneic and allogeneic donors is removed from the donor on the day of transplantation and immediately given to the recipient.

How is the marrow collected?
In all cases, the marrow is collected from the donor in the operating room, under general or epidural anesthesia. This is done through multiple bone marrow aspirations from the donor's hip. The procedure usually takes $1\frac{1}{2}$ to 2 hours.

The marrow is filtered to remove bone and fat particles and other debris. Then it's mixed with heparin and a preservative to prevent coagulation and keep the marrow viable. After the procedure, pressure dressings are applied to the donor sites and pain relievers are given as needed.

SELF-HELP

Recovering from a bone marrow transplant

After you've been discharged from the hospital, follow these important guidelines.

Take special precautions
- Before leaving the hospital, you or your caregiver will be taught to manage the central venous catheter and to administer medications correctly. Make sure you follow these instructions carefully at home.
- Be sure you and your caregiver know the signs and symptoms of complications. Report these to the doctor promptly.

Other points to remember
- Keep emergency phone numbers (doctor, ambulance, emergency squad) handy.
- Keep follow-up appointments so your progress can be monitored and late-occurring complications can be identified and treated.

transplant, chemotherapy is also given to suppress the person's immune system so that the new marrow can begin to function.

What happens during the procedure?

Before the actual transplant, bone marrow must be removed from the donor. This is known as *bone marrow procurement* or *harvesting*. After the marrow is obtained, it's administered to the recipient. (See *Bone marrow procurement,* page 437.)

On the day of the transplant, the previously procured bone marrow is given at the bedside just like a blood transfusion. Once in the person's circulation, the transplanted marrow migrates to the bone marrow cavities, where the new cells begin to grow and produce new blood cells.

What are the possible complications?

The most common complications of bone marrow transplantation are bleeding, infection, and a condition known as *acute* or *chronic graft-versus-host disease.* Graft-versus-host disease occurs only in allogeneic bone marrow transplants. It occurs when the T-lymphocytes (special cells that are part of the body's defense mechanism) in the donor marrow attack specific target organs of the recipient.

What happens after the procedure?

Reverse isolation is maintained. Visitors to the person's room wear sterile gowns, masks, gloves, and shoecovers to prevent bringing infectious organisms into the environment. (See *Recovering from a bone marrow transplant.*)

12

*T*REATING CANCER

DRUG THERAPIES

CHEMOTHERAPY

In chemotherapy, drugs are used to attack cancer cells that are rapidly dividing and to either kill them or render them incapable of further division. Cancer, however, occurs in more than 200 forms. Because of this diversity, doctors use many types and combinations of chemotherapy drugs. Treatment can consist of one drug type (single-drug chemotherapy) or multiple drugs (combination chemotherapy). It may be done as the only treatment or used with surgery or radiation therapy.

Why is this treatment done?
- To eradicate cancer completely
- To control cancer with the expectation that it will recur and progress in the future
- To relieve symptoms caused by the cancer, such as pain

When shouldn't this treatment be done?
Because chemotherapy typically lowers blood counts, it should not be given to persons with blood counts below designated levels. Also, persons with fevers should not receive chemotherapy.

What happens before the treatment?
A doctor or nurse will tell you or family members how to reduce or control side effects of the treatment.

What happens during the treatment?
Chemotherapy can be done in a hospital, office, clinic or, at times, a person's home. Treatments are scheduled to allow recovery of healthy tissues and minimize side effects. These drugs may be given orally or injected into a muscle, a blood vessel, the tissue under the skin, the bladder or spinal fluid. Some may be applied to the skin.

At times, drugs may be given with a portable, battery-operated pump. Small enough to hook onto a belt, the pump allows you to continue daily life while receiving chemotherapy.

Managing common side effects of chemotherapy

Chemotherapy can often cause unpleasant side effects. Fortunately, you can sometimes prevent them. Other times, you can take steps to make yourself more comfortable. Follow the advice below.

Hair loss

- Chemotherapy drugs can affect all hair on the body and head. Effects may range from thinning to complete hair loss. Hair may regrow in a different color and texture.
- Know that hair loss is usually temporary.
- Some people prefer to have their hair cut short to make thinning hair less noticeable.
- To help minimize hair loss, wash your hair with a mild shampoo and avoid frequent brushing, combing, use of rollers, or permanent waving.
- Wear a hat, scarf, toupee, or wig.
- For support, contact local services, such as those offered by the American Cancer Society and the Look Good, Feel Better program.

Lack of appetite

- Good nutrition is important even though you have a poor appetite.
- Eat small, frequent meals and take high-calorie supplements.

Bone marrow depression (leukopenia, thrombocytopenia, anemia)

- Immediately report fever, chills, sore throat, lethargy, unusual fatigue, or unusually pale skin to your doctor.
- Avoid exposure to persons with infections for several months.
- You and your family shouldn't receive immunizations during or shortly after chemotherapy because an exaggerated reaction may occur.
- Take precautions to prevent bleeding. Use extra care with razors, nail trimmers, dental floss, toothbrushes, and other sharp or abrasive objects.

Avoid digital exams, rectal suppositories, and enemas. Increase your fluid intake to prevent constipation.
- Take vitamin and iron supplements.
- Avoid activities that could cause injury and bleeding. Report episodes of bleeding or bruising to the doctor.
- Eat high-iron foods, such as liver and spinach.
- Be aware that follow-up blood studies are important even after completion of treatment.

Diarrhea and abdominal cramps

- Learn how to use antidiarrheal medications, and report diarrhea to the doctor.
- Maintain an adequate fluid intake and follow a bland, low-fiber diet.
- Practice good perianal hygiene to help prevent tissue breakdown and infection.

Nausea and vomiting

Take medication to control nausea and vomiting and let the doctor know if it's ineffective. Follow the nutrition plan given to you by the doctor.

Mouth sores

- Good mouth care — meticulous flossing and brushing — is essential.
- Prevent injury to the oral cavity by avoiding smoking, alcohol, spicy foods, and extremely hot or cold foods or liquids.
- Examine your mouth daily (or have a family member do this), and promptly report any changes.
- If you have dentures, leave them out as much as possible and clean them several times a day.

What are the possible complications?

Chemotherapy drugs are powerful and can cause severe complications. One common complication, called *myelosuppression,* reduces the numbers of circulating blood cells. When chemotherapy lowers the number of white blood cells, a condition known as *leukopenia,* you're at risk for infection. When it reduces the numbers of platelets (which help blood clotting), you have a greater risk of severe bleeding. When it reduces the number of red blood cells, you can develop anemia. (See *Managing common side effects of chemotherapy,* page 441.) The time of deepest reduction of blood counts varies with each drug.

Some chemotherapy drugs cause damage if they leak outside the vein. Others cause psychological complications, such as depression.

What happens after the treatment?

A doctor or nurse will teach you and your family how to reduce or control the side effects of chemotherapy.

BIOTHERAPY

Biotherapy involves the use of drugs known as *biological response modifiers.* Used mostly in cancer treatment, these drugs modify the interaction between a tumor and normal cells. How they work isn't fully understood. Although several biological response modifiers have been approved by the Food and Drug Administration, many more are still being studied. These drugs can be used alone or with other chemotherapy drugs.

What are biotherapy drugs used for?

- To eradicate or control cancer
- To lessen the side effects of other therapies, such as chemotherapy or radiation

What are some commonly used biotherapy drugs?

The most commonly used drug is erythropoietin (Epogen, Procrit), which stimulates the production of red blood cells in persons who are anemic.

Another common biotherapy drug is filgrastim (Neupogen), which stimulates the production of a specific group of white blood cells known as *neutrophils*. Neutrophils are responsible for removing and destroying bacteria in the blood.

What happens during the therapy?

- A nurse usually administers biotherapy in a hospital, ambulatory care, office or clinic, or home setting.
- You must give written consent for treatment with investigational drugs.
- Most biotherapy drugs are given by injection. The dosage and route depend on your type of cancer.
- You and your caregivers need to learn how to deal with the expected side effects and which signs and symptoms must be reported to the doctor.

What are the possible complications?

Side effects and complications of biological response modifiers are numerous and varied. They vary according to the drug used; the dosage, route, and the person's physical status; as well as the type and extent of the disease. Most side effects are reversible when drug therapy is discontinued. Common complications include:

- fatigue
- lack of appetite
- general body discomfort
- hematologic changes.

RADIATION

RADIATION TREATMENTS

Discovered in the 1890s, radiation offers one of the oldest treatments for cancer. Radiation therapy directs high levels of radiation at cancer cells, destroying their ability to grow and multiply.

Before an operation, radiation can shrink a tumor and allow its total removal. After an operation, it can destroy any cancer cells that were undetected during surgery. It can also relieve pain and enhance the person's quality of life in terminal cancer.

Radiation treatments may be delivered externally or internally. External radiation is more widely used.

The treatment uses X-rays or gamma rays that emit a beam of electrons at the target area. Recent advances in radiation therapy include large-field, large-dose radiation, such as half-body treatments. Large-field, large-dose radiation provides an effective, well-tolerated treatment for people with cancer that's spread. Total skin electron therapy, another advancement, radiates the entire skin surface and has been successful in managing extensive skin disease. Hyperfractionation, an experimental approach that attempts to achieve better tumor control, delivers more than one radiation treatment per day.

Why is this treatment done?

Radiation is used to destroy or slow the development and growth of cancer cells.

When shouldn't this treatment be done?

Radiation therapy shouldn't be used to treat pregnant women and should be used cautiously in people with blood disorders whose blood counts may be further lowered by radiation.

What happens before the treatment?

- Men who want to have children are told to deposit sperm in a sperm bank before therapy begins. Radiation can affect fertility.
- Women are informed that pelvic radiation can decrease hormone levels, leading to infertility and missed menstrual cycles.
- The radiation therapist may mark the exact areas of treatment on the person's skin with a pen or dye. The person shouldn't remove these markings until after the completion of therapy.

What happens during the treatment?

During a radiation treatment, you lie still on a table or floor (in the case of large-dose radiation) while a large machine, usually overhead, directs radiation at the target site for the ordered time — usually 1 to 2 minutes.

What are the possible complications?

Radiation therapy damages normal cells along with cancer cells. Normal cells have a greater ability to recover from radiation than cancer cells; however, many complications do occur. The complications or side effects depend on the site receiving the radiation. Such complications include digestive disturbances, headaches, reduced sperm count, decreased hormone levels, and reduced white blood cell and platelet counts. You may also suffer feelings of isolation.

What happens after the treatment?

The full benefit of radiation treatment may not occur for up to several months. (See *Recovering from radiation therapy*.)

RADIOACTIVE IMPLANTS

A radiation source — usually iodine 125 or iridium 192 — implanted directly into a tumor site delivers a high dose of radiation to the tumor while exposing healthy surrounding tissue to little radiation. Thus, this therapy (also called *brachytherapy* or *implant, intracavity*, or *interstitial therapy*) has an important advantage over conventional external radiation therapy.

Recently, radioactive implants have been combined with induced hyperthermia (a high body temperature) to treat brain tumors in the hope of prolonging the person's survival.

Why is this treatment done?

Radioactive implants inhibit the growth of a tumor or possibly decrease its size while sparing surrounding healthy tissue.

People who are considered ineligible for this therapy are those whose brain tumors are diffuse, occur at multiple sites, and are larger than 6 centimeters in diameter or those whose tumors are located in the brain stem, cerebellum, or thalamus.

Because people are considered radioactive while the implants are in place, their contact with caregivers must be limited.

What happens before the treatment?

You're told that you'll be in isolation while the implants are in place but that help will be nearby.

SELF-HELP

Recovering from radiation therapy

After receiving treatment, follow these important guidelines.

Care for your skin
- Use mild soap.
- Avoid irritating the radiated area with perfume, powder, or other cosmetics.

Other instructions
- Report side effects to the doctor.
- Keep follow-up appointments with your doctor.
- Consider joining a support group, such as the local chapter of the American Cancer Society.

Recovering from radioactive implant therapy

After you have been discharged from the hospital, follow these important guidelines.

Report symptoms
- Stay alert for seizures or changes in your level of consciousness, behavior, vision, muscle strength, or sensation. If these symptoms occur, call the doctor at once (or have a family member do so).
- Notify the doctor of a continued headache or a change in your headache, a sustained high fever, severe nausea or vomiting, a stiff neck, or sensitivity of your eyes to light.
- Learn how to recognize symptoms of wound infection, and report an infection to your doctor immediately.

Other instructions
- Take all medications as prescribed. Don't abruptly discontinue any medication.
- Increase your physical activity as you feel up to it, but avoid heavy lifting. Discuss with your doctor specific activities of concern.
- Keep all follow-up appointments for computed tomography scans.

What happens during the treatment?

To begin intracranial brachytherapy, the neurosurgeon places you in a stereotactic head frame while you're under a local anesthesic and mildly sedated. You're then taken from the operating room for a detailed computed tomography scan (commonly known as a CAT scan) of the head. Measurements from the scans are used to determine the three-dimensional coordinates of the tumor; the neurosurgeon makes the determination in consultation with a radiation oncologist and physicist.

After the planning is complete, you return to the operating room for insertion of catheters into which the radiation sources will later be instilled. The catheters are inserted and blank sources placed in them. After you're stabilized, you're taken for another CAT scan to verify the placement of the catheters and blank sources. After this confirmation, the blank sources are removed and replaced by the radioactive sources. Insertion of the sources may be performed by either the radiation oncologist or the neurosurgeon, who takes standard radiation precautions.

During radiation therapy, which may last 3 to 7 days, you're placed in a private room with limited nursing interventions. Depending on the radioactive source implanted, your nursing care may be carried out from behind a lead shield, with the use of lead aprons, or with only a lead helmet worn by you. The amount of time people may spend in the room per day also depends on the type of radioactive isotope used.

After the radiation dose is delivered, the radioactive implants are removed at the bedside. You then receive another CAT scan to assess the preliminary effects of therapy. You're no longer considered radioactive, and routine nursing care may be administered.

What are the possible complications?

Significant complications have been reported during therapy and have occasionally required early removal of the implants. Complications include worsening of neurologic deficits, increased intracranial pressure, seizures, and infection.

What happens after the treatment?

Visitors to your room will have to follow radiation safety procedures. No children or pregnant women are allowed to visit you. (See *Recovering from radioactive implant therapy.*)

OTHER TREATMENTS

LEUKAPHERESIS

Leukapheresis refers to the large-scale collection or removal of any of the three major types of white blood cells: monocytes, granulocytes, and lymphocytes. The primary function of monocytes and granulocytes is phagocytosis, whereas lymphocytes produce antibodies and play a key role in the immune system.

Typically, the leukocyte count (percent of white blood cells in total blood volume) is less than 1%, but some disorders can stimulate massive leukocyte production. When the leukocyte count exceeds 20%, significantly increased viscosity of the peripheral blood reduces pulmonary and cerebral blood flow. The leukocytes also compete with tissue for oxygen in the microcirculation. This condition, known as *leukostasis,* may result in tissue hypoxia and organ dysfunction.

Two methods can be used to achieve cell depletion: manual or automated apheresis. Manual apheresis is the removal of a volume of blood not exceeding 15% of the person's total volume. It may be used for people with extremely poor venous access or for children whose safe extracorporeal volume is less than the amount removed by an automated device. Manual removal is also an option when automated cell separators are unavailable.

Automated apheresis by computerized cell separators is safer and more efficient than manual apheresis; this method is also faster, removes more undesired cells and fewer desired cells, and reduces the risk of misidentification of blood components. However, venous access and the large volume of extracorporeal blood required to prime the disposable set can be limiting factors. The cost of automated apheresis, which is substantial, can also limit its use.

Why is this procedure done?

- To remove leukocytes, reducing the complications of leukostasis
- To alter immune responsiveness

What happens before the procedure?

Usually you're served a balanced, low-fat meal within a few hours of the procedure. Additional oral fluids are encouraged.

Recovering from leukapheresis

Leukapheresis has no long-term effects; home care instructions are required only if you're released from care immediately after apheresis. If you have chronic leukemia and you're undergoing leukapheresis to modify immune responsiveness, you may be treated as an outpatient. Follow these guidelines.

Take special precautions

• Leave the bandage in place for 2 to 3 hours. If bleeding occurs, apply pressure to the venipuncture site and elevate the arm until bleeding stops.

• Avoid lifting heavy objects and strenuous exercise for several hours.

Other instructions

• Eat a low-fat diet before each leukapheresis procedure.

• Drink extra fluids and eat a well-balanced meal after leukapheresis.

• Report any side effects to the doctor.

What happens during the procedure?

Leukapheresis must be performed by an apheresis specialist, typically a registered nurse or medical technologist. The procedure may be performed at the bedside or in the apheresis unit. After venous access is achieved in manual apheresis, the blood is aspirated into a syringe or allowed to flow by gravity into a plastic bag. The bag is disconnected from you and placed in a high-speed centrifuge for separation of plasma, red blood cells, platelets, and white blood cells. The white cell layer (buffy coat) is extracted manually, and the remaining portion of the blood is returned to the person. This process can be repeated until a desired degree of depletion is obtained.

In automated apheresis, the blood is withdrawn by a large-gauge catheter into a sterile plastic kit that has been placed in a blood cell separator. The blood flows into the device under negative pressure and enters a centrifuge, where separation of the blood elements takes place. The desired cell type (lymphocyte, monocyte, or granulocyte) is selectively removed and placed in a collection container. The remaining portion of the blood is returned to the person.

The degree of cell depletion achieved with apheresis depends on the volume of blood processed. An automated apheresis procedure processing 5 liters of whole blood can reduce the white blood cell count by 20% to 50%.

The apheresis specialist monitors you during the procedure. Upon completion, the venipuncture sites are wrapped with a pressure dressing.

What are the possible complications?

The most common complications of routine apheresis are dizziness, low blood pressure, slowing heart rate, fainting, seizures, hematoma formation at the venipuncture site, and discomfort. Leukemia patients with symptoms of leukostasis often develop complications associated with anemia and thrombocytopenia.

What happens after the procedure?

• The dressing is left intact for 3 to 4 hours.

• You're encouraged to drink fluids to ensure hemostatic balance. (See *Recovering from leukapheresis.*)

13

TREATING INFECTIONS

DRUG THERAPIES

PENICILLINS

Because of their effectiveness, safety, and low cost, penicillins are among the most widely used drugs for fighting bacterial infections. They consist of extracts and semisynthetic derivatives of several strains of the Penicillium mold. Penicillin derivatives differ in the types of bacteria they can kill and their ability to resist stomach acid.

What are penicillins used for?
Penicillins are given to treat bacterial infections.

What are some commonly used penicillins?
- amoxicillin, known by the brand names Amoxil and Polymox
- ampicillin, known by the brand names Amcill, Omnipen, Polycillin, and Principen
- bacampicillin, known by the brand name Spectrobid
- cloxacillin, known by the brand names Cloxapen and Tegopen
- dicloxacillin, known by the brand name Dynapen
- methicillin, known by the brand name Staphcillin
- nafcillin, known by the brand names Nafcil, Nallpen, and Unipen
- oxacillin, known by the brand names Bactocill and Prostaphlin
- penicillin G benzathine, known by the brand name Bicillin LA
- penicillin G potassium, known by the brand names Pentids and Pfizerpen
- penicillin G procaine, known by the brand name Wycillin
- penicillin G sodium, known by the brand names Penicillin G Sodium for Injection and (in Canada) Crystapen
- penicillin V potassium, known by the brand names Pen Vee K, V-Cillin K, and Veetids
- piperacillin sodium, known by the brand name Pipracil
- ticarcillin, known by the brand name Ticar

What are the possible side effects?
- Hypersensitivity reactions, ranging from rash and itching to serum sickness and serious systemic allergic reactions

- Sore mouth or tongue, furry tongue, vomiting, cramping, diarrhea
- Irritability, hallucinations, seizures

What are the guidelines for taking penicillins?

- Watch for signs of penicillin allergy, such as rash or itching, which may develop within 20 minutes (or sometimes after several days). Be especially alert for difficulty breathing, choking, dizziness, anxiety, weakness, and sweating. Report such symptoms to your doctor immediately.
- Don't take any other medication without first checking with your doctor.
- Tell your doctor if you've ever had an allergic reaction to any antibiotic.
- If you have a history of severe penicillin reaction, wear a medical identification bracelet or necklace.
- Take all of your medication, even if you feel better. Stopping the drug early can lead to a relapse.
- If you miss a dose, take it as soon as possible. Then space the remaining daily doses closer together to make up for the missed dose. Penicillins are most effective if your body has a steady amount.
- Avoid orange juice, other acidic juices, and vitamin C supplements while taking oral penicillin; they reduce the drug's effectiveness.
- If you develop diarrhea, check with your doctor or pharmacist before taking any drugs for diarrhea.
- Call your doctor if symptoms don't improve within a few days.

> *Penicillins are most effective if a constant serum concentration is maintained.*

CEPHALOSPORINS

Chemically related to penicillin, cephalosporins are a group of antibiotics. Dozens of different cephalosporins are available. Differences among them relate to their bacterial sensitivity, their duration of action, and routes of administration.

What are cephalosporins used for?

Cephalosporins are widely used to treat bacterial infections of the skin, bones, joints, and urinary and respiratory tracts.

What are some commonly used cephalosporins?

The cephalosporins are grouped by generation.

First generation
- cefadroxil, known by the brand names Duricef and Ultracef
- cefazolin, known by the brand names Ancef and Kefzol
- cefprozil, known by the brand name Cefzil
- cephalexin, known by the brand names Keflex and Keftab
- cephalothin, known by the brand name Keflin
- cephapirin, known by the brand name Cefadyl
- cephradine, known by the brand names Anspor and Velocef

Second generation
- cefaclor, known by the brand name Ceclor
- cefamandole, known by the brand name Mandol
- cefoxitin, known by the brand name Mefoxin
- cefuroxime, known by the brand names Ceftin, Kefurox, and Zinacef

Third generation
- cefixime, known by the brand name Suprax
- cefoperazone, known by the brand name Cefobid
- cefotaxime, known by the brand name Claforan
- ceftazidime, known by the brand names Fortaz and Tazidime
- ceftizoxime, known by the brand name Cefizox
- ceftriaxone, known by the brand name Rocephin

What are the possible side effects?
- Mild rashes, fever
- Blood disorders
- Kidney problems
- Nausea, vomiting, diarrhea, abdominal pain

What are the guidelines for taking cephalosporins?
- Tell your doctor if you develop signs of a new infection, such as diarrhea, vaginal itching, or a sore mouth.
- Immediately report signs of an allergic reaction (rash, hives and, possibly, fever) or decreased urination to your doctor.
- Take your medication on an empty stomach unless doing so causes an upset stomach.

- Avoid drinking beer, wine, or other alcoholic beverages. Some cephalosporins react with alcohol, causing flushing, nausea, and palpitations.
- Complete the full course of therapy (usually 7 to 10 days).

AMINOGLYCOSIDES

These powerful antibiotics are typically used only for serious bacterial infections. Because they're poorly absorbed from the digestive tract, these drugs must be given by injection for many infections. However, the drugs also come in forms that can be applied to the skin or eye.

Some aminoglycosides may be given orally in order to clean the intestine before surgery. When given orally, little drug is absorbed into the bloodstream. The drug remains within the intestine and kills the bacteria that normally reside there.

What are aminoglycosides used for?
Aminoglycosides are used to treat severe gram-negative infections caused by susceptible organisms.

What are some commonly used aminoglycosides?
- amikacin, known by the brand name Amikin
- gentamicin, known by the brand names Garamycin or Jenamicin
- kanamycin, known by the brand names Kantrex or Klebcil
- neomycin, known by the brand name Mycifradin
- netilmicin, known by the brand name Netromycin
- streptomycin
- tobramycin, known by the brand name Nebcin

What are the possible side effects?
- Hearing damage
- Kidney damage
- Nausea, vomiting, diarrhea
- Local reactions at the injection site
- Persistent dizziness
- Visual disturbances
- Blood disorders

If you're receiving aminoglycosides by injection in the hospital, expect the doctor to order frequent blood tests to ensure adequate blood levels and avoid toxicity.

What are the guidelines for taking aminoglycosides?

- Tell the doctor or nurse if you notice visual or hearing disturbances, if you feel dizzy or weak, or if you have joint pain, nausea, rash, or signs of infection.
- Drink plenty of fluids to reduce the risk of kidney damage.

What else you should know

If you're receiving aminoglycosides by injection in the hospital, expect the doctor to order frequent blood tests to ensure adequate blood levels of the drug.

MACROLIDES

Erythromycin, a macrolide antibiotic, is one of the most widely prescribed medicines in the world. Effective and inexpensive, it has a low incidence of allergic reactions and toxicity. Newer macrolides have been developed that need to be taken only once or twice a day. This dosing schedule promotes compliance with therapy.

What are macrolides used for?

Macrolides are used to treat bacterial infections.

What are some commonly used macrolides?

- azithromycin, known by the brand name Zithromax
- clarithromycin, known by the brand name Biaxin
- erythromycin, known by the brand names E-Mycin, Eryc, Erythrocin, and Pediamycin

What are the possible side effects?

- Rash and itching
- Sore mouth or tongue, furry tongue
- Vomiting, cramping, diarrhea

What are the guidelines for taking macrolides?

- Don't take any other medication, including nonprescription drugs, without first checking with the doctor. Certain macrolides may impair the body's ability to metabolize drugs, thereby increasing the risk of drug interactions.

- Tell the doctor if you have ever had an allergic reaction to any antibiotic.
- Take all of your medicine, even if you feel better. Discontinuing the drug early puts you at risk for a relapse.
- If you're taking erythromycin and miss a dose, take the missed dose as soon as possible. Then space the remaining daily doses closer together to make up for the missed dose.
- If you experience diarrhea, check with the doctor or pharmacist before taking antidiarrheal medication.

What else you should know
- Call the doctor if your symptoms don't improve within a few days.
- Certain tablets may have a special coating; these should not be crushed or chewed. If you have trouble swallowing the tablets, check with the doctor or pharmacist; there may be another form of the drug that's easier to swallow.

*T*ETRACYCLINES

Tetracycline antibiotics help fight many bacterial infections. Because they can kill a wide variety of bacteria, doctors may prescribe them without knowing exactly which bacteria is causing the infection.

Although usually given orally, some tetracyclines may be given as eye ointment.

What are tetracyclines used for?
Tetracyclines are used to treat bacterial infections.

What are some commonly used tetracyclines?
- doxycycline hyclate, known by the brand names Doxy-Caps and Vibramycin
- minocycline, known by the brand name Minocin
- oxytetracycline, known by the brand name Terramycin
- tetracycline, known by the brand names Achromycin V and Sumycin

Preventing tetracycline malabsorption

If you experience gastrointestinal upset during tetracycline therapy, you might be inclined to drink a glass of milk or take a stomach-soothing product such as an antacid. Unfortunately, taking milk or an antacid with tetracyclines significantly reduces the blood level — and therefore the effectiveness — of these drugs. The calcium, magnesium, or aluminum in these substances interacts with tetracycline to form insoluble complexes.

Prevent stomach upset

To prevent gastrointestinal upset while promoting proper drug absorption, take each dose with a full glass of water on an empty stomach. Be aware that the following foods or drugs interfere with tetracycline absorption:

- milk
- calcium supplements
- antacids that contain calcium, magnesium, or aluminum
- iron preparations, such as vitamins containing iron
- other products that contain magnesium, including sodium bicarbonate and milk of magnesia
- Colestid.

Take any of these at least 1 hour before or 2 hours after taking tetracycline.

What are the possible side effects?

- Liver problems
- Sensitivity to light, severe skin problems
- Light-headedness, dizziness
- Nausea, vomiting, loose stools, diarrhea, hairy tongue
- Increased urine output

What are the guidelines for taking tetracyclines?

- Avoid taking your medication with dairy products, antacids, iron preparations, multivitamins with iron, magnesium or zinc supplements, or laxatives. These substances bind to tetracyclines in the digestive tract and prevent their absorption. (See *Preventing tetracycline malabsorption.*)
- If you experience a sore mouth, black hairy tongue, or rectal and perineal itching, call your doctor.
- Also call the doctor if you develop diarrhea. Don't self-treat diarrhea with nonprescription drugs.
- Take tetracycline at least 1 hour before meals or 2 hours after them. To avoid getting an upset stomach, take the drug with a glass of water.
- Avoid intense or prolonged exposure to sunlight. If exposure is unavoidable, wear protective clothing and use a sunscreen.

SULFONAMIDES

Sometimes called *sulfa drugs,* the sulfonamides were among the first bacteria-killing drugs used. Today, they're frequently used to treat infections of the respiratory and genitourinary tracts.

What are sulfonamides used for?
Sulfonamides are used to treat bacterial infections.

What are some commonly used sulfonamides?
- cotrimoxazole, known by the brand names Bactrim and Septra
- sulfadiazine, known by the brand name Microsulfon
- sulfamethoxazole, known by the brand name Gantanol
- sulfasalazine, known by the brand name Azulfidine
- sulfisoxazole, known by the brand name Gantrisin

What are the possible side effects?
- Nausea, vomiting, diarrhea, hepatitis
- Headache, seizures, hallucinations, dizziness, tingling in the extremities
- Blood disorders
- Blood in the urine, kidney or bladder disorders, urine crystal formation
- Rash, severe skin problems, sun sensitivity

What are the guidelines for taking sulfonamides?
- Take the drug on an empty stomach, and drink plenty of fluids throughout therapy.
- Tell the doctor immediately if you develop a rash.
- Tell the doctor about all of the drugs you are taking, including nonprescription drugs. Don't take any other drugs without checking with the doctor.
- Tell the doctor if you have ever had an allergic reaction to a drug.
- You must complete the full course of prescribed therapy, even after symptoms disappear.
- Call the doctor if you develop a sore throat, fever, mouth ulcers, or jaundice.
- Drink at least eight 8-ounce (240-milliliter) glasses of water daily to prevent formation of urine crystals.

What else you should know

Avoid prolonged exposure to sunlight because photosensitivity reactions may occur. Wearing protective clothing and applying a sunscreen to exposed areas when outdoors will help prevent these reactions.

ANTIFUNGALS

These drugs treat fungal infections. Those fungal infections that affect internal body structures are serious and potentially life-threatening. Some fungal skin infections may be treated with creams and ointments. However, they can be difficult to treat and may require prolonged therapy.

What are antifungals used for?

Antifungals are used to treat a wide range of fungal infections.

What are some commonly used antifungals?

- amphotericin B, known by the brand name Fungizone
- fluconazole, known by the brand name Diflucan
- flucytosine, known by the brand name Ancobon
- griseofulvin, known by the brand names Fulvicin-U/F, Grifulvin V, and Grisactin
- ketoconazole, known by the brand name Nizoral
- miconazole, known by the brand name Monistat
- nystatin, known by the brand names Mycostatin and Nilstat

What are the possible side effects?

- Nausea, vomiting, diarrhea, loss of appetite
- Blood disorders
- Skin reactions, serious skin toxicity, rash, phototoxicity
- Liver or kidney problems
- Heart rhythm disturbances
- Fever, headache, dizziness

What are the guidelines for taking antifungals?

- Mycostatin is essentially nontoxic and very well tolerated. The other antifungals, however, must be used with caution.

- Don't take any other drug, including nonprescription drugs, without first checking with the doctor. Be sure to tell the doctor about any other medicines you are taking.
- Nizoral requires an acidic environment for absorption. Some people do not have enough stomach acid because of their illness and may require the administration of dilute hydrochloric acid to achieve the proper stomach pH.
- Watch for drug side effects such as itching, rash, nausea, vomiting, or headache.
- Promptly call your doctor if you have a persistent fever, chills, headache, nausea, or vomiting.
- Notify your doctor right away if you start to urinate less.
- Take Nizoral with food.
- Follow instructions for all lab tests as scheduled to detect any blood, kidney, or liver complications.

*A*NTIVIRALS

Viral infections are difficult to treat. That's because virus particles are small, simple proteins and many viruses use the host's cells to replicate. Viruses are generally treated using oral or intravenous drugs.

Each antiviral drug is used to treat a different virus. The drug acyclovir, for instance, treats herpes simplex virus Type 1 and Type 2 and herpes zoster varicella (shingles) infections. Another drug, amantadine, can treat or prevent influenza A virus. Two other drugs, foscarnet and ganciclovir, treat cytomegalovirus retinitis in AIDS patients.

In infants and children, the drug ribavirin treats respiratory syncytial virus. The drug vidarabine is used to treat herpes simplex virus encephalitis, herpes simplex virus infections in newborns, and herpes zoster in immunocompromised patients.

Zidovudine has become a mainstay in treating human immunodeficiency virus (HIV) infection and AIDS. Two other drugs, didanosine and zalcitabine, are usually reserved for AIDS patients who are unresponsive to zidovudine or unable to tolerate it.

Each antiviral is used for the treatment of a different viral infection.

What are antivirals used for?
Antivirals are used to treat various viral infections.

What are some commonly used antivirals?

- acyclovir, known by the brand name Zovirax
- amantadine, known by the brand name Symmetrel
- didanosine, also known as ddI, or known by the brand name Videx
- foscarnet, known by the brand name Foscavir
- ganciclovir, known by the brand name Cytovene
- ribavirin, known by the brand name Virazole
- vidarabine, known by the brand name Vira-A
- zalcitabine, also known as ddC, or by the brand name Hivid
- zidovudine, also known as AZT, or by the brand name Retrovir

What are the possible side effects?

Acyclovir

- Inflammation at the injection site
- Headache, lethargy, tremors, confusion, hallucinations, agitation, seizures, coma
- Nausea, vomiting
- Skin rash, hives

Amantadine

- Irritability, insomnia, light-headedness, difficulty concentrating, nervousness
- Loss of appetite, nausea
- Purplish red, netlike, blotchy marks on the skin

Didanosine

- Headache
- Diarrhea, nausea, vomiting, abdominal pain
- Pancreatitis (which may be fatal)
- Peripheral neuropathy (persistent tingling or pain in the extremities)

Foscarnet

- Anemia, blood disorders

Ganciclovir

- Anemia, blood disorders

Ribavirin

- Anemia
- Conjunctivitis, eyelid rash or redness of the eyelids
- Worsening of respiratory problems

Vidarabine

- Tremors, dizziness, hallucinations, confusion
- Loss of appetite, nausea

Zalcitabine

- Headache
- Diarrhea, nausea, vomiting, abdominal pain
- Pancreatitis (which may be fatal)
- Peripheral neuropathy (persistent tingling or pain in the extremities)

Zidovudine

- Anemia, blood disorders

What are the guidelines for taking antivirals?

- Be sure to tell your doctor about all of the other medications you are taking, including nonprescription medicines. Don't take any other medications without first checking with your doctor.
- For best absorption, take Symmetrel after meals.
- Elderly patients are more susceptible to neurologic side effects of Symmetrel. Take the drug in two daily doses rather than a single dose to reduce the incidence of these effects.
- If you are taking Symmetrel and insomnia occurs, take the drug several hours before bedtime. Watch for dizziness, and take care to prevent falls. Rise slowly from a sitting or lying position.
- If you are taking Videx or Hivid, peripheral neuropathy is a major side effect. Report numbness, tingling, or pain in the feet or hands immediately.
- Pancreatitis may occur in as many as 9% of patients taking Videx; it occurs in less than 1% of patients taking Hivid. Report abdominal pain, nausea, or vomiting.
- If you are taking Retrovir, expect the doctor to closely monitor your blood count to detect early signs of toxicity.
- If you are taking Zovirax for herpes lesions, avoid sexual contact while herpes lesions are present. This medication does not cure herpes, but it will prolong the intervals between outbreaks.
- Understand that neither Retrovir, Videx, nor Hivid cures HIV infection. If you have HIV infection, avoid sexual contact or use a latex condom to help prevent spreading the infection to others.
- If you are taking Videx, it's important to chew the tablets thoroughly and drink at least 1 ounce of water with each dose. The tablets

Recovering from incision and drainage

After leaving your doctor's of-fice, follow these important guidelines.

Use care with dressings
- If you must change the dress-ing at home, follow your doc-tor's instructions.
- Remember that cleanliness, hand washing, and proper dis-posal of soiled dressings are important.

Other points to remember
- If the doctor orders warm soaks to promote further drain-age, be sure to do them as in-structed.
- Report redness, warmth, swelling, excessive pain, fever, or changed appearance of drainage to your doctor.
- Take the antibiotics and analgesics as ordered by your doctor.

contain buffers that raise the pH of the stomach; the drug would be rapidly degraded in stomach acid without this buffering action.

What else you should know

Many antivirals are highly toxic drugs. The doctor may order fre-quent blood tests in order to detect the early signs of toxicity so that therapy can be modified to prevent further systemic damage.

SURGERIES

INCISION AND DRAINAGE

This procedure, called an *I&D,* drains accumulated pus from an in-fected area through a surgically created incision.

Why is this procedure done?
An I&D treats localized pus-filled infections. It's done when a local-ized infection does not clear up after antibiotic treatment.

What happens before the procedure?
The doctor sterilizes the incision site.

What happens during the procedure?
The doctor, usually in the office, makes an incision directly over the pus-filled area, spreading the skin's edges to allow drainage of pus. He or she may take a culture sample. After the pus drains, the doctor leaves the cavity open to promote healing. If the cavity is large, it may be packed with gauze to provide further drainage and to ensure heal-ing from within. Finally, the doctor applies a sterile dressing.

What are the possible complications?
Complications rarely occur, but infection may become problematic.

What happens after the procedure?
Local pain diminishes quickly. Aspirin is recommended for pain. (See *Recovering from incision and drainage.*)

MASTOIDECTOMY

Mastoidectomy is a surgical procedure used to remove the mastoid process or the mastoid cells of the temporal bone. There are four types of mastoidectomies: mastoidectomy, radical mastoidectomy, modified-radical mastoidectomy, and mastoid tympanoplasty.

The extent of mastoid involvement, the condition of the small bones of the middle ear, the tympanic membrane, and the presence of a mass of dead tissue in the middle ear will determine which procedure is performed.

Why is this procedure done?

Mastoidectomy is performed to remove parts of the mastoid cells that are invaded by infection or dead tissue mass and to clean the remaining bone.

What happens before the procedure?

The surgeon may order your hair shaved up to 1 inch (2.5 centimeters) around your ear.

What happens during the procedure?

After you receive a general anesthetic, the surgeon will select either a curved incision made behind the ear or an incision made through the ear canal. This exposes the bone and the mastoid.

When an acute infection is limited to the mastoid cells, a mastoidectomy is performed. All infected cells are removed and the remaining area is cleaned. Special care is taken not to injure the facial nerve that passes through the temporal bone. Radical mastoidectomy is indicated when disease has spread to the middle ear as well. If the tympanic membrane is perforated as a result of increased pressure in the middle ear, a combined mastoidectomy and tympanoplasty is performed. A modified-radical mastoidectomy may be performed to remove a dead tissue mass. This procedure leaves the tympanic membrane and the middle ear structures intact. The surgeon may insert some packing and, possibly, a drain; close the incision; and apply a dressing.

SELF-HELP

Recovering from mastoidectomy

After you've been discharged from the hospital, follow these important guidelines.

Take special precautions
- Avoid driving, blowing your nose, and heavy lifting for 1 week after surgery.
- Open your mouth when you sneeze to prevent unnecessary pressure buildup.

Other instructions
- Comply with recommended drug therapy and with wound care and ear care treatments.
- Keep your ear dry using a cotton ball with mineral oil or Vaseline on the visible portion of the cotton ball.
- If you have ear packing, be aware that it will be removed by the surgeon in 3 to 5 days.
- Keep follow-up medical appointments.

What are the possible complications?

Facial nerve paralysis is a serious complication after mastoidectomy. It is due to possible erosion of the bone that protects the nerve. Other complications include infection, vertigo, meningitis, or brain abscess. The use of antibiotics greatly reduces the risk of postoperative infection.

What happens after the procedure?

- You lie on the affected side to promote drainage.
- The nurse administers pain medication and sedatives to control pain and restlessness.
- You may need assistance when getting out of bed to minimize dizziness. (See *Recovering from mastoidectomy*.)

TREATING EYE DISORDERS

DRUG THERAPIES

MIOTICS

Miosis occurs when the sphincter muscle of the iris contracts, causing the pupil of the eye to decrease in diameter. When the pupil is constricted, drainage from within the eye is enhanced, and the pressure within the eye decreases.

Drugs that cause miosis are called *miotics*. There are two major types of miotics: cholinergics and cholinesterase inhibitors (sometimes called *anticholinesterase drugs*). Both of these classes of drugs have the same effect: They mimic or enhance the action of acetylcholine on the structures of the eye. Cholinergics mimic the action of acetylcholine; cholinesterase inhibitors prevent the breakdown of naturally occurring acetylcholine, thereby enhancing and prolonging its action.

What are miotics used for?
Miotics are used to reduce the pressure within the eyeball.

What are some commonly used miotics?
Cholinergics
- acetylcholine, known by the brand name Miochol
- carbachol, known by the brand names Carbacel and Isopto Carbachol
- pilocarpine, known by the brand names Isopto Carpine, Ocusert Pilo, and Pilocar

Cholinesterase inhibitors
- demecarium, known by the brand name Humorsol
- echothiophate, known by the brand name Phospholine Iodide
- isoflurophate, known by the brand name Floropryl
- physostigmine, known by the brand names Eserine Salicylate and Isopto Eserine

What are the possible side effects?
- Eye pain, blurred vision, poor vision in low light, twitching of the eyelids, redness, burning, or tearing of the eye

- Headache
- Nausea, vomiting, diarrhea, cramps
- Frequent urination
- Excessive salivation
- Sweating
- Asthmatic attacks, difficulty breathing.

What are the guidelines for taking miotics?

- Carefully take the drops as instructed. Don't touch the tip of the dropper to the eye or surrounding tissue. Apply light finger pressure to the region below the eye for 1 minute after instillation to reduce systemic absorption.
- If you are using the Ocusert Pilo system, replace the system every 7 days as directed. If it falls out of your eye, rinse it in cool tap water and reposition it in your eye. Don't reuse a system that has been deformed.
- If you're using myotics and develop excessive salivation, diarrhea, weakness, or other signs of toxicity, stop taking the drug immediately and contact the doctor.
- Blurred vision caused by these drugs usually diminishes with continued use. However, if these drugs cause poor night vision, avoid driving or operating machinery after dark.
- Tell your doctor if you've ever had heart failure, bronchial asthma, peptic ulcer, an overactive thyroid, or Parkinson's disease.

What else you should know

- Miotics (especially Pilocar) are used to treat acute angle-closure glaucoma, but they have been largely replaced by beta-adrenergic blockers in the initial treatment of chronic open-angle glaucoma. Miotics are also often used following eye surgeries.
- Be sure to report for all follow-up appointments. Close monitoring is necessary to check for the effectiveness of treatment.

If you're using myotics and develop excessive salivation, diarrhea, weakness, or other signs of toxicity, stop taking the drug immediately and contact the doctor.

CARBONIC ANHYDRASE INHIBITORS

Glaucoma is a condition in which pressure within the eye is higher than normal. Although the causes of glaucoma are many, the end result is the same: Untreated glaucoma can lead to blindness.

Carbonic anhydrase inhibitors are among the many drugs used to treat glaucoma. They reduce intraocular pressure by decreasing the production of aqueous humor, the specialized fluid contained within the eye. They also cause some minor metabolic changes in the body's acid-base balance, and they cause a small increase in urine output. These effects also indirectly lower the pressure within the eye. Interestingly, these effects make Diamox a useful drug for treating acute mountain sickness.

Carbonic anhydrase inhibitors are commonly used with other antiglaucoma drugs. Although carbonic anhydrase inhibitors are administered orally, Diamox, the most widely used drug in this class, may also be given by injection.

What are carbonic anhydrase inhibitors used for?

- To reduce aqueous humor production, thus lowering pressure within the eye
- To prevent or treat acute mountain sickness
- To enhance the effectiveness of other drugs in certain forms of epilepsy
- To promote a mild increase in urine output

What are some commonly used carbonic anhydrase inhibitors?

- acetazolamide, known by the brand names Ak-Zol, Diamox, and Storzolamide
- dichlorphenamide, known by the brand name Daranide
- methazolamide, known by the brand name Neptazane

What are the possible side effects?

- Blood mineral imbalances, acid-base imbalances
- Blood disorders
- Malaise, loss of appetite, fatigue, weakness, drowsiness
- Nausea, vomiting
- Increased urine flow, kidney stones

What are the guidelines for taking carbonic anhydrase inhibitors?

- Because gastrointestinal symptoms commonly occur with carbonic anhydrase inhibitors, take the drug with food.

- Take a missed dose as soon as you remember, unless it's within 2 hours of the next scheduled dose. In that case, omit the missed dose and maintain your regular schedule. Never take a double dose.
- If you're taking a sustained-release form of the drug, don't crush or chew the capsule; swallow it whole. Crushing or chewing damages the integrity of the timed-release formulation.
- This drug may cause potassium loss. Tell the doctor if you experience fatigue, muscle cramps, and increased thirst. Eat foods high in potassium, such as bananas and avocados.
- Contact the doctor if you experience depression, difficult or painful urination, lower back pain, a sore throat, fever, or a skin rash.
- This drug may cause drowsiness. If it does, avoid driving or other potentially hazardous activities that require alertness.

What else you should know

This drug may increase urine output, especially at the beginning of therapy. To avoid disturbing your sleep, take the last dose no later than 6 p.m.

MYDRIATICS

Mydriasis occurs when the pupil of the eye is dilated. Because the diameter of the pupil is controlled by both the adrenergic and cholinergic nervous systems, there are two different classes of drugs that can be used to cause mydriasis.

The adrenergic nervous system causes mydriasis. Drugs that mimic the effects of norepinephrine can increase the size of the pupil.

The cholinergic nervous system acts to decrease pupil size (miosis).

What are mydriatics used for?
- To dilate the pupil and block the ability to focus
- To facilitate eye exams
- To treat certain types of eye inflammation

What are some commonly used mydriatics?
Adrenergics
- apraclonidine, known by the brand name Iopidine
- dipivefrin, known by the brand name Propine

- epinephrine, known by the brand names Epitrate, Epifrin, and Epinal
- phenylephrine, known by the brand names Ak-Dilate and Neo-Synephrine

Anticholinergics
- atropine, known by the brand names Atropisol and Isopto Atropine
- cyclopentolate, known by the brand names Ak-Pentolate and Cyclogyl
- homatropine, known by the brand names I-Homatrine and Isopto Homatropine
- scopolamine, known by the brand name Isopto Hyoscine
- tropicamide, known by the brand names Mydriacyl and Tropicacyl

What are the possible side effects?
- Blurred vision, eye dryness, sensitivity to light, redness and itching of the eye, allergy
- Skin flushing
- Rapid heart rate
- Fever
- Dizziness, irritability, confusion, sleepiness, hallucinations, seizures, and behavioral changes in children

Because mydriatics will temporarily blur vision, avoid driving or operating machinery until your vision clears.

What are the guidelines for taking mydriatics?
- Tell the doctor if you experience eye pain, blurred vision, and headache when the drug dilates the pupil. Also report if you feel an increase in your heart rate, flushing, and dry skin.
- Take the drug as directed. Don't touch the tip of the dropper or tube to the eye or the surrounding tissue.
- Reduce systemic effects by applying light finger pressure on the lower eyelid for 1 minute after instillation.
- Because mydriatics will temporarily blur vision, avoid driving or operating machinery until your vision clears.
- If you become sensitive to light, wear dark glasses when outdoors in the daytime.

VASOCONSTRICTING EYEDROPS

These eyedrops are commonly available without a prescription. They're used to relieve the itching and redness associated with eye irritation and inflammation caused by pollen-related allergies, colds, dust, smog, swimming, and contact lenses. They also provide relief from eyestrain caused by reading or driving.

What are vasoconstricting eyedrops used for?
They're used to temporarily relieve eye itching and redness.

What are some commonly used vasoconstricting eyedrops?
- naphazoline, known by the brand names Ak-Con, Allerest, Clear Eyes, Lubricating Eye Redness Remover, and Naphcon Forte
- oxymetazoline, known by the brand names OcuClear and Visine L.R.
- phenylephrine, known by the brand names Ak-Nefrin, Isopto Frin, Ocu-Phrin Sterile Eye Drops, and Prefrin Liquifilm

What are the possible side effects?
- Mild, transient eye stinging
- Headache, dizziness, excessive drowsiness
- Irregular heartbeat

What are the guidelines for taking vasoconstricting eyedrops?
- Stop using the drug if you experience headache, dizziness, an irregular heartbeat, or excessive drowsiness.
- Follow the label instructions for using the drug. Don't touch the tip of the dropper to the eye or surrounding tissue. Apply gentle pressure to the inside corner of the eye for 1 minute after administration to minimize systemic effects.
- Don't use the solution if it changes color or becomes cloudy.
- Don't take these drugs if you have glaucoma. Check with your doctor before taking these drugs if you have an overactive thyroid, heart disease, high blood pressure, or diabetes.
- Never use in infants or children without checking with a pediatrician.

What else you should know

▪ Don't use the drug for more than 4 days. Longer use may actually worsen eye irritation as well as increase the risk of side effects.

▪ Don't exceed the recommended dose. Doing so can worsen eye irritation and inflammation.

SURGERIES

RADIAL KERATOTOMY

This surgical procedure is performed to correct myopia, a refractive error in which light rays come to a focus in front of the retina. Radial keratotomy involves creation of small radial incisions in the cornea. These incisions flatten the cornea to help properly focus light on the retina.

The degree of myopia — or nearsightedness — is measured in diopters (unit of measurement of refractive power of lenses or prisms). Because radial keratotomy can reduce myopia by only 4 diopters, this procedure will not help highly myopic persons.

Why is this procedure done?

Radial keratotomy is performed to correct nearsightedness in people with myopia (ranging from 2 to 8 diopters) whose vision with glasses or contact lenses is unsatisfactory.

Disadvantages of this procedure are its unpredictability and instability. This procedure is controversial in the ophthalmic community for those reasons.

What happens before the procedure?

▪ You'll have had an ophthalmologic exam to evaluate visual acuity and refraction, the thickness and curvature of the cornea, endothelial cell count, intraocular pressure, and axial length of the eye.

▪ The nurse cleans your face with an antiseptic solution and administers a sedative to help you relax.

▪ You're told to remain still during the 3 to 8 minutes the operation takes.

What happens during the procedure?

Radial keratotomy is commonly performed in an outpatient surgical setting. After giving you a sedative and topical anesthetic eyedrops, the surgeon measures corneal thickness using an ultrasonic pachometer. Then, using a calibrated diamond knife, the surgeon makes eight or more incisions into the cornea in a radial pattern. A topical antibiotic solution and a cycloplegic agent are then applied. An eye patch may be applied for 24 hours.

What are the possible complications?

Because keratotomy has been widely used only since the 1970s, its long-term effects aren't known. Complications include overcorrection or undercorrection of the vision problem as well as corneal perforation, which usually heals on its own.

What happens after the procedure?

After you recover from the local anesthetic, you may experience some discomfort for 10 to 18 hours. The nurse will give you analgesics as prescribed by the doctor. (See *Recovering from radial keratotomy.*)

CATARACT REMOVAL

A cataract is a clouding of the normally transparent crystalline lens of the eye. Surgical removal of the cloudy lens is the treatment of choice. (See *Comparing methods of cataract removal,* page 474.)

Why is this procedure done?

Cataract removal is performed to remove a cloudy lens that prevents light rays from reaching the retina. Traditionally, the procedure was not performed until vision became seriously impaired. Today it can be done as soon as the person notices vision impairment.

What happens before the procedure?

- You must not eat or drink after midnight the night before surgery.
- You'll receive medication that will dilate the eye, antibiotics to reduce the risk of infection, and a sedative for relaxation during the procedure.

 SELF-HELP

Recovering from radial keratotomy

After you've been discharged from the hospital, follow these important guidelines.

Cope with common side effects

- Be aware that your eyes may be more sensitive to light and you may have a foreign body sensation in your eye. However, know that these effects usually subside in 1 to 2 months.
- In bright sunlight, wear dark sunglasses or glasses with polarizing lenses.
- Avoid night driving if you're bothered by glare from oncoming headlights.

Take special precautions

- Avoid wearing eye makeup until the cornea has healed (approximately 1 month).
- If eyedrops are prescribed, be sure to use them.
- Protect the affected eye from soap and water when showering and bathing.
- Avoid contact and water sports until the doctor gives permission.
- Because your vision may fluctuate, avoid potentially hazardous activities that require clear vision (such as driving) until your symptoms subside.

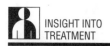

Comparing methods of cataract removal

A cataract is a clouding of the lens of the eye that impairs vision. Cataracts can be removed by intracapsular or extracapsular techniques.

Intracapsular extraction

In this technique, the surgeon makes a partial incision at the superior limbus arc and then removes the lens with either a specially designed forceps or a cryoprobe; the latter freezes and adheres to the lens, facilitating its removal.

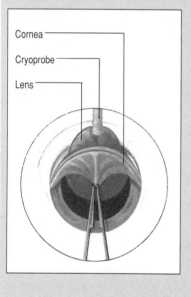

Cornea
Cryoprobe
Lens

Extracapsular extraction

In this technique, the surgeon may use irrigation and aspiration or phacoemulsification.

Irrigation and aspiration

The surgeon makes an incision at the limbus, opens the anterior lens capsule with a cystotome, and expresses the lens. The surgeon then irrigates and suctions the remaining lens cortex.

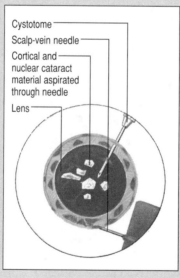

Cystotome
Scalp-vein needle
Cortical and nuclear cataract material aspirated through needle
Lens

Phacoemulsification

In this method, the surgeon uses an ultrasonic probe to break the lens into minute particles. The surgeon then aspirates these particles with the probe.

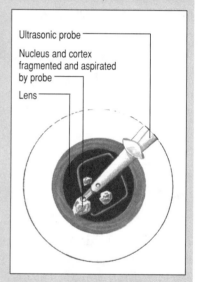

Ultrasonic probe
Nucleus and cortex fragmented and aspirated by probe
Lens

What happens during the procedure?

Cataract extraction may be done in the hospital as a short-stay procedure or in an ophthalmologist's office-based surgical facility.

Usually, the procedure is done under local anesthesia. You'll be in a state of conscious sedation, awake but with diminished motor activity and response to pain. The procedure can also be performed under general anesthesia.

The doctor dilates the pupil to facilitate cataract removal. He or she uses one of two techniques to remove the lens and then may insert one of many types of lens implants.

What are the possible complications?

Formation of a second membrane that becomes opaque and results in reduced vision is the most common complication. It can be corrected easily in the doctor's office with a laser. Other complications include infection, retinal detachment, glaucoma, and hemorrhage.

What happens after the procedure?

- The doctor will instill antibiotic medications before applying a patch and a shield to your affected eye.
- The affected and unaffected eye can work together after cataract surgery with lens implantation. After the eye has healed (approximately 2 months), the doctor will prescribe glasses for reading and any remaining astigmatism.
- If the procedure is performed in an ophthalmologist's surgical facility, you'll be observed for 2 to 3 hours and then sent home. (See *Recovering from cataract surgery*.)

CORNEAL TRANSPLANT

This procedure, also called a corneal *keratoplasty*, replaces a damaged part of the recipient's cornea with healthy corneal tissue from a recently deceased human donor. A corneal transplant can take one of two forms: a full-thickness (penetrating) keratoplasty, involving excision and replacement of all corneal layers, or a partial-thickness (lamellar) keratoplasty, which removes and replaces only the outer layers of corneal tissue. Full-thickness keratoplasty, by far the more common procedure, produces a high degree of clarity and restores vision in 95% of cases. A lamellar transplant is performed rarely and selectively.

Because the cornea doesn't recover as rapidly as other parts of the body, healing may take up to a year. Typically, sutures remain in place and vision isn't completely functional until healing occurs.

 SELF-HELP

Recovering from cataract surgery

After you've been discharged from the hospital, follow these important guidelines.

Take special precautions

- Avoid activities that raise intraocular pressure and place pressure on the sutures: heavy lifting, bending, straining during defecation, and vigorous coughing or sneezing. Sleep on your back or on the nonsurgical side and avoid strenuous exercise for 6 to 10 weeks.
- Contact the doctor immediately if you notice sudden eye pain, bleeding, increased discharge, or decreased vision or if you see light flashes or floaters. These symptoms may signal complications.

Other instructions

- Use eyedrops and ointments and change the eye patch. Use medications as prescribed.
- Wear dark glasses to reduce discomfort in bright light.
- Keep all follow-up appointments to monitor the results of surgery and to detect complications.

Why is this procedure done?

Corneal transplants are performed to replace damaged or opaque corneal tissue with a clear, healthy corneal graft. They help restore corneal clarity lost through injury, inflammation, ulceration, or chemical burns. This procedure is also used to correct corneal dystrophies and abnormal thinning and bulging of the central portion of the cornea.

What happens before the procedure?

The procedure is explained and you sign a consent form.

What happens during the procedure?

A transplant is usually performed under local anesthesia and takes 1 to 2 hours. You must remain still until the surgery has been completed.

In a full-thickness or penetrating keratoplasty, the surgeon cuts a "button" from your diseased opaque cornea and replaces it with a precisely sized button obtained from healthy donor corneal tissue. The donor button is anchored in place with extremely fine sutures. To end the procedure, the surgeon patches your eye and tapes a shield over it.

In a partial-thickness or lamellar keratoplasty, the surgeon excises only the superficial layers of corneal tissue in both the donor and your corneas. The donor graft is then sutured in place. As in the full-thickness procedure, the surgeon patches your eye and applies a rigid shield. (See *Comparing corneal transplants.*)

What are the possible complications?

Graft rejection, which occurs in about 15% of cases, may happen at any time during your life. Uncommon complications include wound leakage, loosening of the sutures, dehiscence, and infection.

What happens after the procedure?

- You'll be given analgesics to relieve dull aching. A bandage and protective shield will be placed over your eye.
- You may get a sedative to reduce eye pressure.
- To avoid increased pressure in your eye, you'll be told to lie on your back or on your unaffected side, with the bed flat or slightly elevated. Rapid head movements, hard coughing or sneezing, squinting or rubbing eyes, bending over, and other activities that could increase

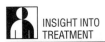
INSIGHT INTO
TREATMENT

Comparing corneal transplants

A corneal transplant may involve replacement of the entire cornea or simply a thin layer of corneal tissue. In a full-thickness transplant, the surgeon removes the corneal disk, which measures 7 to 8 millimeters, and replaces it with a matching "button" from a donor. In a lamellar, or partial-thickness transplant, the surgeon removes superficial corneal tissue only and replaces it with donor tissue.

FULL-THICKNESS TRANSPLANT

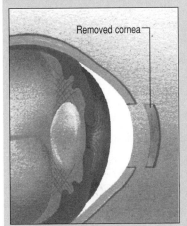

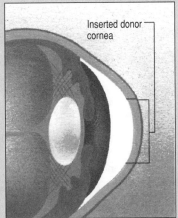

LAMELLAR TRANSPLANT

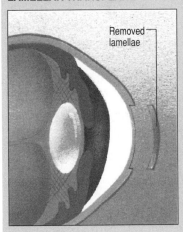

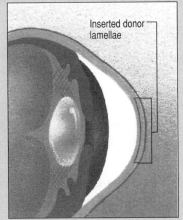

SELF-HELP

Recovering from a corneal transplant

After you've been discharged from the hospital, follow these important guidelines.

Know what to expect
Be aware that sensitivity to light is a common problem that decreases gradually as healing progresses. To ease discomfort, wear dark glasses in bright light.

Other instructions
▪ Avoid activities that increase eye pressure, such as extreme exertion, sudden jerky movements, lifting or pushing heavy objects, and straining during bowel movements.
▪ Make sure you and family members learn how to recognize signs and symptoms of graft rejection (cloudiness, drainage, and decreased vision). Immediately notify the doctor if any of these problems occur. Rejection can occur many years after surgery, so you should check the graft daily for the rest of your life.
▪ Instill your prescribed eyedrops.
▪ Wear an eye shield when sleeping.
▪ Keep regular follow-up appointments with your doctor.

pressure in your eye must be avoided. (See *Recovering from a corneal transplant.*)
▪ You'll need help in standing or walking until you adjust to vision changes.

TRABECULECTOMY

A surgical filtering procedure, trabeculectomy removes part of the trabecular meshwork of the eye to allow water in the eye to bypass blocked drainage channels and flow safely away from the eye. An iridectomy is performed at the same time to prevent the iris from blocking the new opening and obstructing the flow of water from the eye.

Why is this procedure done?
It's the treatment of choice in primary and secondary open-angle glaucoma. It's done:
▪ to create a new path for water to drain from the eye
▪ to prevent the buildup of intraocular pressure.

What happens before the procedure?
▪ You're told that this procedure will probably prevent further visual impairment but that it can't restore vision that's already lost. It will temporarily affect depth perception and peripheral vision on the operative side.
▪ The prescribed antiglaucoma drugs will be administered until you go to the operating room.
▪ Avoid any activities that could increase intraocular pressure, such as bending, vigorous coughing or sneezing, or straining during bowel movements.

What happens during the procedure?
After you've received a local anesthetic, the surgeon makes an incision in the white part of the eye and removes a portion of the trabecular meshwork. The surgeon then performs a peripheral iridectomy to create a filtering bleb, or opening for water to drain, under the conjunctiva. An antibiotic ointment is then applied before your eye is patched.

SELF-HELP

Recovering from trabeculectomy

After you've been discharged from the hospital, follow these important guidelines.

Report symptoms
Immediately report sudden onset of severe eye pain, light sensitivity, excessive tearing, inflammation, or vision loss.

Take safety precautions
- Avoid activities that increase intraocular pressure, such as excessive fluid intake, heavy lifting, and undue straining.
- Avoid driving and other potentially hazardous tasks that require normal vision until the doctor gives you permission.
- Be aware that vision changes can pose safety hazards. To compensate for loss of depth percep-

tion, use up-and-down head movements. To help counteract peripheral vision loss, turn your head fully to view objects on your side.

Other instructions
- Avoid wearing constrictive clothing around your neck or torso because it can increase intraocular pressure.
- Take prescribed drugs regularly because glaucoma isn't curable.
- Keep regular medical follow-up appointments for monitoring of peripheral vision and intraocular pressure. Urge family members to have regular eye exams because glaucoma is usually familial.

What are the possible complications?
Complications of trabeculectomy include a temporary rise in intraocular pressure, collapse of the filtering bleb, severe inflammatory reaction, infection, early cataract formation, and blood in the eye.

What happens after the procedure?
The nurse covers your eye with a patch or shield. Periodic tonometry measurements will be taken, and you'll experience blurred vision. (See *Recovering from trabeculectomy*.)

VITRECTOMY

This microsurgical procedure removes part or all of the vitreous humor (the transparent gelatinous substance that fills the cavity behind the lens of the eye). The surgical instruments used have advanced fiber-

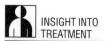

INSIGHT INTO
TREATMENT

Understanding vitrectomy

The illustration below demonstrates the placement of vitrectomy instruments during this surgical procedure.

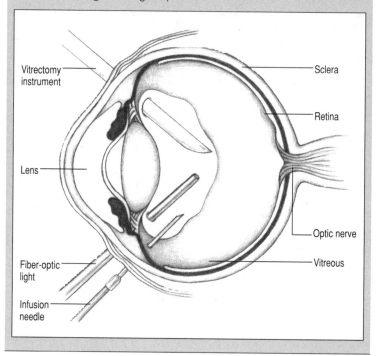

optic and laser delivery systems. This procedure is usually done in
combination with other eye surgeries. (See *Understanding vitrectomy*.)

Why is this procedure done?
- To remove vitreous opacities
- To allow access to the retina
- To allow removal of foreign bodies

What happens before the procedure?
- You receive mydriatic and cycloplegic drugs to dilate the pupil and,
perhaps, antibiotics to prevent infection.
- Preparation for surgery may include facial washing (with antiseptic
soap) and eyedrops the morning of surgery.

What happens during the procedure?

An eye surgeon who specializes in vitreous humor or retinal disorders typically does this procedure. It may be done under local or general anesthesia and usually takes 2 to 3 hours; it's typically performed on one eye at a time. The surgeon makes two incisions in the sclera — one for the insertion of vitrectomy instruments and the other to provide an opening for the fiber-optic light — and then cuts and aspirates the membranes and vitreous humor and infuses saline solution into the vitreous cavity to maintain intraocular pressure. Air or sulfur hexafluoride gas may be injected to hold the retina in place until a firm adhesion develops. Finally, antibiotics are administered and both eyes are patched. You're typically discharged within 3 to 5 days.

What are the possible complications?

Complications of vitrectomy include endophthalmitis (requiring intravitreous and systemic antibiotics and possibly a second vitrectomy), iatrogenic cataracts (requiring later removal), vitreous hemorrhage (which may clear spontaneously or may require laser photocoagulation), and retinal detachment (which may require scleral buckling).

What happens after the procedure?

- You may experience temporary decreased vision until your eye is healed. After laser treatment, your peripheral vision may be permanently impaired. Because you're using only one eye, depth perception will be a problem.
- If you received injections of air or gas during surgery, you must maintain a certain position, usually face down, to keep the gas bubble in place over the retina. If air was infused, this may take several days; if gas was infused, 7 to 10 days. You must maintain this position for several days, but you'll be allowed to sit upright for meals and to stand to use the bathroom. (See *Recovering from vitrectomy.*)

 SELF-HELP

Recovering from vitrectomy

After you've been discharged from the hospital, follow these important guidelines.

Take special precautions

- Don't stoop, lift heavy objects, exercise strenuously, or dive into water. You may read, watch TV, walk up and down stairs, and take walks.
- Sleep with your head elevated on several pillows, as recommended by the surgeon, to prevent further bleeding.
- If a gas bubble was injected into your eye, avoid air travel until the bubble is completely absorbed.
- Use eyedrops for up to 6 weeks to prevent infection and inflammation.

Other instructions

- Wear dark glasses if your eyes are sensitive to light.
- Schedule a follow-up appointment after discharge from the hospital.

SCLERAL BUCKLING

Used to repair retinal detachment, scleral buckling is the use of external pressure on the separated retinal layers to bring the choroid (a membrane that partially covers the eye between the retina and the sclera) into contact with the retina. This forms a scar tissue that binds the

Recovering from scleral buckling

After you've been discharged from the hospital, follow these important guidelines.

Take special precautions
• Avoid strenuous activity or situations in which jostling or eye injury could occur (for example, being in a crowded room).
• Don't do any heavy lifting, straining, or strenuous activity that increases intraocular pressure.
• Avoid rapid eye movement, as occurs during reading, until the doctor gives permission.
• Wear sunglasses during the day and an eye shield at night.

Report potential problems
• Notify the doctor if you experience symptoms of recurring detachment: floating spots, flashing lights, or progressive shadow.
• Report fever, eye pain, or drainage.

Other instructions
• Use prescribed dilating, antibiotic, or corticosteroid eyedrops.
• Remember that meticulous cleanliness is essential to avoid infection.
• Keep all follow-up medical appointments to check for further retinal detachment, glaucoma, and other complications.

layers together. It also prevents fluid from seeping between the detached layers of the retina and causing further detachment and possible blindness. When the break or tear is small enough, laser therapy, diathermy, or cryotherapy may be used to seal the retina.

Scleral buckling is successful in about 95% of people. Its effectiveness depends on the cause, location, and duration of detachment. If the retinal macula is detached, visual acuity may still be poor after surgery.

Why is this procedure done?

Scleral buckling is performed to seal retinal breaks and reattach the retina. It is used to repair detachments caused by holes or tears, fibrous tissue formation, and intraocular inflammation with a build-up of fluid beneath the retina.

What happens before the procedure?

The surgeon dilates your pupil with medication to allow access to the internal eye.

What happens during the procedure?

After you receive a local anesthetic, the surgeon makes an incision in the eye membrane, exposes the sclera, and then tags the rectus muscles with sutures to aid positioning of the eye.

The surgeon then locates the retinal tear and marks its position on the sclera with either heat or cold treatment. This forms a scar at the site of the retinal hole. As the scar heals, it should keep the retina in place.

In some procedures, the surgeon sutures a scleral silicone sponge over the retinal hole. In others, he or she dissects the scleral bed. Then the surgeon drains the subretinal fluid to allow the retina to contact the thin membrane that covers the white of the eyeball.

The surgeon inserts antibiotic ointment or drops into the eye and applies a patch.

What are the possible complications?

The two most common complications of scleral buckling are glaucoma and infection. In about 20% of persons, the retina fails to reattach, possibly requiring a repeat surgery.

What happens after the procedure?

- You'll need assistance with meals and walking.
- You must not rub or squeeze your eyes or squint. This can rupture the suture line or cause retinal detachment.
- You'll use eyedrops to keep the pupil dilated and antibiotics and corticosteroids to reduce inflammation and infection. If your eyelid or conjunctiva swells, ice packs are applied. (See *Recovering from scleral buckling.*)

*E*YE MUSCLE SURGERY

Eye muscle surgery corrects defects in the strength or placement of the eye muscles. Such defects cause misalignment of the eye and other visual problems. Eye muscle surgery adjusts the pull that the muscles exert on the affected eye and helps restore proper vision.

Two types of eye muscle surgery may be performed. Resection, which is the most common procedure, shortens and strengthens eye muscles. Recessive surgery, the other procedure, weakens the muscles by repositioning them. One or both techniques may be used to carefully position the eye back into proper alignment.

Eye muscle surgery is most commonly performed in children, but it may also be therapeutic for adults. It's usually successful in restoring binocular vision but may be repeated if the corrected eye drifts out of alignment.

Why is this procedure done?

- To correct crossed eyes
- To straighten the eyes for cosmetic reasons

What happens before the procedure?

- You must have nothing to eat or drink for 8 to 12 hours before surgery.
- You or a responsible family member will sign a consent form.

What happens during the procedure?

You receive a deep general anesthetic. This allows your eyes to return to their primary position before surgery begins.

Recovering from eye muscle surgery

After discharge from the hospital, follow these important guidelines.

Know what to expect
- Be aware that your conjunctiva will be red for 1 to 2 weeks.
- Know that double vision may persist for several months. To monitor this condition, keep follow-up appointments with the doctor.

Other instructions
- Notify the doctor if increased eye redness, fever, or eye discharge occurs.
- Avoid vigorous sports until the doctor gives permission.
- Shield your eyes from light by wearing sunglasses or a wide-brimmed hat or cap.
- Be sure you (or your child) does the recommended eye exercises.

In recessive surgery (a weakening procedure), the surgeon detaches the muscle from the eye, frees any attachments, and allows the muscle to retract. Then he or she reattaches the muscle to the eye at a measured distance behind the original insertion site.

In resection surgery (a strengthening procedure), the surgeon detaches the muscle from the eye, stretches it longer by a measured amount, and then reattaches the muscle to the eye at the original insertion site.

The greatest advance in eye muscle surgery in the last 10 years is "adjustable sutures." During eye muscle surgery, the muscles are reattached with a special knot in the suture that can be tightened or loosened to change the eye position as necessary when you're awake. The surgeon concludes either procedure by closing the conjunctiva and applying antibiotic ointment.

What are the possible complications?
Complications of eye muscle surgery are rare but may include minor infection and minor bleeding.

What happens after the procedure?
- The doctor may order orthoptic exercises to help train your eyes to work together and enhance restoration of binocular vision.
- You may return to normal daily activities when fully recovered from the anesthetic. (See *Recovering from eye muscle surgery.*)

TARSORRHAPHY

Tarsorrhaphy is the intermarginal closure of the eyelids with sutures. It may be a temporary or a permanent procedure. Tarsorrhaphy is now rarely performed because of the availability of eyedrops and contact lenses to lubricate and protect the eye.

Why is this procedure done?
- To protect the eye from exposure
- To correct deformity of the eyelid

SELF-HELP

Recovering from tarsorrhaphy

After you've been discharged from the hospital, follow these important guidelines.

Take special precautions

- Avoid rubbing the affected eye. If tearing occurs, dab, rather than wipe, the tears.
- Notify the doctor if the affected eye becomes irritated or if a foreign particle becomes lodged in it. Don't try to treat these conditions yourself.
- Don't wear eye makeup until the doctor gives permission.
- Avoid driving and other potentially hazardous tasks that require normal vision until the doctor gives permission. If you must drive, be sure to compensate for vision changes. For instance, turn your head farther or rely more on the car's mirrors.
- Turn your head fully when crossing the street to make up for decreased peripheral vision.

Prevent accidents at home

- Place dishes and beverages on the unaffected side because peripheral vision loss may interfere with eating. To avoid spills when pouring liquids, touch the pouring container to the receiving container. When setting objects down, release them only after they've contacted the surface.
- Keep pathways in your home clear of obstacles. Ask family members to inform you if they rearrange furniture.
- Use caution when assessing the height of stairs or curbs. Reduced depth perception may impair your judgment.

Other points to remember

- Take an analgesic, such as Tylenol (acetaminophen), to relieve mild discomfort. Contact the doctor if pain is severe or persistent.
- If you've had a temporary tarsorrhaphy, be aware that the doctor will remove the sutures in 2 weeks.

What happens before the procedure?

You sign a consent form.

What happens during the procedure?

Tarsorrhaphy is usually performed as an outpatient procedure. After administering a local anesthetic, the surgeon sutures the eyelids closed, leaving small openings for drainage of secretions. An antibiotic ointment is then applied, and the eye is patched.

What are the possible complications?

Complications of tarsorrhaphy are few and minor. They include superficial infection and eyelid swelling. (See *Recovering from tarsorrhaphy.*)

Instilling eyedrops after tarsorrhaphy

Before instilling eyedrops, verify the contents of the bottle and the strength of the medication. Also check the expiration date. Then follow these directions.

Use proper technique
- Wash your hands.
- Have the person lie down and turn the head sideways so gravity will pull the drops down and into the eye. If you're putting drops in the right eye, turn the person's head to the right; if you're putting them in the left eye, turn it to the left.

Find the small opening
- Identify the small opening at the inner corner of the eyelid. Then squeeze the prescribed number of drops into the opening, taking care not to touch the eyelid with the dropper.
- Have the person stay in position for 60 seconds after instillation so that the drops will flow inside the opening.

Remove excess medication
Finally, using a tissue, gently remove excess medication. Wash your hands again.

What happens after the procedure?

You'll need help to get up and walk around until you adjust to the altered vision. (See *Instilling eyedrops after tarsorrhaphy.*)

LASER SURGERY

Laser is an acronym for *l*ight *a*mplification by *s*timulated *e*mission of *r*adiation. An invaluable tool during surgery, a laser generates an intense beam of light. At times referred to as a "scalpel of light," the laser can cut, coagulate, or vaporize tissue. The intense beam can be focused on a very fine spot for extreme precision or defocused (the beam enlarged to affect a wider area) to coagulate or vaporize tissue.

Advantages of laser surgery include the following: noncontact capabilities, the assurance of dry fields (coagulation of the capillary beds prevents oozing into the field) and sterility (the intense heat generated by the laser provides constant sterilization), precise control of the spot size of the beam, and added accessibility (allowing the use of endoscopes to replace open surgical procedures). Laser tissue interaction also aids healing by minimizing swelling while decreasing pain after the procedure. (See *Other uses of laser surgery.*)

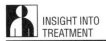
INSIGHT INTO
TREATMENT

Other uses of laser surgery

Laser surgery is used for a wide range of procedures, from simple wart removal to complex intra-abdominal procedures. The following list categorizes specific uses of laser surgery according to medical specialty.

Gynecology
- Cervical procedures
- Removal of warts
- Tubal microsurgery
- Endometrial ablation
- Endometriosis

General surgery
- Laparoscopic cholecystectomy
- Liver resections
- Other laparoscopic procedures
- Incisional and excisional soft-tissue procedures

Gastroenterology
- Treatment of esophageal lesions
- Rectal lesions
- Bleeding
- Esophageal varices
- Ulcers

Urology
- Treatment of urethral stenosis
- Superficial bladder tumors
- Interstitial cystitis
- Transurethral resection and removal of warts

Pulmonary
- Treatment of endobronchial stenosis
- Removal of endobronchial lesions
- Photoradiation of endobronchial cancer

Otolaryngology
- Treatment of tracheal stenosis
- Vocal cord lesions
- Pharyngeal papilloma
- Otoplasty
- Incisional and excisional work in head and neck surgery

Ophthalmology
- Posterior capsulotomy
- Vitrectomy
- Cytocoagulation
- Treatment of diabetic retinopathy
- Glaucoma
- Retinal tears
- Iridectomy

Dermatology
- Removal of port wine stains
- Telangiectasia
- Hemangioma
- Melanoma

- Tattoo removal
- Excision of skin tumors
- Incisional and excisional soft-tissue procedures

Cardiology
- Laser-assisted balloon angioplasty
- Investigational procedures

Dentistry
- Frenectomy
- Gingivoplasty
- Treatment of aphthous ulcers
- Vascular lesions

Neurosurgery
- Treatment of brain tumors
- Spinal cord tumors
- Percutaneous diskectomies

Orthopedics
- Methyl methacrylate removal
- Meniscectomy
- Investigational procedures in other joints

Oncology
- Investigational photoradiation of tumors

Why is this procedure done?

The numerous uses for laser therapy range from a simple wart removal to a complex intra-abdominal procedure. It's used in a wide variety of medical specialties to treat various conditions. It's done:

- to cut, coagulate, or vaporize tissue

SELF-HELP

Recovering from laser surgery

After you've been discharged from the hospital, follow these important guidelines:

• Be aware that recovery from laser surgery resembles recovery from conventional surgery, except that healing may be faster with less pain.

• After a lung or mouth procedure, expect a smoky taste in your mouth. Also, you may cough up small amounts of blackened tissue.

Remember that lasers are not a cure-all. Many laser procedures merely eliminate discomfort.

• to reduce or remove tumors and lesions
• to seal a source of bleeding.

What happens before the procedure?

The laser procedure itself requires no specific preparations.

What happens during the procedure?

Laser procedures are performed by a trained doctor or dentist. They may not require anesthesia depending on the type of laser used and the specific procedure being performed.

To cut tissue, the laser is focused in a precise beam. Laser technology can be used with or without microscopes and together with or separate from conventional surgical methods.

What are the possible complications?

Laser surgery is associated with the same complications that follow conventional surgery (hemorrhage, infection, perforation) as well as some that are uniquely associated with lasers. Fire is a potential complication due to the intense heat from the laser beam. Airway fire and lung explosion, which can result from contact with a flammable breathing tube or oxygen, is a tragic complication that is avoidable when safety precautions are enforced. Eye damage from exposure to the laser beam can result in painful or permanent injury.

What happens after the procedure?

The doctor prescribes analgesics. (See *Recovering from laser surgery.*)

OTHER TREATMENT

REMOVING FOREIGN OBJECTS

Dust, dirt, eyelashes, and airborne particles can come in contact with the conjunctiva or cornea, causing a person to have a foreign object sensation. Removing the object from the eye, eyelid, or conjunctiva is a first-aid procedure that sometimes can be performed by the person. If the object is embedded in the cornea, removal must be done by an ophthalmologist.

Why is this procedure done?

Removing a foreign object from the eye is done to decrease pain, prevent damage from abrasion, and reduce the risk of infection.

What happens before the procedure?

- If the foreign body is lodged in your cornea, an anesthetic will be placed in the eye to reduce discomfort.
- Don't rub your eye because this will cause further damage, making removal more difficult. A protective shield is placed over the eye to prevent you from rubbing it until you can be examined by the ophthalmologist.

What happens during the procedure?

If a foreign particle is lying on the surface of the conjunctiva, you'll tilt your head back and move your eyes away from the site of the particle. Your eyelids should be held open to prevent blinking. Then another person should gently touch the particle with the tip of a wet cotton-tipped applicator and lift it from the eye, taking care not to drag the applicator across the surface of the cornea.

If the foreign object is not visible, the lid should be inverted. You should look downward as another person grasps the eyelashes of your upper lid and gently exerts pressure in the midportion of the upper lid with a wet cotton-tipped applicator. If a foreign object is present, it can be easily seen and removed with the applicator.

Corneal foreign bodies can frequently be removed by holding the eye open and flushing the cornea with a steady stream of sterile ophthalmic irrigating solution. Aim the stream at the corner of the eye and allow it to run over the cornea. Repeat the irrigation until the foreign body is removed. Then dry the eye with a cotton ball, wiping from the inner to the outer corner of the eye.

Embedded foreign bodies should be removed by an ophthalmologist after instillation of topical anesthetic eyedrops. Iron and steel foreign bodies will leave a rust ring around the foreign body site. This is removed by using a speed spatula or appropriate instrument. Antibiotic eyedrops should be instilled and continued for several days to prevent infection of the damaged cornea. The eye is patched for several hours as well.

SELF-HELP

Recovering from foreign object removal

After the particle is removed from your eye, follow these important guidelines.

Apply ointment as prescribed
- To apply antibiotic ointment, pull down the lower lid and apply the ointment along the entire length of the conjunctival sac.
- Don't touch the tip of the tube to your eye or eyelid.

Other instructions
- Wear an eye patch for 24 hours after the foreign body is removed.
- Wear sunglasses for increased comfort.
- Contact your ophthalmologist if your eye pain doesn't subside in 24 hours, if your vision worsens, or if you notice eye discharge, increased redness of the eye, blurred vision, or sensitivity to light.

What are the possible complications?

Deeply imbedded corneal foreign objects can leave corneal scars that can cause impaired vision. Corneal infections can lead to more serious ocular infections. Using topical anesthetic eyedrops for pain control after the foreign body is removed may delay healing.

What happens after the procedure?

- After removal of an embedded particle, sit quietly for a few minutes with your eyes closed.
- Wear glasses, goggles, or safety glasses when working. (See *Recovering from foreign object removal*.)

15

TREATING EAR, NOSE, & THROAT DISORDERS

DRUG THERAPY

DECONGESTANTS AND ANTIHISTAMINES

Histamine is a naturally occurring substance that's important for the body's immune response. After exposure to an allergy-triggering substance, specialized cells release histamine, which acts to open blood vessels and makes it easier for specialized blood cells to reach their target and destroy invading allergy-triggering susbstances. Unfortunately, many of the unpleasant effects of allergies — including watery eyes and stuffy nose — can be attributed to the actions of histamine in the eyes or respiratory tract.

Decongestants relieve nasal stuffiness by acting on blood vessels in the respiratory tract. By narrowing these blood vessels, they alleviate the stuffy feeling in the nasal and upper airway passages and make it easier for the person to breathe.

Antihistamines relieve allergic symptoms by blocking the effects of histamine. Most antihistamines also have a drying effect — called an *anticholinergic effect* — which also helps to relieve symptoms. This anticholinergic effect is responsible in part for the drowsiness that often accompanies antihistamine therapy. Interestingly, most nonprescription sleep aids are antihistamines.

Recently, scientists have developed a series of antihistamines that don't enter the nervous system and so don't cause drowsiness. These drugs have been named the *nonsedating antihistamines.*

Most antihistamines are given orally; some, including brompheniramine, diphenhydramine, chlorpheniramine, and promethazine, can also be given by injection into a muscle. Such injection brings rapid relief of allergic symptoms but may cause local stinging and burning or other side effects.

Decongestants and antihistamines are often combined in cold and allergy medications to relieve a wide range of symptoms.

What are decongestants and antihistamines used for?
- To decrease allergic reactions and decrease allergy symptoms (antihistamines)
- To decrease nasal stuffiness (decongestants)

What are some commonly used decongestants and antihistamines?

Decongestants

- ephedrine (generic)
- pseudoephedrine, known by the brand names Decofed, Dorcol Children's Decongestant, Robidrine, and Sudafed
- phenylpropanolamine, known by the brand name Phenyldrine

Nonsedating antihistamines

- astemizole, known by the brand name Hismanal
- loratadine, known by the brand name Claritin
- terfenadine, known by the brand name Seldane

Other antihistamines

- azatadine, known by the brand name Optimine
- brompheniramine, known by the brand names Bromphen, Codimal-A, and Dimetane Extentabs
- chlorpheniramine, known by the brand names Chlor-Pro, Chlor-Trimeton, and Teldrin
- clemastine, known by the brand name Tavist
- cyproheptadine, known by the brand name Periactin
- dexchlorpheniramine, known by the brand names Dexchlor, Polaramine, and Polargen
- diphenhydramine, known by the brand names Benadryl, Benylin, Sleep-Eze 3, and Sominex
- methdilazine, known by the brand name Tacaryl
- promethazine, known by the brand names Phenazine, Phenameth, and Phenergan
- trimeprazine, known by the brand name Temaril
- tripelennamine, known by the brand name PBZ
- triprolidine, known by the brand names Actidil and Myidyl

What are the possible side effects?

Decongestants

- Restlessness, irritability, insomnia
- Palpitations

Nonsedating antihistamines

- Headache
- Increased appetite, weight gain
- Visual disturbances
- Cough

- Hair loss, rash, itching
- Abdominal pain, dry mouth
- Abnormal heart rhythm (with high doses)

Other antihistamines
- Drowsiness, fatigue, confusion, dizziness
- Stomach distress, dry mouth, nausea, vomiting

Drowsiness is common with antihistamine therapy. Avoid hazardous tasks that require alertness until the central nervous system response is clearly established.

What are the guidelines for taking decongestants and antihistamines?

- Take the drug exactly as directed. Tolerance to the drug may develop, as evidenced by decreased effectiveness over time. If this happens, don't increase the dose. Call the doctor.
- Take a missed dose as soon as possible, unless it's within 2 hours of the next dose (or within 12 hours if taking an extended-release product). Don't double the dose.
- Drowsiness is common with many antihistamines. So, avoid hazardous tasks that require alertness until your reaction to the drug is clearly known. Caffeine-containing beverages may combat drowsiness, but avoid drinking alcohol or taking sedatives unless directed otherwise by the doctor. Ice chips, sugarless gum, or hard candy may relieve dry mouth. If you get an upset stomach, take the drug with food or milk.
- If you're taking a decongestant, avoid excessive amounts of caffeine-containing coffee, colas, and other beverages because these may make you jittery. Notify the doctor if symptoms don't improve in a week.

What else you should know
- Tell your doctor if you have problems with urine retention or an enlarged prostate because these drugs may worsen urine retention. Decongestants should be avoided if you have high blood pressure because they may cancel out the effects of medication or further raise blood pressure.
- Although many of these drugs are available without prescription, check with your doctor or pharmacist if you're taking any other medication.

SURGERIES

Myringotomy and Ear Tubes

Myringotomy is a surgical incision in the tympanic membrane (eardrum) performed to relieve pain and prevent membrane rupture by allowing drainage of pus or fluid from the middle ear. It's most commonly performed on children with acute middle ear infection.

Myringotomy may be performed on one or both ears. After myringotomy, a pressure-equalizing tube may be inserted through the incision to allow fluid to drain. Myringotomy usually provides almost instant relief, and the incision typically heals in 2 to 3 weeks. (If tubes have been inserted, they remain in place for about 6 months or until they spontaneously fall out.)

Why is this procedure done?
- To relieve pain and drain fluid from the middle ear
- To aerate the middle ear when eustachian tube dysfunction prevents it
- To obtain infected material for lab testing

What happens before the procedure?
The person or a responsible family member will sign a consent form.

What happens during the procedure?
- First, a local anesthetic is administered to an adult or older child. However, if the person is a young child, is uncooperative, or has severe middle ear infection, he or she may receive a light general anesthetic. (An infant may receive no anesthetic.)
- After the anesthetic takes effect, the doctor makes a small slit in the eardrum. Afterward, the doctor may insert a tube to allow continuous drainage, equalize pressure within the middle ear, and let the eustachian tube recover.
- A larger U-shaped incision, used when pus or thick drainage is present, permits more drainage. The surgeon may then irrigate the middle ear or apply gentle suction to remove persistent drainage. If the drainage is excessive, the doctor may apply a small piece of sterile cotton loosely in the external ear canal.

How to care for a child with ear tubes

When tubes are inserted in your child's ears, you'll need to follow these important guidelines.

Check the drainage

- If a cotton ball is placed in the ear to absorb drainage, wash your hands before and after changing the cotton ball. Dispose of old cotton by placing it in a small paper or plastic bag before throwing it in the trash. Notify the doctor if drainage lasts more than 1 week or changes color or character. Call the doctor if your child has any ear pain or fever, which may signal a blocked tube or reinfection.
- Expect considerable drainage through the tubes.

Other instructions

- Keep water out of the ear canal until the eardrum is intact. Do this by rolling absorbent cotton in Vaseline to form a plug, and then insert the plug in the outer part of the ear before showering or washing your child's hair.
- Sometimes the tubes fall out. Look for them to be small, white, spool-shaped, and plastic. Notify the doctor if the tubes fall out.
- If the doctor has ordered antibiotic eardrops, use them as prescribed and continue them for several days after the drainage stops.

- If the person requires a bilateral myringotomy, the procedure is repeated on the other ear.

What are the possible complications?

Myringotomy can cause minor complications, such as bleeding during tube insertion if the ear canal is inadvertently scratched and scars or sclerotic patches on the eardrum. When tubes are inserted, ear discharge can become chronic. The tubes may become blocked and need to be reinserted. Another complication associated with tube insertion is contamination from water entering the middle ear under pressure.

What happens after the procedure?

If the doctor has placed sterile cotton in the external ear canal, this should be changed when it becomes moist to prevent a secondary infection. The ear may drain for 2 to 3 days after the procedure. (See *How to care for a child with ear tubes.*)

STAPEDECTOMY

Stapedectomy is the surgical removal of all or part of the stapes, the innermost of the three sound-conducting bones of the middle ear, and its replacement with a tiny prosthesis (artificial body part). It's usually performed to restore hearing due to a condition called *otosclerosis,* in which an overgrowth of spongy new bone causes the stapes to become immobile. Because otosclerosis usually occurs in both ears, stapedectomy is usually performed twice — first in the ear with the greatest hearing loss and then, a year or more later, in the other ear.

Why is this surgery done?

Stapedectomy is performed to remove all or part of the stapes and restore hearing.

When shouldn't this surgery be done?

Stapedectomy shouldn't be performed in people with external or middle ear infection and inner ear disease. It shouldn't be performed cautiously, if at all, in people with complete hearing loss in the other ear because of the risk of complications.

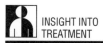

INSIGHT INTO
TREATMENT

Understanding types of stapedectomy

Stapedectomy may be total or partial, depending on the extent of otosclerotic growth. It may also be performed using various techniques. Two types of stapedectomy are shown here.

NORMAL MIDDLE EAR

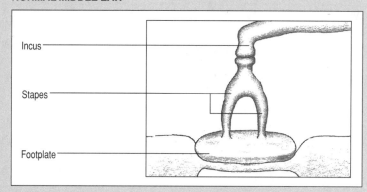

Incus

Stapes

Footplate

PARTIAL STAPEDECTOMY
Wire-Teflon prosthesis

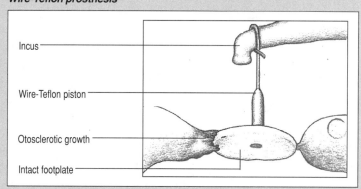

Incus

Wire-Teflon piston

Otosclerotic growth

Intact footplate

TOTAL STAPEDECTOMY
Vein graft and strut prosthesis

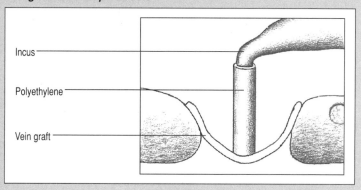

Incus

Polyethylene

Vein graft

SELF-HELP

Caring for yourself after a stapedectomy

When you've been discharged from the hospital, follow these important guidelines.

Know when to call your doctor
- Inform your doctor immediately if you experience fever; pain; pus-filled drainage; prolonged dizziness; a constant, loud buzzing or ringing; significant decrease in hearing; or sudden hearing loss. These signs may indicate infection or displacement of the prosthesis (artificial body part).
- Take your medications. Report any signs of respiratory infection to your doctor immediately.

Protect your ear
- Protect your ear from cold drafts for 1 week and avoid contact with people who have colds, the flu, or other contagious illnesses.
- Postpone washing your hair for 1 to 2 weeks; then, for the next 4 weeks, avoid getting water in your ears. Place a cotton ball in the ear canal and apply

Vaseline over the cotton to form a seal when washing your hair.
- Don't swim for 6 weeks and wear a sweatband to prevent perspiration from getting into the ear during hot weather or exercise.
- To prevent displacement of the prosthesis, avoid blowing your nose for at least 1 week after surgery. Keep your mouth open when you sneeze. Avoid blowing up balloons and playing wind instruments for 1 month, and avoid air travel for 6 months.

Other points to remember
- Ear drainage may be reddish brown, but usually becomes clear and disappears within 1 to 2 weeks.
- Your taste sensation will be slightly altered for several weeks or months because the nerve for taste passes through the ear.
- Hearing may improve or fade at times during the first 3 weeks after surgery. It's normal to hear cracking, popping, and echoing sounds (as if your head is "in a barrel").

What happens before the surgery?
- The nurse may wash your hair or shave around your ear. Eardrops, ointments, irrigations, and hot or cold compresses may be administered to decrease any inflammation and relieve discomfort.
- Ear wicks will be loosely inserted into your external ear to remove any drainage.

What happens during the surgery?
You receive a general or local anesthesic. The surgeon may perform a total or a partial stapedectomy, depending on the extent of otosclerotic growth. (See *Understanding types of stapedectomy,* page 497.)

What are the possible complications?
Complications include sudden hearing loss, which can occur if the prosthesis slips into the vestibule or if fibrosis develops at the site. Other possible complications include transient dizziness, nausea,

and vomiting. Facial nerve paralysis can result from the surgery or the local anesthetic. Rejection of the graft or prosthesis or complete closure of the oval window (an opening in the inner ear that's closed by the base of the stapes) may allow inner ear fluid to leak. You may also develop ringing in the ears, vertigo, and fluctuating hearing loss.

What happens after the surgery?

- Your hearing may not improve for several weeks after the surgery because ear packing and swelling may mask any initial improvement. The packing is usually removed after 1 week; if absorbable gelatin foam is used, it will dissolve and doesn't require removal.
- Depending on the surgeon's orders you'll lie on the operated ear to facilitate drainage, on the opposite ear to avoid graft displacement, or in the most comfortable position. Moving slowly and without bending when changing position will help to prevent dizziness and nausea. (See *Caring for yourself after a stapedectomy.*)

RHINOPLASTY AND SEPTOPLASTY

Commonly called a *nose job,* a rhinoplasty is a surgical procedure that changes the nose's external appearance. It corrects congenital or traumatic deformity. Septoplasty corrects a deviated septum, preventing nasal obstruction, thick discharge, and secondary throat, sinus, and ear problems. These procedures may be performed together or independently.

Why is this surgery done?
- To correct a deformity and enhance the appearance of the nose
- To correct a deviated septum and restore easy breathing

What happens before the surgery?
For rhinoplasty, the surgeon will explain the extent of the procedure and how your nose should look after surgery.

What happens during the surgery?
In both procedures, you receive topical and local anesthetics. During a rhinoplasty, the surgeon fractures the nasal bones, removes excess

SELF-HELP

Caring for yourself after rhinoplasty and septoplasty

After you've been discharged from the hospital, follow these important guidelines.

Protect your nose
- Don't blow your nose for at least 10 days after the nasal packing is removed, or your nose may bleed. If you need to clear your nose, sniff gently.
- If you have a bandage or an external splint in place, don't manipulate it or you may cause misalignment or bleeding.
- Avoid bending or heavy lifting for 1 to 2 weeks as recommended by your doctor.

Other instructions
- If the doctor orders inhalation treatments to reduce swelling and prevent crusting, place a bowl of hot water in front of you and drape a towel over your head, creating a tent. Breathe in the warmed air.
- If the doctor prescribes nose drops, this is how you should take them: Lie flat on your back, instill the drops, and remain on your back for 5 minutes until they're absorbed by the swollen tissues.
- Take antibiotics and pain relievers as prescribed.
- Report severe pain, bleeding, or fever to your doctor (who will rule out a nasal septal hematoma).

tissue, and then repositions the bones. The surgeon makes an incision in the groove between the upper and lower nasal cartilages and trims the soft tissue to reshape the tip of the nose, and may also insert a cartilage implant if necessary.

During a septoplasty, the surgeon makes an incision inside the nose. The surgeon cuts the deviated cartilage into pieces or incises and repositions it. Alternatively, in a procedure known as *submucous resection,* the cartilage is removed entirely except for a small wedge that supports the nose.

After either procedure, the doctor inserts nasal packing.

What are the possible complications?
Although both procedures are generally well tolerated, they can cause swelling, heavy bleeding from the nose, and septal hematoma (blood around the septum). Other complications include nasal skin necrosis, infection, and septal perforation.

What happens after the surgery?
- For both rhinoplasty and septoplasty, you'll have nasal packing. This, along with swelling, may produce an uncomfortable sensation of facial fullness.
- The doctor will remove the packing 24 to 48 hours after surgery.

- You'll need to rinse your mouth every 2 to 4 hours. You can resume a normal diet the next day. (See *Caring for yourself after rhinoplasty and septoplasty.*)

TONSILLECTOMY AND ADENOIDECTOMY

Tonsillectomy is the surgical removal of the palatine tonsils; adenoidectomy is the surgical removal of the pharyngeal tonsils. Both procedures were once performed routinely on school-age children but are now less commonly used. Instead, antibiotics are prescribed to treat tonsils and adenoids enlarged by bacterial infection.

Tonsillectomy is most commonly performed on children over age 3. In rare circumstances, an adult may require this procedure. Adenoidectomy is performed almost exclusively in children because adenoid tissue usually shrinks by adolescence.

Why is this surgery done?
Tonsillectomy is performed to remove the palatine and pharyngeal tonsils when enlarged tonsillar tissue obstructs the upper airway. Tonsillectomy is the preferred treatment for peritonsillar abscess and chronic tonsillitis that causes more than seven acute attacks within 2 years. Adenoidectomy may be performed to prevent recurrent middle ear infection, although some experts dispute its effectiveness.

When shouldn't this surgery be done?
Tonsillectomy and adenoidectomy shouldn't be performed on people with acute tonsil infection, active tuberculosis, hemophilia, or leukemia. They shouldn't be performed in persons with cleft palate because removal of this tissue allows air to escape through the nose and may create severe speech problems.

What happens before the surgery?
- The child and family will tour the operating and recovery rooms. Hospital routines are explained to the child.
- If the child is scheduled for an adenoidectomy, speech and articulation will be evaluated. A speech therapist is sometimes consulted.

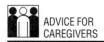
ADVICE FOR CAREGIVERS

Caring for your child after tonsillectomy and adenoidectomy

After your child is discharged from the hospital, follow these important guidelines.

Watch for and report problems
Report any bleeding or fever immediately. Watch for frequent swallowing, especially during sleep. The risk of bleeding continues until 7 to 10 days after surgery, when the white membrane formed at the operative site begins to slough off.

Avoid injuries
- Don't let your child participate in any vigorous activity for 5 to 7 days after discharge. A child typically returns to school after 10 to 14 days. Keep your child away from people with colds or other contagious illnesses for at least 2 weeks.

- Make sure your child brushes his or her teeth gently. Avoid vigorous brushing, gargling, and irritating liquids for several weeks.

Other instructions
- Limit your child's diet to liquids and soft foods for 1 to 2 weeks to avoid dislodging clots or causing bleeding. Drink plenty of fluids to avoid dehydration and soothe the throat.
- Minor discomfort, such as ear pain (especially on swallowing), a sore throat, and voice changes, may persist for 1 to 2 weeks after surgery. Avoid medications that contain aspirin. Instead, use Tylenol (or another drug containing acetaminophen).

- The child will be checked for the presence of loose teeth, which can become dislodged during surgery.

What happens during the surgery?
Both surgeries may be performed either in the hospital or as outpatient procedures. For tonsillectomy, a child typically receives a general anesthetic. An adult may receive a local anesthetic. In an adenoidectomy or adenotonsillectomy, the child receives a general anesthetic. Adenoidectomy is usually performed before tonsillectomy.

What are the possible complications?
The most serious complication of these surgeries is bleeding, which may occur within 24 hours after surgery or up to 10 days later, when the healing tissue formed at the operative site begins to slough off. Other complications include pain that interferes with the person's ability to drink and problems with airway obstruction caused by swelling or accumulated secretions.

What happens after the surgery?

▪ Fluids are offered to soothe the throat. The person starts with ice chips, and progresses to ice pops and clear cold fluids.

▪ An ice collar or cool compresses are applied to relieve sore throat. (See *Caring for your child after tonsillectomy and adenoidectomy*.)

LARYNGECTOMY

Laryngectomy is the removal of all or part of the larynx or voice box. The various types of laryngectomy differ mainly in the anatomical structures that are surgically removed, depending on the extent of underlying disease. However, radiation is now replacing some procedures because both treatments have similar survival rates and radiation leaves the person with a better voice quality.

The prognosis after laryngectomy, though generally good, reflects the extent of the disease at the time of surgery. After laryngectomy and radiation treatment, the 5-year survival rate is about 80% to 85% for cancer without vocal cord fixation, 75% for cancer with cord fixation, and 50% for cancer that's spread to the cervical lymph nodes.

Why is this surgery done?

Laryngectomy is performed to treat laryngeal cancer.

What happens before the surgery?

▪ The doctor explains the procedure, describing the expected voice quality and extent of speech the person will have after the operation.

▪ The person is told that he or she will have a feeding tube in the nose for 7 to 10 days after the surgery.

▪ The person is helped to develop a communication system for use after surgery. If the person will be unable to speak after surgery, he or she may use a communication system such as flash cards, paper and pencil, or a magic slate. A speech pathologist will evaluate the person.

What happens during the surgery?

The person receives a general anesthetic. The surgeon chooses the specific procedure based on the type and site of the tumor, the extent and location of tumor spread, and vocal cord mobility. The most

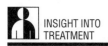

INSIGHT INTO
TREATMENT

Understanding types of laryngectomy

Although laryngoscopic surgery may be used to remove an early localized glottic (vocal cord) tumor, other techniques must be used to remove more widespread tumors. These are explained below.

Total laryngectomy

Used to remove a large glottic or supraglottic tumor with vocal cord fixation, this procedure involves removal of the true vocal cords, false vocal cords, epiglottis, hyoid bone, cricoid cartilage, and two or three rings of the windpipe.

Neighboring areas may also be removed, depending on the extent of the tumor. A permanent tracheotomy is performed, creating a stoma (a surgically created opening) in the larynx that leaves the person unable to speak.

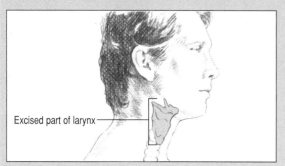

Excised part of larynx

Horizontal supraglottic laryngectomy

Performed to remove a large supraglottic tumor, this procedure excises the top of the larynx (the epiglottis, the hyoid bone, and the false vocal cords), leaving the true vocal cords intact. Although there's no laryngectomy stoma, a temporary tracheotomy may be performed to ensure a patent airway until swelling subsides. The person's voice is unaffected by this procedure, but removal of the epiglottis may cause difficulty swallowing.

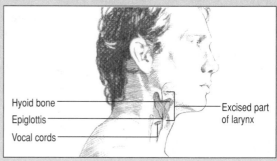

Hyoid bone
Epiglottis
Vocal cords
Excised part of larynx

common procedures used are total laryngectomy, horizontal supraglottic laryngectomy, vertical hemilaryngectomy, and laryngofissure. (See *Understanding types of laryngectomy.*)

What are the possible complications?

Many complications can result from laryngectomy. Immediately after surgery, respiratory distress or, rarely, bleeding into the wound or formation of a blood blister may occur. Other complications include infection or presence of pus and swelling. Later complications include pneumonia, incomplete filling of the lung, and formation of an abnormal passage from the throat to the skin.

Vertical hemilaryngectomy

Used to remove a widespread tumor, this procedure involves removal of half the thyroid and subglottis, one false vocal cord, and one true vocal cord. The area is then rebuilt with strap muscles. The person doesn't have a laryngectomy stoma, but his voice may be hoarse after the operation.

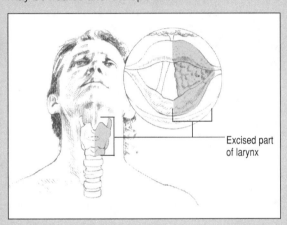

Excised part
of larynx

Laryngofissure

This procedure removes a glottic tumor limited to one vocal cord. To perform laryngofissure, the surgeon incises the thyroid cartilage and removes the affected vocal cord.

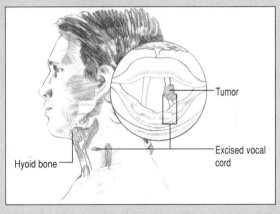

Tumor

Excised vocal
cord

Hyoid bone

What happens after the surgery?

▪ If the person has a total laryngectomy, he or she will breathe through a stoma (a surgically created opening) in the neck. He or she won't be able to smell, blow the nose, whistle, gargle, sip, or suck on a straw. The person will expel secretions through the stoma, which will need suctioning periodically. The person will be able to perform his or her own stoma care and suctioning. (See *Caring for yourself after a laryngectomy,* page 506.)

▪ The person will be fed through the nasal tube for 7 to 10 days and will then begin receiving oral feedings (thick, easy-to-swallow fluids, such as gelatin or ice cream).

SELF-HELP

Caring for yourself after a laryngectomy

After you've been discharged from the hospital, follow these important guidelines.

Learn about stoma care

- Be aware that the nurse or another health care professional will teach you how to care for the stoma (a surgically created opening) in your windpipe as soon as possible after the operation. You won't be discharged from the hospital until you know how to do it. If you had a total laryngectomy, a speech pathologist will work closely with you.
- When cleaning your stoma, don't use tissues, loose cotton, or soap because these may obstruct your airway. Wear a bib or dressing over your stoma to act as a filter and to warm incoming air. Avoid swimming and getting water in your stoma. You'll need to humidify your home, especially during the winter.
- You'll be taught how to perform tracheostomy care using a germ-free technique. To do that, clean the inner cannula of your tube with hydrogen peroxide and water daily. This helps maintain a patent airway and prevents infection. You must suction the outer cannula to keep your airway patent whenever you feel congested or your breathing sounds raspy or wheezy, or when excess mucus forms. Also, watch for bloody secretions, which may indicate injury.

Other instructions

- Learn the signs and symptoms of later complications, such as pneumonia and incomplete expansion of your lungs, wound infection, and bleeding.
- Inform the doctor promptly if you develop symptoms of a respiratory infection, such as a fever, cough, yellow or green drainage from the stoma, pain, or redness around the stoma.
- Keep follow-up medical appointments to monitor for recurrence of cancer.
- Contact organizations such as the International Association of Laryngectomees and the American Cancer Society to learn about support groups in your area.

- The nurse will encourage the person to frequently cough, turn, and do deep-breathing exercises. If the person has a tracheostomy, it will be suctioned regularly until he or she can do it.

RADICAL NECK DISSECTION

Radical neck dissection is a surgical procedure performed on the head and neck to remove the cervical chain of lymph nodes, the sternocleidomastoid muscle, the layer of tissue surrounding the muscle, and the internal jugular vein. It may be performed alone or with other head and neck surgery such as a total laryngectomy.

This procedure causes dramatic changes in the person's appearance that may cause profound emotional reactions. It may also cause difficulty eating and, when performed with a laryngectomy, inability to speak. The person undergoing radical neck dissection will need a strong support system to successfully adapt to a new self-image.

Why is this surgery done?
- To remove cancerous tissue from the tongue, tonsil, lip, nasopharynx, or thyroid
- To prevent or treat cancer that's spread to the cervical lymph nodes

What happens before the surgery?
- The person is told to expect the presence of tubes and drains and treatment in the intensive care unit immediately after surgery. He or she will be unable to talk if a laryngectomy or tracheotomy is performed.
- If the person is scheduled for a total laryngectomy with a radical neck dissection, he or she is told that there will be a stoma (a surgically created opening) in the throat. The person will use alternative means of communicating after surgery, such as paper and pencil, flash cards, chalkboard, or magic slate.

What happens during the surgery?
After the person receives a general anesthetic, the surgeon makes large incisions in the neck, unfolding skin flaps that allow access to the involved area. The surgeon then removes muscle and its covering, including the cervical chain of lymph nodes, the internal jugular vein, and the sternocleidomastoid muscle. The spinal accessory nerve is severed, but the carotid artery and the vagus nerve are spared. If necessary, the surgeon may perform a laryngectomy or a tracheotomy at this time. Next, the surgeon may insert drains, protect the carotid artery with a dermal or muscle pedicle graft, and then carefully position skin flaps over the dissected area. The flaps are stitched closed before a bandage is applied to the person's neck.

What are the possible complications?
Radical neck dissection can cause several life-threatening complications, including carotid artery rupture and heavy bleeding, aspiration and airway obstruction, development of an abnormal passage from the throat to the skin, infection, necrosis, and collapsed lungs. Other complications include facial swelling, damage to the larynx resulting

Recovering from radical neck dissection

After you've been discharged from the hospital, follow these important guidelines.

Help relieve shoulder discomfort

Use massage and muscle-strengthening exercises to relieve shoulder discomfort, which may last for months after surgery. Don't lie on the affected side and don't lift more than 2 pounds (about 1 kilogram) with that arm.

Other instructions

- If you've also had a laryngectomy, you and a family member must learn how to care for a stoma (a surgically created opening) and tracheostomy. Contact a speech therapist.
- Keep follow-up appointments so the doctor can check for possible recurrence of cancer.
- If necessary, seek counseling along with family members. A community support group also may be helpful.

in vocal impairment, skin sloughing, shoulder droop due to nerve damage, erosion of the skin and major vessels due to suction tube placement, and Frey's syndrome (excessive sweating of the cheek after eating, which usually occurs when the parotid gland is also removed).

Radical neck dissection may cause facial disfigurement, leading to changes in the person's self-perception. As a result, the person may have intense emotions such as anger, grief, and denial or may feel depressed, withdrawn, and unable to cope.

What happens after the surgery?

- The person's head is elevated 30 to 45 degrees in bed to reduce tension on the incision, ease drainage, and decrease swelling.
- The person needs help to change position because he or she will be unable to support his or her own head and neck. (See *Recovering from radical neck dissection.*)

NASAL POLYPECTOMY

This surgery removes nasal polyps, which are fluid-filled sacs originating from the sinus mucosa. They occur in individuals who have allergic or chronic rhinitis (inflammation of the nose). Multiple polyps are common; they can occur on both sides of the nasal cavity.

Removal of nasal polyps eliminates obstruction of the sinus openings. However, because polyps have a strong tendency to recur after surgical removal, more extensive sinus surgery may later be required.

Laser polypectomy is another technique used to remove polyps within the nasal cavity. This method is less invasive and reduces the person's discomfort.

Why is this surgery done?

- To reestablish the normal flow of mucus from the sinuses
- To prevent recurrent or chronic infection
- To eliminate airway obstruction

What happens before the surgery?

Steroid drugs are administered to decrease inflammation and polyp size.

What happens during the surgery?

The surgeon administers a local or a general anesthetic, depending on the extent of disease, then places a wire snare around the base of the polyp and removes it. If laser polypectomy is the chosen technique, the surgeon uses a laser beam to cut and vaporize tissue.

What are the possible complications?

Complications are rare but may include bleeding and infection.

What happens after the surgery?

- The head of the bed is elevated to reduce swelling.
- The nurse administers pain relievers. (See *Recovering from a nasal polypectomy*.)

OTHER TREATMENTS

HEARING AIDS

A hearing aid is an electronic device that, when placed in the ear, improves hearing in people with certain types of hearing loss. Powered by a replaceable battery, a hearing aid consists of a microphone, an amplifier, a receiver, and an ear mold. The microphone picks up sound and converts it to electrical energy. The amplifier magnifies this energy electronically, and the receiver converts it back to sound waves, which the ear mold directs into the person's ear.

Why are hearing aids used?

Hearing aids amplify sound for people with hearing loss. Typically, an audiologist administers hearing tests and, after determining the type and extent of hearing loss, selects the appropriate hearing aid.

What types of hearing aids are available?

Four types of hearing aid are commonly available: behind-the-ear, eyeglass, in-the-ear, and body aids. A behind-the-ear hearing aid, the most commonly used type, consists of a short curved plastic tube that connects the unit (which rests behind the ear) to an ear mold. In an

SELF-HELP

Recovering from a nasal polypectomy

After you've been discharged from the hospital, follow these important guidelines.

Take it easy

- The doctor may advise you not to return to work for up to 10 days if your work is physically strenuous.
- Avoid heavy lifting or straining. Don't blow your nose. Sneeze with your mouth open. This will prevent unnecessary pressure and reduce the chance of bleeding.

Other instructions

- Wear the nasal dressing until drainage subsides, possibly as long as 10 days.
- Use saline nasal spray.
- Follow-up care is important. If bleeding or other complications occur, be sure to call your doctor.

SELF-HELP

Using a hearing aid

When you start to use your hearing aid, follow these important guidelines.

Learn to use the hearing aid properly
- Consistently use the hearing aid at the prescribed setting. Increase amplification, if necessary, to improve hearing.
- Use the hearing aid's on-off switch and volume control and learn how to change the battery.
- Store the hearing aid in a dry place when you're not using it. Don't get it wet. Inspect the unit daily for a cracked case, corroded battery contacts, frayed wires, or a blocked ear mold. Except for an in-the-ear hearing aid, the ear mold can be cleaned with warm, soapy water after disconnection from the unit.
- Don't use hairspray when wearing the aid because it may damage the microphone. Never insert sharp objects, such as needles or pencil points, into the unit.
- If the hearing aid seems to be malfunctioning, check the battery first. Contact the audiologist or hearing-aid dealer if the hearing aid continues to malfunction.

Other points to remember
- Your family needs to be patient and to speak in a normal voice as you adjust to the hearing aid. Tell them that they should get your attention before speaking and, if possible, eliminate background noise. They should repeat messages, if necessary, and reword them.
- Consider contacting an organization that offers help for the hearing-impaired such as the Alexander Graham Bell Association for the Deaf.
- You may want to get other hearing devices, such as a loop system to clarify sound on the television set, a coupler for the telephone to improve clarity, and a battery tester.
- Routinely check your ears for excessive earwax, which may muffle sounds. If you have this problem, your ears may have to be irrigated by a doctor or nurse.

eyeglass hearing aid, a similar unit, the components are contained in the eyeglass temple. An in-the-ear hearing aid, the most compact device, consists of a single piece fashioned like an ear mold, which houses the microphone, amplifier, and receiver. A body hearing aid, most suitable for the person with severe or profound hearing loss or with limited manual dexterity, has a larger microphone, amplifier, and power supply than the other types of hearing aid and produces less distortion. It's built into a case that can be clipped to the person's pocket or worn on the body. A long wire connects the unit to an ear mold.

Some newer hearing aids contain computer chips that allow them to be programmed by an audiologist. These programmable aids can be finely adjusted to better compensate for a person's hearing loss.

An estimated 22 million Americans with hearing disorders wear some sort of hearing aid. Other assistive devices are available, including amplified telephone receivers, flashing lights to replace doorbells and telephone rings, vibrators that respond to sound, headphones for television sets, and teletypewriters.

What are the possible problems?

Hearing aids are usually beneficial and have few disadvantages. The body hearing aids pick up the sound of the person's clothing rubbing against his or her body. Behind-the-ear hearing aids eliminate this problem but are less durable and more prone to acoustic feedback. All hearing aids require a period of adjustment because the person may hear background noises that he or she hasn't heard in years. All types that depend on batteries require that the person keep an extra supply of batteries on hand. (See *Using a hearing aid*.)

NASAL PACKING

Nasal packing, which consists of gauze or other material, is inserted into the nasal cavity to control severe bleeding.

Depending on the bleeding site, nasal packing can be inserted into either the front or back of the nose. Packing in the front of the nose may be an absorbable gauzelike material that can remain in place for 3 to 5 days. If this type of packing fails to control the bleeding, the doctor may use antibiotic-impregnated petroleum gauze strips that are layered in tiers in the nasal cavity. This type of packing is typically removed after 48 hours.

Packing in the back of the nose is commonly inserted when packing in the front doesn't stop the bleeding or when the doctor can't identify the bleeding vessel in the back of the nasal passage. Many times, such bleeding can't be seen due to the location, especially if the nasal septum is deviated. Packing in the back of the nose typically remains in place for 4 days.

The doctor will first try to control the bleeding by cautery with silver nitrate pledgets, by using electrocautery, or by applying an anesthetic that acts to temporarily constrict blood vessels. If these methods fail to control the bleeding, nasal packing is used.

An alternative to nasal packing is the use of a nasal balloon catheter. Once inflated, the balloon exerts pressure on the bleeding site in the back of the nose. Single-balloon or double-balloon catheters may be used.

Why is this procedure done?

Nasal packing is used to control severe nosebleeds that are uncontrollable by other treatments.

What happens before the procedure?

▪ The doctor or nurse explains the procedure to you. You'll have to breathe through the mouth, which will make your mouth dry, but mouthwash may relieve it.

▪ You're told that pain medication will be available to relieve the headache that often accompanies nasal packing.

▪ The nurse administers a sedative or tranquilizer.

What happens during the procedure?

To insert nasal packing into the front of the nose, a doctor may place an absorbable packing moistened with a drug that constricts blood vessels into the nasal cavity. If this doesn't control the bleeding, the doctor then places antibiotic-impregnated petroleum gauze strips horizontally in the front of the nostrils until the nasal passage is completely packed.

To insert nasal packing into the back of the nose, the doctor first anesthetizes the nose, then passes a small catheter through the nose into the throat, where it's grasped by forceps and pulled out through the mouth. The pack is usually a roll of gauze or a tampon that has three black silk sutures tied around it. One string is tied to the catheter tip that is coming out of the mouth; then the catheter and string are pulled out through one side of the nose. This is repeated through the other side of the nose. When the pack is in position, the two strings coming out of the front of the nose are tied around a roll of gauze placed in front of the nostrils; the third string, which is left hanging from the mouth, is taped to the cheek.

Alternative methods to control bleeding in the back of the nose include insertion of a urinary catheter or a nasal balloon catheter. (See *Understanding nasal balloon catheters.*)

What are the possible complications?

Possible complications of nasal packing include lack of oxygen and shock from blood loss and breathing problems. In the person who's sedated for packing in the back of the nose, aspiration and airway obstruction may also occur. Less frequent complications include sinus infection, middle ear infection, and pressure necrosis. Nasal balloon catheters have similar complications. In addition, balloon

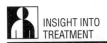
INSIGHT INTO
TREATMENT

Understanding nasal balloon catheters

To control bleeding in the back of the nose, the doctor may insert a nasal balloon catheter instead of nasal packing. These catheters are self-retaining and disposable and include either a single balloon or double balloon. These balloons are inflated with saline solution, not air, because air will leak slowly.

Single-balloon catheter
The single-balloon catheter includes a balloon that, when inflated, compresses the blood vessels and a soft, collapsible outside bulb that prevents the catheter from slipping out of place.

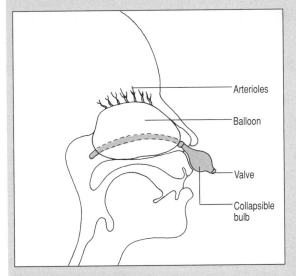

Double-balloon catheter
The double-balloon catheter includes a balloon that goes in the back of the nose and that, when inflated, secures the catheter in the throat; a balloon in the front of the nose that, when inflated, compresses the blood vessels; and a central airway that helps the

person breathe more comfortably. Each balloon is inflated independently.

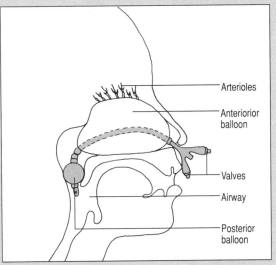

To use either type of balloon catheter, the doctor lubricates the catheter with an antibiotic ointment and inserts it through the person's nostril, then inflates the balloon by instilling saline solution into the appropriate valve. (If a double-balloon catheter is used, the doctor will inflate the balloon in the back of the nose first.) The doctor may secure the catheter by taping its tip to the outside of the person's nose.

deflation may dislodge clots and nasal debris into the throat, which could prompt coughing, gagging, or vomiting.

What happens after the procedure?
- You're told to report any fresh blood in the back of your throat or blood you cough up.

SELF-HELP

Recovering from nasal packing

After you've been discharged from the hospital, follow these important guidelines:

- Avoid blowing your nose for 2 to 3 days. It could cause bleeding. Expect slight oozing of blood-stained fluid from your nose for the next few days. Report any heavy bleeding.
- Use a humidifier (cool mist) at home to help prevent crusting inside the nose.
- Avoid activities that may promote nosebleeds.

- An intravenous line is maintained.
- Mouthwashes or ice chips to moisten your mouth and pain medication are provided.
- If a nasal balloon catheter is in place, the doctor may order the balloon deflated for 10 minutes every 24 hours to prevent damage to nasal tissue.
- While the nasal packing is in place, you're usually placed on a liquid diet. The nasal packing causes a partial vacuum of the nasal passage, which makes swallowing difficult. (See *Recovering from nasal packing*.)

NASAL IRRIGATION

Nasal irrigation is the instillation of water or saline solution into the nasal cavity to drain mucus or debris.

A layer of mucus is formed by the mucous membrane that lines the nasal cavity and acts as a filter to remove bacteria, viruses, and particles from the air when it enters the nose. Cilia (hairlike projections) continually vibrate and assist with filtering by direct contact with the mucous layer. Continuous ciliary propulsion pushes the mucus toward the sinus opening and down into the back of the throat. When normal ciliary function fails, nasal deposits may impede sinus drainage and air flow and cause headaches, infections, and unpleasant odors.

Nasal irrigations may be performed manually with a bulb syringe or oral irrigating device. Irrigating solutions should always be warm; solutions that are too hot or cold may irritate the nasal mucosa.

Why is this procedure done?
- To facilitate the cleaning of the mucous membranes of the nasal cavity and paranasal sinuses
- To soothe irritated mucous membranes
- To aid breathing
- To treat nasal polyps, nasal septal deviation, cystic fibrosis, allergic nasal inflammation, nasal injury, chronic sinus infection, swollen mucous membranes, and granulomatous diseases
- To treat persons who've been long-term users of inhalants (such as cocaine or nose drops containing phenylephrine chloride) and those

who regularly inhale occupational toxins or allergens (paint fumes, sawdust, pesticides, or coal dust)

When shouldn't this procedure be done?

Nasal irrigation should not be performed on people with an absent gag reflex because the fluid can enter the windpipe. Nasal irrigation sometimes isn't performed in people who've had recent sinus surgery, severe destruction of the sinuses, or a history of frequent nosebleeds.

What happens before the procedure?

You're told to keep your mouth open and not speak or swallow during the irrigation. If you do, it could force infectious material into the sinuses or eustachian tubes.

What happens during the procedure?

This procedure may be performed by the nurse or you can do it yourself. Sit upright with your head bent forward over a basin or sink and well flexed on your chest. A warmed solution is introduced into the nostril by either a bulb syringe or an oral irrigating device (such as the Water-Pik). Both types of devices facilitate the drainage of mucoid debris and loosen nasal crusting. Each nostril is irrigated alternately until the return irrigant runs clear. Nasal irrigation can safely be performed twice daily unless it causes excessive irritation; if so, one irrigation daily is adequate. (See *How to perform nasal irrigation,* page 516.)

Nasal irrigation is usually performed with saline solution, which mimics the body's own fluid. You may use a commercially prepared isotonic solution (such as Ocean, Ayr, or NaSal) or prepare your own solution by adding half a teaspoon of salt for every 8 ounces (240 milliliters) of warm water. The amount of solution used for irrigation varies depending on the amount of crusted mucus. A typical irrigation requires 17 to 34 ounces (500 to 1,000 milliliters).

What are the possible complications?

Complications associated with nasal irrigation include irritation of the nasal mucous membranes resulting from too-frequent irrigation or extreme temperatures of the solution. Fluid can also enter the windpipe; this is rare but can occur in people with an absent gag reflex.

SELF-HELP

How to perform nasal irrigation

Following these tips will help you perform nasal irrigation at home.

Equipment

You need a bulb syringe or an oral irrigating device (such as the Water-Pik), rigid or flexible disposable irrigation tips, saline solution, plastic sheet, apron or towels, facial tissues, bath basin, and gloves. Warm the solution to about 105° F (40.5° C) and then warm the bulb by drawing up and expelling some irrigating solution. If you're using an oral irrigating device, plug it into an electrical outlet and run 8 ounces (240 milliliters) of solution through the tubing to clear previous solutions and warm the tubing. Then, fill the reservoir of the device with warm saline solution.

Procedure

Begin by assuming a comfortable upright position with your head bent over the basin and well flexed on the chest.

The nose and ear should be on the same vertical plane. You're less likely to breathe in the irrigating solution when holding the

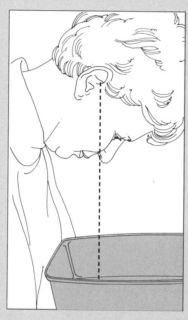

head in this position. Moreover, this position should keep the irrigant from entering the eustachian tubes. You should also keep your mouth open and breathe rhythmically during the irrigation.

To use a bulb syringe, fill the bulb syringe with irrigating solution, insert the tip about ½ inch (1.3 centimeters) into the nostril,

and then squeeze the bulb until a gentle stream of warm irrigant washes through your nose. Forceful squeezing should be avoided to prevent driving debris from the nasal passages into the sinuses or eustachian tubes.

To use an oral irrigating device, insert the catheter tip into your nostril about ½ to 1 inch (1.3 to 2.5 centimeters) and then turn on the irrigating device. You should start with a low-pressure setting and then increase the pressure as needed to obtain a gentle stream of irrigating solution.

Points to remember

With either type of irrigating device, both nostrils should be irrigated and the returning irrigant should be inspected.

Report changes in color, viscosity, or volume or the presence of blood or necrotic tissue to your doctor.

You should wait for a few minutes after the irrigation and then blow excess fluid from both nostrils at once. Then clean the device with disinfectant.

What happens after the procedure?

You clean the device. To clean the electronic device, about 8 ounces of 0.25% acetic acid solution is run through the irrigating tip and tubing. You or the nurse should shake the excess moisture from the parts and allow them to dry thoroughly. If using a bulb syringe, draw the acetic acid solution into the bulb and swirl and expel the solution; this is repeated two or three times.

TREATING SKIN DISORDERS

DRUG THERAPIES

TOPICAL ANTI-INFECTIVES

Topical anti-infective drugs are used to prevent or treat bacterial, viral, or fungal infections of the skin. The choice of the drug depends on the type of infection that's present.

Topical anti-infectives are useful for minor abrasions or cuts; however, when there is swelling, redness, or other signs of moderate to severe infection, systemic anti-infectives may be necessary because penetration of the skin by these drugs is limited.

The topical antiviral ointment acyclovir is used to treat initial episodes of genital herpes and in immunocompromised persons who have mucocutaneous herpes simplex virus infections that aren't life-threatening. Acyclovir is for use on the skin only and shouldn't be applied to the eye.

The bacteria-fighting drugs bacitracin, gentamicin, neomycin, chloramphenicol, chlortetracycline, erythromycin, mupirocin, and tetracycline are used to treat local bacterial infections caused by susceptible organisms.

Silver sulfadiazine treats or prevents wound infections in persons with burns. It shouldn't be used to treat people with poor kidney or liver function.

Topical antifungal drugs (miconazole, econazole, ciclopirox, tolnaftate, ketoconazole, clotrimazole, haloprogin, and nystatin) are effective against skin fungi and yeasts. These antifungals may be formulated as aerosol powders or spray solutions, topical powders, creams, or gels.

What are topical anti-infectives used for?

Topical anti-infectives are used to prevent infection in minor skin abrasions, cuts, and scratches.

What are some commonly used anti-infectives?

For bacterial skin infections

- bacitracin, known by the brand name Baciguent
- chloramphenicol, known by the brand name Chloromycetin
- clindamycin, known by the brand name Cleocin T Gel

- erythromycin, known by the brand names Akne-Mycin, EryDerm, Erygel, and Staticin
- gentamicin, known by the brand names Garamycin and G-Myticin
- mafenide, known by the brand name Sulfamylon
- metronidazole, known by the brand name MetroGel
- mupirocin, known by the brand name Bactroban
- neomycin, known by the brand name Myciguent
- silver sulfadiazine, known by the brand names Silvadene and Thermazene
- tetracycline, known by the brand names Achromycin and Topicycline

For fungal skin infections
- amphotericin, known by the brand name Fungizone
- ciclopirox olamine, known by the brand name Loprox
- clotrimazole, known by the brand name Lotrimin
- econazole, known by the brand names Ecostatin and Spectazole
- haloprogin, known by the brand name Halotex
- ketoconazole, known by the brand name Nizoral
- miconazole, known by the brand names Micatin and Monistat-Derm
- nystatin, known by the brand names Mycostatin and Nilstat
- oxiconazole, known by the brand name Oxistat
- sulconazole, known by the brand name Exelderm
- tolnaftate, known by the brand names Aftate, NP-27, Tinactin, and Ting

For viral skin infection
- acyclovir, known by the brand name Zovirax

What are the possible side effects?
- Local burning sensation, local rashes, itching
- Allergic reactions

What are the guidelines for using topical anti-infectives?
- Apply the medication according to the doctor's or pharmacist's instructions. The specific procedure will depend on the type of medication prescribed. Typically, a ½-inch (1.3-centimeter) ribbon of cream is used for every 4 square inches (26 square centimeters) of body surface; aerosols are sprayed onto the affected area from a distance of 6 to 10 inches (15 to 25 centimeters); spray solutions are released

from a distance of 4 to 6 inches (10 to 15 centimeters); and topical powders are dusted lightly onto the affected area and gently rubbed in.

- Keep the affected areas clean and dry for maximum drug effectiveness. Clean crusted or oozing lesions before applying the drug and to treat these areas frequently.

What else you should know

- Don't expect immediate improvement, but inform the doctor if the infection worsens or if there is any evidence of new blistering, burning, peeling, swelling, or excessive redness.
- Continue the full course of treatment, even if symptoms have cleared within a few days. Symptoms of infection will reappear if the drug is discontinued prematurely.
- Return for all follow-up appointments. The doctor will need to test the affected area after completion of therapy to check for any remaining infection or overgrowth of new fungi or bacteria.

Continue the full course of treatment, even if symptoms have cleared within a few days. Symptoms of infection will reappear if the drug is discontinued prematurely.

PEDICULICIDES

These drugs treat lice. They're available in various forms, including shampoos, creams, lotions, gels, and topical solutions. Typically, treatment with pediculicides requires two applications: the first eradicates adult lice; the second, given about 10 days later, kills newly hatched lice.

What are pediculicides used for?
Pediculicides are used to kill lice.

What are commonly used pediculicides?
- lindane, known by the brand names Kildane, Kwell, and Scabene
- crotamiton, known by the brand name Eurax
- pyrethrins, known by the brand names A-200, Barc, Blue, and Rid
- permethrin, known by the brand names Elimite and Nix

What are the possible side effects?
- Itching, irritation, mild redness and swelling, rash or allergic reactions, local burning sensation (common)

- Dizziness and other nervous system effects (lindane)
- Sneezing, sinusitis, wheezing, vomiting, respiratory distress, paralysis if inhaled (pyrethrins)

What are the guidelines for taking pediculicides?

- Although your skin may be irritated by the lice infestation itself, be alert for any new rashes that occur after treatment, and report them to the doctor; they may require additional drug treatment.
- Check other family members for lice because transmission is common.
- When using preparations containing lindane, watch for signs of systemic absorption and central nervous system toxicity, especially in children. Dizziness, muscle cramps, irritability, palpitations, and vomiting are early signs of toxicity.
- When using pyrethrins, watch for signs of respiratory distress caused by inadvertent inhalation of the drug.
- If you're using lindane shampoo, apply it to dry hair, rub it in thoroughly, and leave it in place for 4 minutes. Then apply a little water, work the shampoo into a lather, and rinse your hair thoroughly. Afterward, use a fine-tooth comb to remove nits and nit shells.
- Depending on the type of infestation, pyrethrins may be applied to the scalp, body, or pubic area. If using a gel or solution form, first wash the affected area with warm water and soap or regular shampoo; if using a shampoo, apply it to dry hair and work it into a lather using a small amount of water. Leave all forms of pyrethrins on the affected area for 10 minutes and then rinse thoroughly. Afterward, comb your hair with a fine-tooth comb.
- No matter which pediculicide is used, apply it again after 7 to 10 days to kill any newly hatched lice.
- Don't apply pediculicides on broken skin, the face (especially the eyes), mucous membranes, or the opening of the urethra.
- Don't use lindane during or immediately after a bath or shower.
- Apply pyrethrins in a well-ventilated area.
- If a rash or an irritation develops during application, wash the medication off and notify the doctor. Itching may persist for several weeks after successful treatment and may be treated with topical corticosteroids.

What else you should know

- Pediculicides are generally safe, causing only local stinging and burning. Occasionally, they cause a severe rash. However, they should be applied cautiously, especially in children, because systemic absorption can cause central nervous system side effects.

- Take steps to prevent reinfestation: clean the house thoroughly and vacuum upholstered furniture, rugs, and floors; scrub the toilet seat thoroughly; wash all recently worn clothing, bed linens, and towels in hot water or have them dry-cleaned; and wash hairbrushes and combs in hot, soapy water for 5 to 10 minutes. Hats, combs, and hairbrushes should never be shared.

SURGERIES

CRYOSURGERY

Cryosurgery is the destruction of tissue by the application of extreme cold. This procedure is often performed in the doctor's office. It can be done simply, with a cotton-tipped applicator dipped into liquid nitrogen and applied to the lesion, or it may involve use of a complex cryosurgical unit.

The success of cryosurgery depends on the type of skin problem, the extent and depth of the freeze applied, and the duration between freezing and thawing. A slow thaw destroys lesions most effectively. Liquid nitrogen and nitrous oxide are the most commonly used cryogens, but some cryosurgical units employ carbon dioxide or Freon. Liquid nitrogen is by far the most powerful cryogen and is especially useful for treating cancerous lesions, which resist cold because they contain so many blood vessels. Nitrous oxide is often favored for less extensive procedures because the surgeon can more easily control its effects.

Cryosurgery is used to treat a variety of skin, ophthalmic, and gynecologic conditions.

Why is this procedure done?
Cryosurgery is performed to destroy diseased tissue by the application of extreme cold and to create a scar to seal tears or holes in the retina. Cryosurgery is used to treat a variety of skin, ophthalmic, and gynecologic conditions.

When shouldn't this procedure be done?
Cryosurgery shouldn't be performed in people with disorders that are aggravated by cold temperatures, connective tissue or autoimmune

disease, blood disorders, or the cancerous condition known as *multiple myeloma*. It should also be avoided in persons receiving concurrent dialysis or drug therapy that suppresses the immune system.

What happens before the procedure?

- The doctor or nurse will explain the procedure to you, including the fact that there will be no incision (except for certain procedures on the eye).
- You'll be told to expect to initially feel cold, followed by burning, during the procedure. You'll be warned to remain as still as possible during the procedure to prevent inadvertent freezing of normal tissue.
- You'll sign a consent form.
- If necessary, your eyes or ears will be shielded to prevent damage.

What happens during the procedure?

The surgeon may give a local anesthetic, depending on the type of procedure. When freezing superficial lesions, the surgeon can often determine the correct temperature and depth of freezing simply by palpating and observing the lesion. When treating skin cancers, however, he or she inserts thermocouple needles (needles used to measure temperature differences) into the base of the tumor and a tissue temperature monitor to ensure that the tissue at the deepest part of the lesion has been adequately frozen.

The surgeon uses the cotton-tipped applicator or the cryosurgery unit to freeze the lesion and may refreeze a tumor several times to ensure its destruction.

If cryosurgery is used to treat retinal disease, the person will receive topical anesthetic eyedrops, and the pupils will be well dilated. A cryoprobe is then used to freeze affected tissue. The affected eye is patched until the anesthesia has worn off. However, if cryosurgery is used to treat posterior retinal disease, an incision is required to enable eye rotation with exposure of the white outer coat of the eye.

What are the possible complications?

Complications of cryosurgery are usually minor and may include reduction of the coloring of the skin and infection. Rarely, the procedure may damage blood vessels, nerves, and tear ducts. Any procedure requiring cryosurgery carries a risk of infection.

SELF-HELP

Recovering from cryosurgery

When you've been discharged from the hospital, follow these important guidelines.

Know what to expect
▪ You may continue to have pain when you're home. Use the pain medication prescribed by your doctor.
▪ If you had skin surgery, you should expect redness and swelling and the formation of a blister. It's important not to touch the blister. It will slough off in 2 to 3 weeks. If it becomes extremely uncomfortable or interferes with daily activities, ask your doctor to decompress it.

Other instructions
▪ If you experience new, intense pain; fever; or drainage of pus, notify your doctor immediately.
▪ If you had skin surgery, clean the area gently with soap and water, alcohol, or a cotton-tipped applicator soaked in hydrogen peroxide. To prevent loss of skin color, cover the wound with a loose bandage when you're outdoors. After the wound heals, apply a sunscreen over the area.
▪ If you had surgery for skin cancer, be sure to have regular checkups because skin cancers may recur.
▪ If you had gynecologic surgery, avoid intercourse for 2 weeks and see your doctor for regularly scheduled physical exams.

What happens after the procedure?

▪ After dermatologic cryosurgery, the nurse will clean the area gently with a cotton-tipped applicator soaked in hydrogen peroxide. Because cryosurgery doesn't cause bleeding, a bandage is not necessary. (See *Recovering from cryosurgery*.)
▪ An ice bag may be applied to relieve swelling and medications are given to relieve pain. Cryosurgery may cause considerable pain, especially if it was performed on or near the lips, eyes, eyelids, tongue, or the soles of the feet.

SKIN GRAFTS

A skin graft consists of either an autograft (in which healthy skin is taken from the person needing the graft) or an allograft (in which healthy skin is taken from a donor). In these procedures, skin is applied to resurface an area damaged by burns, injury, or surgery.

The graft may be one of several types: split-thickness, full-thickness, or pedicle-flap. A split-thickness graft is the type most commonly used for covering open burns. It includes the outer layer of the skin and part of the layer beneath that, and it may be applied as a sheet (usually on the face or neck to preserve the cosmetic result) or as a mesh. A mesh graft has tiny slits that allow the graft to expand up to nine times its original size. Mesh grafts prevent fluids from collecting under the graft and are typically used over extensive, deep burns.

A full-thickness graft includes the outer layer of the skin and all of the layer beneath that. Consequently, it contains hair follicles, sweat glands, and sebaceous glands, which typically aren't included in a split-thickness graft. Full-thickness grafts are commonly used for small burns that cause deep wounds.

A pedicle-flap graft is a full-thickness graft that includes skin and the underlying tissue with its blood vessels to ensure a continued blood supply to the graft. Pedicle-flap grafts may be used during reconstructive surgery to cover previous defects.

Why is this surgery done?

Skin grafts are performed to restore skin integrity to areas that can't heal on their own. Grafts are necessary when stitching the wound together isn't possible or cosmetically acceptable, when it would interfere with function, or when the defect is on a weight-bearing surface.

When shouldn't this surgery be done?

Grafts should not be done if the area lacks a sufficient blood supply; for this reason, they can't be applied directly over bare tendon, bone, cartilage, nerves, large fat deposits, or tissue damaged by X-rays. They sometimes shouldn't be done in people with arteriosclerosis, poor circulation, or previous surgery; however, in these people, skin grafts may be the only treatment available to close a large defect.

What happens before the surgery?

- To preserve potential donor sites, your skin will be carefully cared for. You'll be turned or repositioned every 2 hours and will be given range-of-motion exercises, massage, and a nutritious diet.
- The recipient site is also assessed. The graft's survival depends on close contact with the underlying tissue; ideally, the recipient site should appear healthy and be free of a thick leathery covering, debris, or infection.
- The doctor or nurse will explain the procedure to you and your family, providing realistic expectations. Many people expect to look better immediately after the surgery; however, you won't see the final results for at least a year. Immediately after surgery, normal contours

may be distorted by tissue reaction, suture lines may be red, and the color of the newly transplanted skin may differ somewhat from that of surrounding skin.

- You'll be told what to expect after the procedure. For instance, the graft will be inspected frequently to ensure that it's adhering to the underlying tissue, and your ability to move will be restricted to keep the graft in place. The original, rather bulky, bandage will remain in place for 1 or 2 days.

- The surgeon will decide how the donor and recipient sites are prepared for surgery. The donor site may be washed twice with soap and water, with the final shave and scrub done in the operating room; the recipient site may receive three or more bandage changes before grafting, with the last one including application of a topical antibiotic.

What happens during the surgery?

Grafting may be performed under general or local anesthesia, either in the operating room or at the bedside. Occasionally, grafting may be performed on an outpatient basis for extremely small facial or neck defects.

The thickness of the graft depends largely on the defect to be covered, with thicker grafts used for larger defects. If the blood supply is poor at the recipient site, a thinner graft is used because it requires less time to develop a new blood supply.

Autografts are taken from another area of your body with an instrument known as a *dermatome*. This instrument cuts uniform, split-thickness portions — typically about 0.005 to 0.02 inches thick. The graft is then placed on the damaged site, which must be a clean healing area for development of a new blood supply. The graft survives initially by direct contact with the underlying tissue, receiving oxygen and nutrients from existing lymph, but it eventually will die unless new capillaries develop. In split-thickness grafts, a new blood supply usually develops in 3 to 5 days; in full-thickness grafts, it may take up to 2 weeks. A bulky pressure bandage may be used over the recipient site and will remain in place for 24 to 48 hours.

What are the possible complications?

Complications include graft failure caused by inadequate blood supply, formation of a bruise, poor contact between the graft and the underlying tissue, or infection. Infection of the bloodstream may develop from infected graft or donor sites, especially in the elderly, and in people with reduced immune response or poor circulation.

What happens after the surgery?

- The nurse may cover the donor site with fine-mesh gauze or an ointment-filled bandage and otherwise leave it open to the air. In some cases, the graft will be covered with a synthetic adhesive bandage to promote moist wound healing.
- Meticulous wound care is vital for graft survival. You'll lie so that you're not lying on the graft, and the graft area will be kept elevated and immobilized.
- The donor site will be more painful than the recipient site. You'll be given pain medication.
- The doctor removes the outer pressure bandage on the graft, usually 24 to 48 hours after surgery, and may change the graft bandages on the 3rd to 5th day after surgery to assess the graft.
- The nurse will change the donor site bandage every 6 to 8 hours until oozing stops.
- The donor site may be treated with a heat lamp for 20 minutes three or four times a day.
- The nurse will apply cream daily to the healed donor site to keep it pliable. (See *Caring for yourself after a skin graft.*)
- If your graft or donor site is on your back, you may use a special bed.

DEBRIDEMENT, BATHS, & LIGHT TREATMENTS

DEBRIDEMENT

Debridement is the mechanical, chemical, or surgical removal of dead tissue from a wound. This procedure can be extremely painful, but it's necessary to promote healing and prevent infection of burns, bed sores, and nonhealing surgical or traumatic wounds.

Mechanical debridement includes application of wet-to-dry bandages (bandages that are applied wet and dry on the wound), flushing, hydrotherapy, and bedside debridement. *Chemical debridement* uses enzymes that selectively digest dead cells. These agents also absorb bacteria and thus reduce the risk of infection. *Surgical debridement,*

SELF-HELP

Caring for yourself after a skin graft

When you've been discharged from the hospital, follow these important guidelines.

Help promote healing
- If the grafting was done as an outpatient procedure, limit movement of the graft site to aid healing.
- Don't disturb the bandage on the graft or donor site for any reason. If the bandage must be changed, call the doctor.
- After the bandages have been removed, follow your doctor's instructions for applying cream to the healed graft several times a day. This will keep the skin pliable and aid scar formation.

Other points to remember
- Because sun exposure can affect pigmentation of the graft, limit exposure to direct sunlight and use a sunscreen on all grafted areas.
- Be aware that after scar formation is complete, you may need additional plastic surgery to improve the graft's appearance.

performed under general or regional anesthesia, affords the fastest and most complete debridement. The method selected depends on the type and extent of injury and the person's overall condition.

Why is this treatment done?

Debridement is done to promote wound healing, to prepare the wounded skin area for grafting, and to prevent infection. The use of mechanical, chemical, or surgical debridement depends on the size and extent of the person's wound and the overall condition.

In the simplest type of mechanical debridement, wet-to-dry dressings are applied to partially healed wounds with only slight amounts of dead tissue and minimal drainage; this method's most commonly used to treat bed sores rather than burns. Flushing and wound packing are necessary for deeper wounds to allow proper healing from the inside outward to the skin surface and to prevent abscess formation.

Hydrotherapy, another type of mechanical debridement, is usually performed on people with burns. It allows relatively nontraumatic wound debridement, bandage changes, removal of previously applied topical agents, and general body cleaning.

A third type of mechanical debridement, called *bedside debridement* (not always done at the bedside), can be used in the treatment of burns, bed sores, and nonhealing surgical or traumatic wounds.

Chemical debridement is most often used for bed sores or ulcers occurring from poor circulation and traumatic infected surgical wounds. Sometimes chemical and mechanical debridement are combined by applying bandages saturated with various medications.

Surgical debridement is usually reserved for burns or extremely deep or large ulcers. It is typically performed along with skin grafting.

When shouldn't this treatment be done?

Caution should be used when applying wet-to-dry bandages because they can have a harmful effect on healing tissues. Enzyme debridement should not be used on wounds with exposed bone.

What happens before the treatment?

- The doctor or nurse will explain the procedure to you.
- The nurse will teach you relaxation techniques to aid in controlling pain.
- Your doctor will prescribe pain medication.

What happens during the treatment?

Wet-to-dry bandages are placed in contact with the wound and covered with an outer layer of bandages. As the bandage dries, it sticks to the wound and, when the dry dressing is removed, the attached dead tissue comes off with it.

When a wound is flushed, the solution is instilled with a syringe. The solution should flow from the cleanest part of the wound to the dirtiest to prevent cross-contamination. The flush is repeated until the desired amount of solution has been used or until the fluid comes back clear. After flushing, a wound is usually packed with bandages to absorb additional drainage.

Hydrotherapy

Usually performed by a nurse assisted by a physical therapist, hydrotherapy — also called *tubbing* or *tanking* — involves immersing the person in a tank of warm, chemically treated water that is intermittently agitated. The person soaks for a predetermined time to loosen the old bandages (gentle agitation may be needed), and the burned areas are gently scrubbed to remove medication applied to the top of the wound, drainage, dead tissue, and debris. Debridement is then performed as necessary, usually by a doctor, and the areas are rebandaged.

Bedside debridement

Bedside debridement of a wound involves careful prying and cutting of loosened burned tissue or dead tissue with tweezers and scissors to separate it from the healthy tissue beneath. Depending on the size and severity of the burn, bedside debridement may be performed during hydrotherapy or afterward. One of the most painful types of debridement, it may be the only way to remove dead tissue from a severely burned person. Bedside debridement of bed sores can be performed by specially skilled nurses. If the person is at home, it can be performed there.

Chemical debridement

Chemical debridement is performed by a nurse and is accomplished by first gently flushing the wound with saline solution to remove the previous application and any drainage and dead tissue. The topical debriding agent is then applied to the dead tissue, and the wound is covered with a sterile bandage. Surrounding healthy tissue may require protection from the debriding agent with a skin-toughening agent.

Surgical debridement

Surgical debridement is performed by the doctor in the operating room using one of two procedures, depending on the depth and extent of the wound. In the first, tangential excision, the doctor uses a knife to remove sequential layers of dead tissue until healthy tissue is reached. In the second, fascial excision, the surgeon removes all injured tissue and underlying fat down to the muscle by using a scalpel or laser or by tearing it away.

What are the possible complications?

In any type of debridement, there's a risk of infection. Surgical debridement may cause infection of the bloodstream, if the wound is grossly infected at the time of debridement, as well as bleeding.

In debridement of extensive wounds, fluid and electrolyte imbalance may occur. Also, application of wet-to-dry dressings may lead to destruction of newly healed skin.

What happens after the treatment?

- You'll receive pain medication as necessary.
- Your fluid and electrolyte status will be watched, especially if you have burns.
- The nurse will weigh you daily.
- If a limb was debrided, you'll keep it elevated to increase circulation.
- The nurse will watch you for excessive bleeding and signs of infection after bedside and surgical debridement. (See *Recovering from debridement*.)

THERAPEUTIC BATHS

Balneotherapy, or a therapeutic bath, treats large skin areas and also promotes relaxation. Four types of therapeutic baths are commonly used: antibacterial, colloidal, emollient, and tar. (See *Comparing therapeutic baths*.)

Why is this treatment done?

Therapeutic baths are used to clean the skin, loosen or remove crusts or scales, and relieve itchiness and to deliver medications to the skin

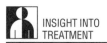

INSIGHT INTO
TREATMENT

Comparing therapeutic baths

TYPE	AGENTS	PURPOSE
Antibacterial	• Acetic acid • Hexachlorophene • Potassium permanganate • Povidone-iodine	To treat infected eczema, dirty ulcerations, boils, and blisters
Colloidal	• Aveeno colloidal oatmeal • Aveeno colloidal oatmeal, oilated • Starch and baking soda	To relieve itchiness and to soothe irritated skin; helpful for any irritating or oozing condition such as allergic eczema
Emollient	• Bath oils • Mineral oil	To clean and hydrate the skin; helpful for any dry skin condition
Tar	• Bath oils with tar • Coal tar concentrate	To treat scaly skin conditions, sometimes in combination with ultraviolet light therapy; loosens scales and relieves itchiness

or hydrate the outermost layer of the skin to allow penetration of medications. Therapeutic baths help treat psoriasis, allergic eczema, scaly dermatitis, blisters, and skin infections.

What happens before the treatment?
The nurse will explain the purpose of the bath to you and answer your questions.

What happens during the treatment?
You'll soak in a medicated bath, in water at approximately 97° F (36° C) for 20 to 30 minutes. (See *Giving yourself a therapeutic bath,* page 532.)

What are the possible complications?
Complications are uncommon but can include dry skin, itchiness, scaling, and cracklike breaks in the skin, depending on the medication added to the bath and how long you soak in it.

Giving yourself a therapeutic bath

When you've been discharged from the hospital, follow these important guidelines.

Prepare the bath correctly
- Therapeutic agents may make the bathtub slippery; therefore, use a bath mat.
- Overly hot water can increase itchiness and scaling; check water temperature with a bath thermometer.
- The average home bathtub holds 150 to 200 gallons of water. You should measure the prescribed medication accordingly and mix the water well to prevent a reaction to the medication.

Protect your skin
- If you have dry skin, remember that soap is drying. Normal skin requires bathing only every other day, with soap applied only to the underarms, groin, and bottoms of the feet.
- Friction during or after the bath can damage your skin. Unless you're being treated for psoriasis, you should wash with bare hands instead of a washcloth. If you have psoriasis, loosen crusts with a washcloth, but only after soaking for 15 or 20 minutes. Gently pat yourself dry with a clean towel, leaving the skin slightly damp.

Other instructions
- If you notice any increase in itchiness, oozing, redness, or scaling, report it to your doctor.
- Make and keep regular follow-up appointments with your doctor.

What happens after the treatment?
You'll dry off quickly by patting gently with a towel until the skin is damp dry. Apply topical medications immediately because they're absorbed easily when the skin is damp.

ULTRAVIOLET LIGHT TREATMENTS

Ultraviolet light, administered through sources that may include projectors, xenon arc lamps, fluorescent bulbs, or lasers, is used to treat various skin disorders. Ultraviolet light decreases the rate of cell division in the outer layer of the skin. New and experimental ultraviolet light treatments (photopheresis and photodynamic therapy) are being used to relieve symptoms and as a potential cure in some cancers.

Ultraviolet light is categorized as ultraviolet A, ultraviolet B, and ultraviolet C light, depending on its wavelength. Ultraviolet C (long waves) light is used in germicidal (germ-killing) lamps but is not used therapeutically because it carries the risk of serious burns and cancer.

Ultraviolet B (middle-length waves) light, the component of sunlight that causes sunburn, has been successfully used in the treatment of psoriasis for over 50 years. Ultraviolet A (short waves) light alone has little effect on normal skin, but certain medications such as psoralens can create an artificial sensitivity to ultraviolet A light. The combination of psoralens and ultraviolet A light is known as *photochemotherapy*.

Why is this treatment done?

Ultraviolet light treatments are used to decrease cell growth, to induce mild exfoliation and clearing of the skin, and to stimulate cells responsible for skin color in depigmented areas. Ultraviolet light treatment is used in people with psoriasis, allergic dermatitis, vitiligo (a pigmentation disorder), and the itchiness that is associated with kidney failure. Photodynamic laser therapy may be used to treat cancers of the esophagus, inner layer of the breathing passages in the lung, throat, bladder, retina, cervix and vagina, head and neck, and in skin lesions.

When shouldn't this treatment be used?

Photochemotherapy and ultraviolet B therapy shouldn't be used in people who have photosensitivity disease, those who take medications that cause sensitivity to light, and in people who have had skin cancer, previous radiation therapy to skin, cataracts, or loss of a lens of the eye due to cataract surgery.

What happens before the treatment?

- The doctor or nurse will explain the treatment. You'll be told that ultraviolet light treatments produce a mild sunburn that will help clear up skin lesions. With ultraviolet B therapy, the redness appears within 4 to 6 hours; with photochemotherapy, it may not become evident for 48 to 72 hours. In either case, it should disappear within another 24 hours. You'll also be informed that mild dryness and exfoliation will follow within 1 to 2 days.
- The doctor or nurse will obtain your medical history. He or she will want to know if you have a history of photosensitivity diseases or skin cancer, or if you've had radiation treatments or are taking medications that cause sensitivity to light.
- If you're receiving photochemotherapy, the nurse will give you the medication psoralens with food 2 hours before the ultraviolet light treatment.

Caring for yourself after ultraviolet light treatments

When you go home, follow these important guide-lines.

Protect yourself against burns

- If you're using a sunlamp, first allow the lamp to warm up for 5 minutes and then limit exposure to the time prescribed. Protect your eyes with goggles and use a dependable timer or have someone else monitor exposure time.
- Never use a sunlamp when tired; falling asleep un-der the warm lamp can cause severe burns.
- If you do get a small burn, apply cool water soaks for 20 minutes or until skin temperature is cool; noti-fy your doctor of larger burns.
- When outdoors, limit exposure to natural light, use a sunscreen with a skin protection factor rating of 15 or greater, and wear a hat, long sleeves, and sun-glasses.

Other instructions

- Use moisturizers and a mild soap to combat dry skin. Avoid hot baths or showers, which also pro-mote dry skin.
- If you're having photochemotherapy, follow the doctor's or nurse's instructions regarding when to take psoralens. If you don't take it exactly as direct-ed, the treatment may cause burns or be ineffective. Also, be sure to wear ultraviolet-opaque sunglasses outdoors for at least 12 hours after taking psoralens.
- Have an annual eye exam to detect possible for-mation of cataracts.
- Check with your doctor before taking any drug, in-cluding aspirin, to prevent heightened sensitivity to light.
- Notify your doctor if you develop any new skin problems.

What happens during the treatment?

Ultraviolet light therapy may be performed in the hospital, in a doc-tor's office, or at home. Typically, the light source is a bank of high-intensity fluorescent bulbs set into a reflective cabinet. The therapy may be delivered in full body cabinets, smaller cabinets (to treat lo-calized lesions), or by natural sunlight. Appropriate dosage is deter-mined according to your skin type and pigmentation.

You undress and put on a gown that bares only the area to be treated; vulnerable areas of the skin are protected by towels and sun-screen. You wear protective goggles. After the prescribed dosage of ultraviolet light has been administered, you may continue daily activ-ities with appropriate precautions to minimize further exposure to ultraviolet light.

What are the possible complications?

Overexposure of the skin to ultraviolet light can result from pro-longed treatment, inadequate distance between you and the light source, use of drugs that make your skin sensitive to light, or sensitive skin. Cataracts and corneal and retinal damage may result if your eyes are not protected during the treatment and for 24 hours after treatment with psoralens. Long-term effects of treatment are essentially the same as those of excessive sun exposure: aging of the skin and an increased risk for skin cancer. (See *Caring for yourself after ultraviolet light treatments.*)

What happens after the treatment?

The nurse will observe the treated area for marked redness, blisters, peeling, or other signs of overexposure 4 to 6 hours after ultraviolet B therapy and 24 to 48 hours after photochemotherapy. If overexposure occurs, ultraviolet treatments are usually stopped for a few days and then restarted at a lower level of exposure.

OTHER TREATMENTS

DERMABRASION

Dermabrasion is the surgical removal of the surface layer of the skin by high-speed sanding to improve many superficial skin problems. Dermabrasion removes the outer layer and part of the layer under that while preserving enough skin for regrowth. In some cases, people require two to three dermabrasion procedures for optimal results.

Careful screening of potential candidates for this procedure is essential. People who have unrealistic expectations shouldn't have dermabrasion. Those who have this procedure must understand its limitations and be able to accept the fact that some skin defects will remain afterward.

Pigment changes following dermabrasion may occur in people with pigmented skin such as brunettes, Asians, and light-skinned blacks.

Why is this procedure done?

Dermabrasion removes minor imperfections from the surface of the skin, improves a person's appearance and thereby boosts self-esteem, and reconstructs a skin area after surgery. Dermabrasion is performed most frequently for scar caused by acne. It's also been useful for removing superficial scars after injury or surgery. Other reasons to have dermabrasion include smallpox scars, removal of decorative or traumatic tattoos, sun damage, and some types of warts.

When shouldn't this procedure be done?

Dermabrasion should not be done in people who have undergone radiation therapy that has weakened underlying skin structure, and in those with uncontrolled diabetes or severe heart and blood vessel disease. It shouldn't be used for at least 6 to 12 months after taking the medication isotretinoin (known by the brand name Accutane) or in a person with a positive blood test for HIV.

What happens before the procedure?

- For screening purposes, the doctor will ask you about your medical history, level of knowledge about the procedure, and expected outcome.
- You'll be informed about the procedure, risks, complications, and possible results.
- Your skin must be free of cosmetics and washed with soap and water or an antimicrobial soap. For men, the area to be abraded must be clean-shaven.
- You'll be asked to bring someone along to provide transportation home.
- You'll sign a consent form.

What happens during the procedure?

Dermabrasion may be performed by a dermatologic surgeon, a plastic surgeon, or a cosmetic surgeon. The dermabrasion may take place in an office, an outpatient clinic, or a hospital operating room.

A sedative is administered either orally or by injection. After the skin is cleaned with an antimicrobial soap, gentian violet is painted on the areas to be planed. This fills and identifies the deepest pits for abrasions. You're asked to hold a cold pack on the area to be planed to lower the temperature of the skin.

A local anesthetic is administered to provide regional numbness. A refrigerant spray may be used to freeze the skin and to harden the surface for improved abrasion. The surgeon then removes the area that is to be abraded with a high-speed diamond fraise or a wire brush. A thick, nonadherent pad is then applied directly to the abraded area to absorb the drainage.

Deep scars that cannot be dermabraded can be excised and sutured closed or later filled with collagen.

What are the possible complications?

Alterations in pigmentation may follow dermabrasion. Reduced pigmentation occurs in about 50% of all dermabrasions. Rare complications include infection and scarring. If you've had herpes simplex (shingles), dermabrasion may reactivate the virus. Because the results of dermabrasion are never perfect, if you're unable to accept the remaining defects, you may develop emotional problems.

What happens after the procedure?

- The nurse will monitor your vital signs.
- The nurse will show you how to care for the wound and identify signs of infection, such as fever or drainage of pus. (See *Caring for yourself after dermabrasion*.)

WOUND FLUSHING

Wound flushing is the application of fluid under pressure to a wound site to clean tissues, remove contaminants, loosen dead tissue, and flush debris and bacteria. Flushing with an antiseptic solution helps the wound heal properly from the inside tissue layers outward to the skin surface. It also helps prevent premature surface healing over an abscess or infected area. After flushing, open wounds usually are packed with gauze to absorb additional drainage.

Wound flushings are usually performed in the hospital but may be required at home for care of chronic, slow-healing wounds. The home environment has fewer bacteria than a hospital or nursing home, so the risk of infection is somewhat lessened during treatment at home.

Choice of the flushing solution is important. An appropriate wound flushing solution has the following characteristics:

- strong enough to remove bacteria and debris
- nontoxic, to avoid tissue damage
- sterile, to minimize risk of infection
- nonirritating and painless to the person because nerve endings may be exposed in the wound.

 SELF-HELP

Caring for yourself after dermabrasion

When you go home, follow these important guidelines.

Protect your skin
- Remove the dressing the day after the procedure and clean the skin with soap and water. The skin should be patted dry, not rubbed, and then covered with an antibacterial ointment.
- Avoid sun exposure for 3 to 6 months and, afterward, use a sunscreen with a skin protection factor of at least 15 when outdoors.

Other points to remember
- Keep in mind that you'll experience swelling, redness, crust formation, and some discomfort and itching after the procedure.
- Make and keep follow-up medical appointments to treat problem areas.

Flushing wounds at home

When you've been discharged from the hospital, follow these important guidelines:
- Observe the instructions you received at the hospital for doing wound flushes at home.
- A visiting nurse may assist you with the wound flushes.
- Notify the doctor promptly if you notice any signs of infection, such as fever, swelling, or drainage of pus.

Why is this treatment done?

Wound flushing is done to enhance wound healing, to reduce the risk of infection, and to treat an established infection. Wound flushing is used primarily in three situations: injury, surgery, and after surgery. Traumatic wounds have a high potential for becoming infected. Flushing is used to reduce the risk of infection in people with crush injuries, bites, and lacerations, for example. During surgery, the wound may be flushed with an antibacterial solution just before closure. After surgery or for people who don't require surgery, open wounds are often flushed to treat or prevent infection — for example, in people with bed sores, abscesses, or infected areas.

What happens before the treatment?

- The doctor or nurse will ask you about allergies, especially to povidone-iodine or other topical medications or solutions.
- The doctor or nurse will explain the procedure, provide privacy, and position you for the flushing procedure, so that the solution will flow away from the wound.

What happens during the treatment?

For repair of lacerations, wound flushing is carried out as part of wound closure, with flushing occurring after the local anesthetic has been given. When performed during surgery, flushing is carried out by the surgeon as part of the operative procedure. Other wound flushings are usually performed by a nurse. At home, the person or a family member may be responsible for wound flushing. (See *Flushing wounds at home.*)

What are the possible complications?

Complications are rare. Careful choice of the solution minimizes wound or skin irritation and cell damage.

What happens after the treatment?

- The nurse or doctor will clean the area around the wound to promote local circulation and help prevent skin breakdown and infection.
- The nurse or doctor may insert packing into the wound, if appropriate, and apply a sterile bandage.
- The nurse will carefully monitor the size and appearance of the wound.

17

TREATING
TRAUMATIC INJURIES

DRUG THERAPIES

VASOPRESSORS

These drugs rapidly raise blood pressure and increase cardiac output, thereby improving circulation to vital organs. In patients with traumatic injuries, vasopressors prevent or treat shock.

Vasopressors are usually administered intravenously in a hospital's critical care unit.

What are vasopressors used for?
- To raise blood pressure
- To increase cardiac output
- To enhance blood flow to the kidneys, preserving kidney function

What are some commonly used vasopressors?
- dopamine, known by the brand name Intropin
- epinephrine, known by the brand name Adrenalin
- norepinephrine, known by the brand name Levophed
- phenylephrine, known by the brand name Neo-Synephrine
- metaraminol, known by the brand name Aramine

What are the possible side effects?
- Decreased urine output
- High blood pressure, heart rate changes, palpitations
- Local tissue breakdown at the infusion site
- Headache, nervousness, restlessness, insomnia
- Nausea, vomiting

What else should you know about vasopressors?
- If possible, tell the doctor about all of the other medications you're taking, including nonprescription medicines.
- If you feel pain or notice swelling, blanching, or discoloration at the injection site, tell the doctor or nurse immediately.
- Expect the doctor and nurse to closely monitor your blood pressure, heart rate, and other vital signs while you're receiving this drug.

CHELATION THERAPY FOR LEAD POISONING

Chelation therapy is the administration of drugs that bind with lead present in the body to facilitate its excretion and reduce its toxic effects. It's commonly used to treat lead poisoning, which is considered the most serious chronic childhood disease in the United States today. Chelation therapy may also be used to bind with other metals, such as iron, arsenic, and mercury.

Several medications are available for chelation therapy. Age, health status, presence of iron deficiency anemia or sickle cell disease, and the environment of the home and any additional addresses of the child are all factors that determine the use and method of chelation therapy.

Chelation therapy isn't a permanent solution to the problem of lead poisoning. Only removal of lead from the child's home or moving the family to lead-safe housing can be considered permanent treatment of the problem.

Why is this treatment done?

Chelation therapy is given to increase excretion of lead from the body. Children with high levels of lead in their blood are candidates for chelation therapy.

When shouldn't this treatment be done?

Chelation therapy using edetate calcium disodium (also known as *Calcium EDTA*) shouldn't be given to children with severe kidney disease and inadequate urine output. Treatment with the medication dimercaprol should only be used in life-threatening situations, such as when the disease affects the brain, and only in children with normal levels of the enzyme glucose-6-phosphate dehydrogenase, because the drug may cause the breakdown of red blood cells in those who are born with a deficiency of this substance. This drug also shouldn't be used in children who are allergic to peanuts or products derived from peanuts.

What happens before the treatment?

- The doctor or nurse will explain the procedure to the child and parents. If the parents will be administering the drug, they'll be informed about the drug treatment program and its possible side effects.
- The doctor or nurse will check the results of liver and kidney function tests before initiation of therapy with edetate calcium disodium.
- The child will need to be in lead-safe housing when receiving edetate calcium disodium because this therapy will increase gastrointestinal absorption of lead if exposure to lead continues during treatment. A social worker is often called upon to help with housing arrangements.

What happens during the treatment?

Four drugs can be used for chelation therapy, including dimercaprol, edetate calcium disodium, succimer, and D-penicillamine. Information about each agent is summarized below.

Dimercaprol

Dimercaprol is usually used with edetate calcium disodium and only in children with very high blood lead levels or those who have symptoms of the disease. Dimercaprol increases the excretion of lead in feces and urine. However, because the primary site of excretion is through the liver, this drug can be used in children with kidney impairment. Dimercaprol is administered by injection into a muscle. Children receiving dimercaprol shouldn't take iron supplements because the combination of medications causes vomiting.

Edetate calcium disodium

This drug can be administered by injection either into a muscle or vein but is usually given into the muscle. Because the injection is quite painful, the medication is mixed with a local anesthetic. Intravenous infusion of edetate calcium disodium is most effective and may be used in adults with lead poisoning.

Administration of edetate calcium disodium without dimercaprol may increase symptoms in people with very high lead levels; therefore, these two drugs are used together in children who have symptoms of lead poisoning and in those with high lead levels.

This drug can be used for outpatient treatment of lead poisoning, but the child must return to the hospital or clinic to receive the medication.

Dimercaprol is given by injection into a muscle. Children receiving the drug should not take iron supplements because this combination causes vomiting.

Succimer

This relatively new drug may be administered orally. It produces excretion of lead in the urine.

When given on an outpatient basis, succimer can be administered by the parent. However, therapy should begin in a hospital setting (especially the first 5 days) until the child's housing is made lead-safe.

D-penicillamine

Although this drug is not yet approved by the Food and Drug Administration as a chelating agent for lead poisoning, some doctors prescribe it. It can be given orally for extended periods (weeks to months) and may be given on an outpatient basis, provided the child is seen regularly by the doctor and remains in lead-safe housing. D-penicillamine has been particularly useful as follow-up therapy after initial treatment of lead poisoning with dimercaprol or edetate calcium disodium.

What are the possible complications?

The most common side effects of dimercaprol are mild temperature elevations, liver enzyme elevation, nausea with occasional vomiting, headache, mild conjunctivitis (an eye infection), tearing, runny nose, and excessive salivation.

High doses of edetate calcium disodium are toxic to the kidneys. Impending kidney failure is reversible once therapy is discontinued and the remainder of the drug is excreted. Abnormal heart rhythms may also occur, especially with rapid intravenous administration.

Succimer can cause drowsiness, dizziness, unusual sensations such as feelings of "pins and needles" in the extremities, nausea, vomiting, metallic taste in the mouth, flulike symptoms, and liver enzyme elevation.

D-penicillamine can cause kidney failure, blood disorders, and allergic reactions. This drug should be used cautiously in people who are allergic to penicillin because cross-sensitivity may occur.

What happens after the treatment?

- The nurse monitors the child for side effects and response to therapy.
- The child is discharged to a lead-free environment. Parents are told to make and keep follow-up appointments with the doctor.

SURGERY

REATTACHMENT AFTER TRAUMATIC AMPUTATION

Reattachment after traumatic amputation is an emergency attempt to reconnect an accidentally severed finger or toe, limb, or other body part. Advances in microvascular surgery have resulted in a reported 80% to 90% success rate in the repair of severed body parts. Even when there is severe injury to the skin, muscle, bone, and blood vessels, repair may be attempted if the nerves are intact or minimally damaged. The person may then regain a significant degree of function in the reattached body part. Unfortunately, only 20% of people whose accidentally amputated body parts might be reattached reach a microsurgeon in time for successful repair.

One of the key factors to successful repair is minimizing the period of time that a body part is without blood supply. Because muscle fibers are sensitive to lack of oxygen and show microscopic damage after 30 minutes without blood flow, successful repair requires that this time be kept to a minimum and that proper care be taken of the body part.

Why is this surgery done?

The surgery reconnects a fully or partially severed body part and restores function greater than that provided by a prosthesis (artificial body part). Reattachment surgery should be considered for all traumatic thumb amputations; multiple finger or toe amputations; all amputations in children; clean amputations at the palm, wrist, or forearm; and any complex injury that may benefit from microvascular surgery. Successful repair has been performed on arms, legs, scalps, ears, and penises.

What happens before the surgery?

- The doctor will evaluate the site of amputation and examine the person for additional injuries and infection. The doctor will also obtain a detailed medical, surgical, and social history, including circumstances surrounding the injury.

- The person will lie on his or her back with the affected arm or leg elevated and in good body alignment.
- The nurse will insert an intravenous catheter for administration of fluids or blood as necessary.
- The nurse will administer pain medication.
- The person will have an X-ray of the body part to evaluate bone damage and a chest X-ray. Also, he or she will have have blood drawn for a complete blood count and studies to evaluate blood clotting and chemistry. The person's blood type will be determined and additional analyses made to obtain suitable blood for transfusion.
- The nurse will cover the wound with a moist sterile pressure bandage and place a light ice bag over it to control bleeding.
- The person will receive antibiotics to prevent infection and a tetanus immunization if he or she hasn't had one within the past 10 years.

What happens during the surgery?

The person will arrive in the operating room with the amputated part preserved in saline solution and packed in ice. The reattachment requires a team of surgeons, nurses, and technicians well versed in microvascular surgery. While one microsurgery team examines, identifies, cleans, and tags structures on the amputated part, another prepares the stump. A vein or tendon graft may be necessary to increase circulation or stabilize the amputated part. Next, the bone is aligned and stabilized, all clots are removed, and the condition of each blood vessel is assessed by a special X-ray procedure. The surgeon then repairs the main nerve trunks and reconnects the body part. Muscles and tendons are repaired, if possible, and all reconnected sites are covered with muscle to allow for optimal capillary and lymph system regeneration.

After loosely stitching the skin, the surgeon may apply partial-thickness skin grafts. The surgeon may also make an opening in the layer of tissue covering muscles so that muscle swelling doesn't cut off circulation. After completing these procedures, the surgeon applies a bandage over the site.

What are the possible complications?

Complications following this procedure include bleeding, infection, and an inability to extend the reconnected part because of shortening of the muscle fibers or scar tissue formation. When body parts are reconnected after prolonged periods without blood supply, there's a

Recovering from reattachment of a body part

When you've been discharged from the hospital, follow these important guidelines.

Take special precautions

- Watch for and report to your doctor any unusual pain, bleeding, or symptoms of infection.
- Keep the repair site clean and dry to avoid skin breakdown, irritation, and infection.
- Don't smoke and make sure those who live with you don't smoke for at least 6 weeks after surgery. Cigarette smoke may cause impaired circulation.

Know what to expect

- Know that to recover use of the repaired part, learn to accept an altered body image, and resume an independent lifestyle, you'll require a lengthy and perhaps difficult rehabilitation.
- Be aware that you may be referred to a support group or a mental health professional to help you develop coping strategies.

higher risk for kidney failure, too much potassium in the blood, and infection.

The person may experience an intolerance to cold in the reattached part, but this usually resolves within 2 years.

What happens after the surgery?

- The nurse will check the reattached part hourly, paying particular attention to blood circulation through it.
- The nurse will monitor the person's vital signs and urine output regularly and administer intravenous fluids, blood, and plasma expanders.
- The nurse will check the person's bandages frequently and report any excessive bleeding or drainage to the doctor. (See *Recovering from reattachment of a body part.*)
- The person will receive antibiotics and pain medication as prescribed by the doctor.

HEAT & COLD TREATMENTS

REWARMING TREATMENTS

Rewarming includes a range of strategies from external application of a hot-water bottle to insertion of a tube in the chest for instillation of a heated solution to treat hypothermia. Hypothermia is defined as a central body temperature below 95° F (35° C). Below this temperature, the body can no longer generate enough heat to sustain essential body functions.

The type of rewarming used depends on the degree of hypothermia and the person's age and general health. In a healthy person with mild hypothermia (temperature of 90° to 94° F [32.2° to 34.4° C]), passive external rewarming, such as the use of blankets, is performed to reduce heat loss by evaporation, convection, and radiation and to allow spontaneous rewarming through generation of body heat.

Active external rewarming, such as use of heating pads or a hypothermia blanket, may be ordered for moderate hypothermia or if passive rewarming fails to raise the temperature at least 1.8° F (1° C) per hour. For severe hypothermia, active rewarming techniques may be used to raise the person's temperature rapidly. Intravenous infusion of warmed fluids, administration of warmed oxygen, or peritoneal dialysis (instillation of warmed solution between the two layers of the membrane that covers the abdomen) may be necessary. In extremely severe hypothermia, a tube may be inserted in the chest to instill heated saline solution into the space between the lungs. Use of a heart-lung machine for blood rewarming may also be initiated.

Why is this treatment done?

Rewarming treatments are used to restore normal temperature in people with a central body temperature below 95° F.

What happens before the treatment?

- If you're alert, the doctor or nurse will explain the treatment to you.
- The nurse will cover you with blankets and wrap a towel around your head.
- The nurse will check your vital signs and, if you have severe hypothermia, monitor your electrocardiogram.
- The nurse will insert an intravenous catheter and possibly a urinary catheter to monitor your urine output.

What happens during the treatment?

For extremely severe hypothermia, the doctor may insert a chest tube and instill warmed saline solution into the space between the lungs. The doctor may also initiate blood rewarming with a heart-lung machine.

In a case of severe hypothermia, warmed intravenous fluids are given to improve circulation, reduce the viscosity of the blood, and improve blood flow to the coronary arteries, reducing the risk of abnormal heart rhythms. Heated, humidified oxygen is given by mask or through a breathing tube; a mechanical breathing machine may be used. Peritoneal dialysis, using a solution that has been warmed to 110° F (43.3° C), may also be instituted.

If there's evidence of frostbite, the body part is handled extremely carefully and quickly immersed in warm water (100° to 108° F [37.8° to 42.2° C]) or wrapped with warmed, moist gauze. (See *Caring for yourself after a rewarming treatment.*)

In a case of mild hypothermia, rewarming is begun with a simple measure such as blankets. If the central temperature doesn't rise at least 1.8° F after an hour, active external warming is begun by placing

 SELF-HELP

Caring for yourself after a rewarming treatment

When you've been discharged from the hospital, follow these important guidelines:
- Take measures to prevent recurrence of hypothermia.
- If you had severe frostbite, you may need physical therapy.
- If you don't have adequate shelter or clothing, contact a social service agency. If the underlying cause is drug or alcohol abuse, you should seek counseling.

a hot-water bottle or an electric heating pad on the blanket and over the chest or by immersing you in a warm-water bath. A hypothermia blanket may also be used.

What are the possible complications?

Complications during rewarming may include life-threatening abnormal heart rhythms and circulatory collapse. Temperature can plummet after treatment is stopped. However, careful application of rewarming techniques and frequent monitoring help avoid such complications.

What happens after the treatment?

Your temperature is carefully monitored. If hypothermia recurs, rewarming procedures are begun again.

HEAT TREATMENTS

Applying heat directly to a person's body raises tissue temperature and increases inflammation by causing blood vessels to expand, increasing nutrition to cells, and helping to remove waste products from cells. Heat increases local circulation and tissue metabolism, reduces pain, provides comfort by promoting muscle relaxation, and decreases congestion in deep internal organs. It also raises the pain threshold of sensory nerve endings and thus may break the pain-spasm-pain cycle with its pain-relieving effects. Heat increases the ability of connective tissue to stretch, thereby preparing stiff joints and tight muscles for activity.

Heat treatments can be superficial or deep. Superficial heat can be applied in many forms, such as chemical hot packs, paraffin, heat lamps, hot-water bottles, heating pads, and warm packs, and can be moist or dry. Dry heat can be delivered at a higher temperature and for a longer time. Moist heat penetrates more deeply than dry heat, doesn't dry the skin, produces less perspiration, and is usually more comfortable for the person.

Deep-heat treatments include ultrasound therapy and a procedure known as *diathermy.* Ultrasound therapy directs sound waves that are absorbed by various tissues and converted into heat energy. Diathermy uses high-frequency electric current. Both ultrasound therapy and diathermy penetrate deeply and significantly elevate tissue temperature. They're valuable for delivering heat to injured soft tissue such as muscle. Ultrasound therapy is currently used more often than diathermy, but both forms of treatment can be useful.

Why is this treatment done?

Heat treatments are given to relieve pain and stiffness, relax muscles, increase range of motion, and promote tissue healing. Heat treatments are commonly used to treat muscle spasms and arthritis and to restore mobility after muscle or joint injury or surgery. They also may be used in combination with other therapies.

When shouldn't this treatment be done?

Heat treatments should be used cautiously in people with decreased sensation in the affected body part, heat intolerance, or impaired kidney, heart, or lung function. People with reduced circulation have a decreased ability to dissipate heat effectively, thereby reducing their tolerance and increasing the risk of heat-induced injury. Ultrasound heat treatments shouldn't be applied over the heart, eye, or a pregnant uterus.

Because heat dilates blood vessels, it shouldn't be used in people who have bleeding disorders and should be avoided after traumatic injury. It should be used with caution in people who take cortisone, which causes capillaries to break easily. Deep-heat therapy shouldn't be used in people with metal implants because of the risk of local tissue damage.

What happens before the treatment?

- The physical therapist or technician will explain the purpose and effects of the treatment to you.
- Your pain level, activity level, circulation, and need for pain medication will be evaluated.
- You'll lie comfortably with only the area to be treated exposed.
- The physical therapist or technician will make sure that your skin is clean, dry, and free of oils and creams.

What happens during the treatment?

Superficial heat treatments may be self-administered or provided by a physical therapist or technician.

With chemical hot packs, the size and shape of the pack used depends on the area being treated. The packs are made of canvas and contain a heat-sensitive chemical. Towels are wrapped around the packs before they are applied. The pack is then placed on you. (You shouldn't lie on the pack to avoid overheating of skin.) The pack is removed when it becomes cool.

Paraffin wax is melted and mixed with mineral oil and then maintained at a temperature of 118.4° to 131° F (48° to 55° C). Your hands or feet are then dipped in and out of the paraffin tank 8 to 10 times to form a solid coating. Then, a plastic bag and toweling are wrapped around the part to retain heat. When the paraffin is cool, it is removed.

With a heat lamp, the heat output is determined by the wattage and the distance of the lamp from the area being treated. In most cases, the physical therapist or technician will allow 14 inches (35 centimeters) between the bulb and your skin for a 25-watt bulb, 18 inches (46 centimeters) for a 40-watt bulb, and 24 to 30 inches (61 to 76 centimeters) for a 60-watt bulb. Only one body part should be heated at a time, and the lamp should be turned off after 10 to 15 minutes for the first treatment and after 20 to 30 minutes for subsequent treatments.

Hot-water bottles are filled one-half to two-thirds full with water that has been heated to 115° to 125° F (46.1° to 51.7° C). The bottle is covered with an absorbent protective cloth and applied to the area to be heated.

Heating pads may be moist or dry. The temperature shouldn't exceed 131° F (55° C). The pad shouldn't be applied longer than 20 to 30 minutes unless specifically prescribed.

A warm pack may be nonsterile material, such as an absorbent towel or a few abdominal pads. Soak the towel or pads in water that has been heated to 131° F (55° C), and apply them to the affected area. Cover with a hot-water bottle or chemical hot pack to maintain the temperature.

Deep-heat treatments require specially skilled personnel and equipment. Ultrasound therapy is delivered to you through a transducer. A coupling medium, such as mineral oil, water, or a commercial ultrasound gel, is applied to the area to be heated and then the ultrasound transducer is applied and activated. Ultrasound heat treatments typically last 5 to 10 minutes. Diathermy supplies heat through a cable electrode. A layer of toweling is placed between your skin and the coils that are wrapped around the desired body part.

What are the possible complications?

Any of the superficial heat treatments can cause redness, blistering, burns, maceration, or reduced blood flow to the treated area if it is exposed to excessive heat or the treatment is continued too long (over 45 minutes). (See *How to give yourself a heat treatment.*)

What happens after the treatment?

- The physical therapist or technician will allow at least 1 hour between treatments to avoid reduced blood flow to the area being treated.
- Your response to the therapy and its effectiveness will be evaluated.

COOLING TREATMENTS

Cooling treatments are fundamental procedures that, despite new high-tech medical therapies, are still commonly used. Cooling treatments include both moist and dry forms. Moist cold, which provides deeper penetration, includes tepid sponge baths, cold compresses for small areas, and cold packs for large areas. In severe hyperthermia, hypothermia blankets (which provide a type of dry cold) may be used. Other dry-cold methods include ice bags or collars and chemical cold packs. Chilled saline enemas may control hyperthermia if other cooling treatments fail.

Why is this treatment done?

Cooling treatments are given to lower body temperature, thereby preventing cellular death and organ damage by decreasing metabolic demands; to relieve local pain by reducing nerve impulse conduction; to prevent swelling and relieve vascular congestion; and to slow or stop bleeding by constricting blood vessels.

Cooling treatments are used to lower body temperature in people with hyperthermia. They're also useful in relieving acute pain and inflammation and are commonly used for initial treatment after eye injuries, strains, sprains, bruises, muscle spasms, and burns. Cooling therapy is also used to treat chronic pain and may be warranted for people with bleeding episodes.

 SELF-HELP

How to give yourself a heat treatment

If you'll be continuing heat treatments at home, a physical therapist will teach you how to perform the treatment. Once you've been discharged from the hospital, follow these important guidelines.

Take special precautions
- Observe the following safety measures: check the equipment carefully before use, don't lie or sleep on or near the heating device (to prevent burns), secure the device with gauze — never with safety pins (heated metal can cause burns or electric shock), and don't expose electrical heating devices to water because of the risk of electric shock.
- Check your skin every 5 minutes during the treatment. Be especially cautious if you have decreased sensation in the area being treated. Report any unusual redness or blistering or any increase in pain or skin injury to your doctor.

When shouldn't this treatment be done?

Cooling treatments should be used cautiously, if at all, in people with impaired circulation, young children, and the elderly because of the risk of tissue damage from reduced blood flow.

What happens before the treatment?

- The procedure will be explained to you. If the treatment is used to relieve pain, you'll be told that the first few treatments may not be noticeably effective, but that repeated treatments can produce significant pain relief (lasting from 15 minutes to several hours).
- If an ice bag or collar is used, it will be filled halfway with crushed ice so it can be molded to conform to your body.
- If using a chemical cold pack, the manufacurer's directions are followed to activate the cold-producing chemicals.
- If using a cold compress or pack, you or the nurse cools a container of tap water by placing it in a basin of ice or by adding ice to the water. The water is chilled to about 59° F (15° C) or as ordered, and the compress or pack is immersed.
- If using a hypothermia blanket, after connecting the blanket to the control unit, the nurse specifies the manual or automatic setting, as needed, and the desired temperature. Next, the unit is turned on and distilled water is added to the reservoir. Then the nurse allows the blanket to cool, and places the control unit at the foot of your bed.
- To give a warm sponge bath, the nurse places a bath thermometer in a basin of warm water, and then adds cool water until the temperature reaches 93° F (34° C).
- To administer a chilled enema, the nurse places the solution container in a basin of ice water until it reaches the prescribed temperature.
- A protective covering is used for all devices.

What happens during the treatment?

A properly prepared and covered ice bag, ice collar, or activated chemical cold pack is placed on the desired site for the required time. For treatment of hyperthermia, the cooling device will be placed on the groin or under the arms. The device is refilled or replaced as necessary.

A cold compress or cold pack is wrung dry, covered with a waterproof cloth, and then applied to you for the required time. The compress or pack is changed as needed to maintain the correct temperature.

A preset and covered hypothermia blanket is placed under you. Your head should not lie on the blanket's cold surface. The rectal temperature probe is inserted and taped in place. The probe's other end is plugged into the blanket's control panel, which will indicate your temperature. If necessary, a sheet or a second hypothermia blanket is placed over you to increase cold transfer.

A warm sponge bath is administered by first sponging each extremity with moist, warm washcloths for about 5 minutes. Then your chest and abdomen are sponged for 5 minutes, followed by sponging of the back and buttocks for 5 to 10 minutes. Throughout therapy, you're covered except for the area being sponged. A covered hot-water bottle is kept at your feet to prevent chills, and a covered ice bag is kept on your head to prevent headache and nasal congestion. Moist washcloths are placed under your arms, over the groin, and behind your knees.

What are the possible complications?

In you're overheated, too-rapid cooling may cause a decrease in your level of consciousness, pupillary response to light, and the amount of blood pumped by your heart. Chills may occur, which are detrimental because they increase metabolism, thereby raising body temperature.

Tissue damage or frostbite may also result from cooling procedures. (See *How to give yourself a cooling treatment.*) Blood clots may result from increased thickness of the blood.

A hypothermia blanket can cause sudden changes in vital signs, increased pressure in the skull, difficulty breathing, decreased urination, or no urination.

What happens after the treatment?

- Your skin is dried.
- Your temperature and other vital signs are monitored for several days after cooling therapy.

 SELF-HELP

How to give yourself a cooling treatment

If you'll be continuing cooling treatments at home, a nurse or physical therapist will teach you how to perform the treatment. Once you've been discharged from the hospital, follow these important guidelines.

Take special precautions
- Don't exceed the recommended duration of treatment because frostbite may result.
- Report to your doctor any change in the symptoms or location of pain as well as any associated blotching, grayness, or blanching.
- Don't put ice directly against your skin because the extreme cold can damage tissue.

OTHER TREATMENTS

AUTOTRANSFUSION

Autotransfusion is a procedure for reinfusing a person's own blood. It can be performed after injury or before, during, or after surgery. Autotransfusion has become popular in recent years because of the AIDS epidemic. Autotransfusion eliminates the danger of transmitting such blood-borne infections as HIV and hepatitis from a blood donor to a blood recipient. It also greatly reduces the possibility of a transfusion reaction.

Moreover, autotransfusion provides an available source of compatible blood, saving time otherwise spent on typing and cross-matching. This feature is especially important in treating injury, where seconds may count. Unlike banked blood, the person's own blood has a near-normal temperature, a high oxygen-carrying capacity, and normal clotting factors. Another positive feature of autotransfusion is its possible acceptance by people whose religious beliefs prohibit the transfusion of a donor's blood.

Why is this procedure done?

Autotransfusion is done to increase circulation through reinfusion of a person's own blood. It can be used for traumatic injuries, most commonly those that cause blood to collect in the chest. Autotransfusion can also be used after primary injury to the lungs, liver, chest wall, heart, blood vessels of the lung, spleen, kidneys, and major veins of the body. However, use of autotransfusion after abdominal vascular injuries is much less common because of the increased risk of fecal contamination.

Autotransfusion before surgery is done primarily for the person with a rare blood type who will undergo major surgery, for the person in whom development of antibodies may complicate future transfusion needs, or for a person who fears exposure to blood-borne infection, such as AIDS or hepatitis, if blood must be transfused after surgery.

Autotransfusion during surgery is performed most often during chest, heart, and blood vessel surgery, but can also be used during hip surgery, spinal fusion, liver resection, and surgery to treat ruptured tubal pregnancy.

Autotransfusion is done to increase circulation through reinfusion of a person's own blood. It can be used for traumatic injuries, most commonly those that cause blood to collect in the chest.

Autotransfusion after surgery is used to replace blood lost during heart surgery. A new method of autotransfusion has recently been developed for use after orthopedic surgery, such as reconstructive procedures of the hip, knee, and spine.

When shouldn't this procedure be done?

Autotransfusion shouldn't be done when blood lost from hemorrhage is contaminated with feces or urine, which makes the person susceptible to bacterial growth, leading to infection of the blood, clotting problems, and movement of small clots through the circulation. Autotransfusion is not recommended for people with clotting defects, malignant tumors, or respiratory infection, or for those with traumatic wounds over 4 hours old because blood degradation occurs rapidly beyond that time. People with a low blood count should not plan to give blood for themselves before surgery.

What happens before the procedure?

- The doctor will give written permission for you to donate blood.
- If possible, you'll take a daily supplement of iron, starting 1 week before the first donation and continuing to hospital admission.
- A hospital staff member or the doctor will notify you of the start date for donation.
- The doctor or nurse will explain the procedure for blood collection and reinfusion to you beforehand.

What happens during the procedure?

Two methods of autotransfusion before surgery include collection of blood for later reinfusion and hemodilution. In the first method, blood for reinfusion is obtained several weeks before the planned surgery. You come to the blood donor center, and the blood is removed from a vein in the arm and stored until you need it. In the second method, hemodilution, your blood is withdrawn immediately before surgery and an equivalent volume of fluid is replaced with a solution suitable for intravenous administration. The collected blood is reinfused as needed during or after surgery.

For blood salvage during surgery, the surgeon uses a suction catheter to remove blood and debris from the surgical field and mixes it with a dilute solution of a medication to prevent clotting. This solution is then filtered and placed in a rotating bowl, which removes the medication to prevent clotting, the debris, and nearly all other blood components except the red blood cells. The red blood cells are then

SELF-HELP

Caring for yourself after autotransfusion

When you've been discharged from the hospital, follow these important guidelines:
- If you had autotransfusion after surgery or trauma and the chest tube site did not heal before discharge, observe the nurse's instructions about care of the incision.
- Be alert for any signs of infection — fever, pain at the insertion site, and redness — and notify your doctor if they occur.

washed, mixed with saline solution, and pumped into a bag for reinfusion. The blood is then reinfused intravenously as needed.

For autotransfusion following heart surgery or injury, the doctor places a tube in your chest and connects it to an autotransfusion device that collects blood from the chest cavity for reinfusion. When sufficient blood has been collected, the blood collection bag is removed from the autotransfusion device, a filter is attached, and the blood is transfused in the typical way.

What are the possible complications?

Autotransfusion has several potential complications, such as the entrance of air into the circulation, clotting disorders, fecal contamination, infection of the blood, damage to red blood cells, a reduced platelet count, and poisoning from the substance added to the blood to prevent clotting. Occasionally, autotransfusion causes transient blood in the urine.

What happens after the procedure?

- The doctor or nurse will check the volume of blood collected and reinfused.
- Your heart and lung function are monitored.
- If you had autotransfusion after heart surgery or injury, the nurse checks you for signs of bleeding if drainage from the chest tube is more than expected, and notifies the doctor. Further surgery or a repeat of the procedure may be necessary. (See *Caring for yourself after autotransfusion.*)
- Your blood count, clotting function, and calcium levels are monitored.
- The nurse observes you for signs of complications and notifies the doctor if these occur.

18

TREATING PAIN

DRUG THERAPIES

Nonnarcotic Pain Relievers

Besides relieving mild pain, nonnarcotic pain relievers also lower fever. Some of them reduce inflammation as well, and relief of swelling may explain some of their effectiveness in relieving pain.

If combined with narcotic pain relievers, these drugs can also relieve moderate to severe pain while allowing a reduced narcotic dosage. Unlike narcotic pain relievers, these drugs don't cause dependence. They're commonly used to treat pain after surgery or childbirth, headache, muscle and joint pain, and menstrual cramps.

What are nonnarcotic pain relievers used for?
- To curb mild pain
- To reduce fever

What are some commonly used nonnarcotic pain relievers?
These pain relievers are divided into three groups: nonsteroidal anti-inflammatory drugs (abbreviated NSAIDs), salicylates, and acetaminophens.

NSAIDs
- diclofenac, known by the brand name Voltaren
- fenoprofen, known by the brand name Nalfon
- flurbiprofen, known by the brand name Ansaid
- ibuprofen, known by the brand names Advil, Midol, Motrin, and Nuprin
- indomethacin, known by the brand names Indameth and Indocin
- ketoprofen, known by the brand name Orudis
- ketorolac, known by the brand name Toradol
- meclofenamate, known by the brand name Meclomen
- mefenamic acid, known by the brand name Ponstel
- naproxen, known by the brand name Naprosyn
- naproxen sodium, known by the brand names Anaprox and Aleve
- piroxicam, known by the brand name Feldene
- sulindac, known by the brand name Clinoril
- tolmetin, known by the brand name Tolectin

Salicylates

- aspirin, known by the brand names Bayer Aspirin, Empirin, and Norwich Aspirin
- choline salicylate, known by the brand name Arthropan
- diflunisal, known by the brand name Dolobid
- magnesium salicylate, known by the brand names Doan's, Magan, and Mobidin
- salsalate, known by the brand names Amigesic, Diagen, Disalcid, and Salflex

Acetaminophens

- acetaminophen-containing drugs, known by the brand names Aceta, Genapap, and Tylenol

What are the possible side effects?

- Heartburn, stomach distress, nausea, abdominal pain
- Ringing in the ears, hearing loss, dim vision, headache, dizziness, confusion, sweating, rapid breathing, and rapid heart rate (from salicylate overdose)
- Fatal liver damage (from acetaminophen overdose)

What are the guidelines for taking nonnarcotic pain relievers?

- Don't use NSAIDs if you have aspirin allergy because many people sensitive to aspirin are also sensitive to NSAIDs.
- If you have a history of eye, kidney, liver, or gastrointestinal disease, check with your doctor before taking any nonprescription pain reliever. Also check with your doctor if you are taking medication for arthritis or blood disorders, or if you are taking blood thinners.
- Immediately report rash, difficulty breathing, confusion, blurred vision, nausea, bloody vomit, or black, tarry stools. These may indicate an overdose, allergic reaction, or gastrointestinal bleeding.
- Avoid alcohol while taking the drug because it may increase the risk of ulcers and bleeding.
- To minimize stomach upset, take the drug with food or a full glass of milk. Afterward, remain upright for 15 to 30 minutes to reduce the risk of the drug irritating the esophagus (the organ that connects your mouth to the stomach). If you feel stomach burning or pain, notify the doctor.

If you have a history of eye, kidney, liver, or gastrointestinal disease, check with your doctor before taking any nonprescription analgesic. Also check with your doctor if you're taking medication for arthritis or blood disorders, or if you're taking blood thinners.

- If you are taking acetaminophen, immediately notify the doctor of any signs of an overdose: nausea, vomiting, abdominal cramps, or diarrhea.
- Some NSAIDs may cause prolonged bleeding time. If you notice excessive bleeding or bruising, call the doctor.
- Dizziness or drowsiness may occur. Avoid driving and other hazardous tasks that require alertness until your response to the drug is known.
- Take a missed dose as soon as you remember. However, if the next dose is less than 4 hours away, skip the missed dose and resume the regular schedule. Never double the dose.
- Always take the tablet or capsule whole; swallow without crushing or chewing. Many of these drugs are prescribed in a sustained-release or specially coated formulation. Crushing, chewing, or otherwise breaking the coating may damage the capsule and release its contents prematurely. This may lead to overdose or possibly increase the risk of stomach irritation. If you have trouble swallowing the drug, check with the doctor or pharmacist. Many nonnarcotic analgesics are available as an oral liquid.

What else you should know

- Long-term abuse of nonnarcotic pain relievers has been associated with kidney and liver problems. Don't take these drugs for longer than a week without first checking with your doctor.
- Aspirin is usually considered the salicylate most likely to cause gastrointestinal side effects.

NARCOTIC PAIN RELIEVERS

Narcotic pain relievers, also known as *opioid pain relievers,* are used to provide relief from moderate to severe pain. They act on specific receptors in the brain and spinal cord to decrease the person's perception of pain.

Narcotic pain relievers can be classified as narcotic agonists or narcotic agonist-antagonists. Agonists produce relief by binding to opioid receptors in the nervous system. Agonist-antagonists also produce relief the same way. However, these drugs block the effects of other narcotics and may cause withdrawal symptoms in narcotic-dependent people.

Narcotic pain relievers can be given orally or may be injected into a muscle or a vein; they may also be directly injected into the spinal cord by the epidural or intrathecal route.

Narcotic agonists may be the drugs of choice for severe chronic cancer pain. The agonist-antagonists are usually only used in persons with moderate to severe postoperative or other short-term pain. They are avoided for long-term use because they have been known to produce hallucinations and other psychological effects; in the narcotic-dependent patient, they may produce withdrawal symptoms.

What are narcotic pain relievers used for?
Narcotic pain relievers curb moderate to severe pain.

What are some commonly used narcotic pain relievers?
Narcotic agonists
- codeine (generic)
- hydromorphone, known by the brand name Dilaudid
- levorphanol, known by the brand name Levo-Dromoran
- meperidine, known by the brand name Demerol
- methadone, known by the brand name Dolophine
- morphine, known by the brand names Astramorph, Duramorph, MS Contin, and Roxanol
- oxycodone, known by the brand name Roxicodone
- oxymorphone, known by the brand name Numorphan
- propoxyphene, known by the brand names Darvon, Dolene, and Doraphen

Narcotic agonist-antagonists
- buprenorphine, known by the brand name Buprenex
- butorphanol, known by the brand name Stadol
- dezocine, known by the brand name Dalgan
- nalbuphine, known by the brand name Nubain
- pentazocine, known by the brand name Talwin

What are the possible side effects?
- Respiratory depression
- Drowsiness, faintness, dizziness, palpitations
- Dry mouth, nausea, vomiting, constipation
- Muscle tremor
- Flushing of the face and neck, sweating

- Cough suppression
- Tolerance and dependence (with prolonged use)

What are the guidelines for taking narcotic pain relievers?

- Tell your doctor if you have a history of respiratory, kidney, or liver disease.
- Make sure your doctor knows about all of the other medications you are taking, including nonprescription drugs. Don't take any other drug without first checking with the doctor.
- To help prevent constipation, take a stool softener. Also eat a high-fiber diet and drink plenty of fluids. Regular exercise may also help prevent constipation.
- Because narcotic pain relievers can cause dizziness, take precautions to avoid accidents. If you have difficulty walking, have someone help you. Get up slowly from a lying or sitting position.
- Practice coughing and deep-breathing exercises to promote ventilation and prevent pooling of secretions, which could lead to respiratory difficulty.
- Take your medication as prescribed. The drug is most effective when taken before pain becomes intense.
- Consult the doctor if the drug becomes less effective in relieving pain. Don't increase the dose or the frequency of administration.
- Take a missed dose as soon as you remember, unless it's almost time for the next dose. Never double the dose.
- Your family should call the doctor immediately if they detect these signs of an overdose: cold, clammy skin; confusion; severe drowsiness or restlessness; slow or irregular breathing; pinpoint pupils; or unconsciousness.
- Avoid alcohol and other central nervous system depressants while taking this medication.
- If you are taking a sustained-release form of the drug, never crush or chew the capsule; doing so may cause the immediate release of a large amount of the medication and cause side effects. If you have trouble swallowing the tablets or capsules, check with the doctor. Many of these drugs are available as an oral solution.

What else you should know

Because narcotic pain relievers can lead to increased tolerance and physiologic and psychological dependence, they shouldn't be used for chronic pain unless it is derived from cancer.

Topical Anesthetics

Topical medications that anesthetize the skin and mucous membranes, these drugs can be applied to the mucous membranes of the rectum, vagina, urethra, and bladder before invasive procedures; some formulations may be incorporated into nonprescription remedies for sunburn, poison ivy, or minor burns and irritation.

Topical anesthetics act locally on the pain receptors found in the skin and mucous membranes. They block the conduction of the pain impulse, providing temporary relief.

What are topical anesthetics used for?

Topical anesthetics produce a local loss of sensation by temporarily blocking conduction of pain impulses.

What are some commonly used topical anesthetics?

- benzocaine, known by the brand name Americaine
- dibucaine, known by the brand name Nupercainal
- lidocaine, known by the brand name Xylocaine
- pramoxine, known by the brand names Prax and Tronothane
- tetracaine, known by the brand name Pontocaine

What are the possible side effects?

- Excitement, seizures, or sleepiness (usually with overdose)
- Rash and other local skin reactions

What are the guidelines for using topical anesthetics?

- Tell your doctor if you have ever had an allergic reaction to an anesthetic.
- Oral use of these drugs may make swallowing difficult. Avoid eating or drinking for 1 hour after application to prevent gagging and minimize the risk of biting the inside of your mouth.
- Discontinue using the drug and contact the doctor if your condition worsens; if it doesn't improve in several days; or if a rash, swelling, or an infection occurs.

What else you should know

- Topical anesthetics are less effective in areas where there is infection. If pain is caused by an infection, check with your doctor.

- Use these drugs sparingly. Applying too frequently or in excessive amounts can lead to systemic toxicity. If the local pain is severe, see your doctor.

NERVE BLOCKS

Nerve blocks are used to control moderate to severe pain. The procedure is usually performed by an anesthesiologist. Drugs are injected around nerves that conduct pain impulses into the central nervous system. Because the procedure actually prevents the pain sensation from reaching the brain, the need for systemic pain relievers or narcotics is greatly decreased.

The most common drugs used to perform nerve blocks are local anesthetics, such as bupivacaine, etidocaine, lidocaine, procaine, and tetracaine. If inflammation is present, a corticosteroid may be added. (See *Comparing types of nerve blocks*.)

Nerve blocks may be the treatment of choice for pain relief in some disorders, such as the condition known as *reflex sympathetic dystrophy;* for symptomatic pain relief, such as for the pain of certain cancers; or to provide anesthesia during surgery to a specific area.

Why is this procedure done?
Nerve blocks provide analgesia or anesthesia by interrupting pain pathways.

What happens before the procedure?
- A nurse or doctor will explain the procedure to the person receiving the nerve block, and answer any questions. The doctor will ask the person if he or she has ever experienced any side effects from a local anesthetic.
- The person will report for preliminary testing. Some doctors require bleeding times or blood clotting studies before epidural or intraspinal injections.
- A nurse will take the person's drug history and check for use of blood thinners or aspirin.
- Because the person will be awake during the injection and may feel anxious, the doctor may give the person a sedative to help him or her relax.

Comparing types of nerve blocks

NERVE BLOCK	USES	POSSIBLE COMPLICATIONS
Subarachnoid	▪ Diagnostic purposes before surgery ▪ Pain after an amputation ▪ Abdominal pain ▪ Cancer pain	▪ Weakness, paralysis, meningitis, impaired sensation, nerve damage, inflammation of the covering of the spinal cord, and injury to the spinal cord
Epidural	▪ Radicular or visceral pain ▪ Pain after surgery ▪ Pain after nerve injury ▪ Anesthesia during cesarean section or pain relief during vaginal delivery	▪ Low blood pressure and headache
Paravertebral somatic nerve	▪ To predict results before surgery ▪ Neuralgia ▪ Cancer pain ▪ Pain after nerve injury ▪ Pain from vertebral fracture	▪ Muscle weakness or paralysis ▪ Injection in the neck may cause puncture of the vertebral artery and inability to breathe if the nerve block affects the phrenic nerve ▪ Injection in the upper back may cause collapse of a lung
Sympathetic ganglion nerve	▪ Pain after nerve injury ▪ Neuralgia after shingles ▪ Abdominal pain ▪ Phantom pain ▪ Acute shingles attack	Depending on the location of the block: ▪ Paralysis of the diaphragm or vocal cords and collapse of a lung ▪ Low blood pressure ▪ Bleeding or sexual impotence
Peripheral nerve	▪ Rib fracture or hip pain ▪ Neuralgia after shingles ▪ Pain after surgery ▪ Pain in the outer surface of the thigh from nerve entrapment	▪ Hemorrhage and collapse of a lung
Local infiltration	▪ Inflammation of the cartilage between the ribs ▪ Muscle pain	▪ Usually none

▪ A nurse will tell the person not to move during the injection to confine the local anesthetic and avoid injury. The nurse will also tell the person to report any pain to the doctor.

What happens during the procedure?

The area for the injection is cleaned. The doctor inserts the needle into the appropriate area and may use special visualizing equipment to verify needle placement. Once proper needle placement has been verified, the doctor injects a small test dose.

A nurse observes the person for side effects, such as ringing in the ears, headache, palpitations, changes in breathing pattern, confusion,

SELF-HELP

Recovering from a nerve block procedure

After you've been discharged from the hospital, follow these important guidelines:
- If the area of the nerve block is still numb when you leave the hospital, move the limb every 30 minutes to prevent skin breakdown.
- Avoid falling by moving cautiously.
- Immediately report any bleeding, fainting, difficulty breathing, or decreased motor function to the doctor.

muscle twitching, or taste alteration. If any occur, the doctor will stop the injection.

If no side effects occur, the remainder of the anesthetic is injected, usually in small increments. After completing the injection, the doctor removes the needle and applies pressure over the site. The person remains lying down for the specified time and is then returned to his or her room.

What are the possible complications?

Nerve blocks can cause headache, difficulty breathing, or blood pressure changes. Puncture of a blood vessel can cause bleeding.

Absorption of a sufficient amount of anesthetic into the bloodstream may produce systemic effects, including changes in heart rate or blood pressure, alterations in taste, altered mental status, excitation, and seizures. Most of these reactions occur within 10 minutes of injection. Rarely, injection causes severe allergic reactions.

What happens after the procedure?

- The person is told to report any discomfort.
- After an epidural nerve block, the person will maintain the side-lying position for 30 minutes.
- The person will be told to get up slowly from a lying position and to lie down immediately if he or she feels dizzy. (See *Recovering from a nerve block procedure*.)

PATIENT-CONTROLLED ANALGESIA

Patient-controlled analgesia (also known as PCA) is a method of self-administering medication, commonly via the intravenous route, to provide optimal pain control. Delayed or inadequate administration of pain relievers can cause pain to escalate and become difficult to control. Because the person controls the administration of pain relievers, PCA avoids delayed treatment and decreases anxiety.

Why is this treatment done?

Patient-controlled analgesia enables the person to achieve satisfactory control of pain.

Two systems for self-administered pain relief

The accompanying illustrations show commonly used self-administered pain relief devices.

The first device is a reusable, battery-operated pump that delivers a drug dose when the person presses a call button at the end of a cord.

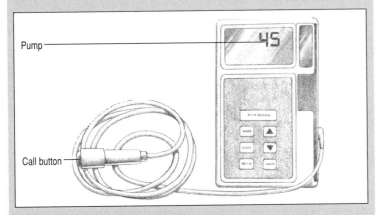

Pump

Call button

The other device is disposable and mechanically operated. It contains an infusor and a unit that's worn like a wristwatch. The person pushes a button on the device to receive the pain medication from a collapsible chamber.

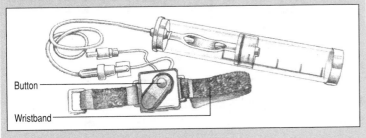

Button

Wristband

What happens before the treatment?

- The doctor will ask the person about any drug allergies.
- A nurse will teach the person or a family member about pain management, how to use the pump, and how to manage side effects. The person will be told to take enough analgesic to relieve acute pain but not enough to induce drowsiness. (See *Two systems for self-administered pain relief.*)

What happens during the treatment?

PCA therapy is ordered by the doctor and initiated by the nurse. The nurse selects an appropriate PCA pump. The PCA pump is programmed to deliver a preset amount of drug, usually a narcotic analgesic, when the person presses a button. The pump can be programmed with a lock-out time (in minutes) to place a safe limit on the time between injections. Certain pumps can deliver a continuous infusion of drug as well as the larger injection, as required.

A nurse will monitor the person for changes in levels of sedation, monitor respirations, and assess the person for constipation and nausea. The nurse will also check for local pain or swelling at the intravenous site.

The nurse will assess for pain control, as described by the person, and adjust analgesia as necessary. If the person reports insufficient pain relief, the nurse will notify the doctor.

What are the possible complications?

Complications are rare but can be related to side effects of the analgesic drug, errors in programming the pump, or pump malfunction.

NERVE STIMULATION

ELECTRICAL NERVE STIMULATION

A useful method for relieving both acute and chronic localized pain, electrical nerve stimulation uses a mild electric current to stimulate nerve fibers and block the transmission of pain impulses to the brain. This method is based on the gate theory of pain, which proposes that painful impulses pass through a "gate" in the spinal cord.

The device, available by prescription, is a portable, battery-powered generator that transmits painless electric current through electrodes placed on the skin at points determined to be related to the pain. Treatments may be given three or four times daily for 30 to 45 minutes, for periods of 6 to 8 hours, or intermittently at the person's discretion. The device is easy for the person to use and permits normal activity.

The newest device, called a "pain suppressor," utilizes electrodes with water as the conducting substance. The electric current, not felt by the person, increases levels of a substance known as *serotonin* in the blood, which enhances the effect of natural pain-relieving substances known as *endorphins*. With this device, treatments are administered only for short intervals several times a day.

Why is this treatment done?

Electrical nerve stimulation is performed to reduce pain by sending electrical impulses to the skin and underlying tissues. The device is used to treat chronic back pain and pain after knee, hip, or lower back surgery. Other uses include dental pain, pain from nerve damage or nerve injury, pain that sometimes follows shingles, musculoskeletal trauma, arthritis, and phantom limb pain (which can occur after amputation of an arm or leg).

When shouldn't this treatment be done?

Electrical nerve stimulation should not be used in people with pacemakers. The electric current may also interfere with electrocardiography, or heart monitoring. The device shouldn't be used for pain of unknown origin because it may mask a new disease. The electrodes should never be placed over the carotid sinus nerves in the neck, over muscles of the throat or voice box, or on the eyes. They should never be placed on a pregnant person's abdomen because safety during pregnancy has not been determined.

What happens before the treatment?

The physical therapist or nurse will show you the device and explain that you'll have electrodes attached to your skin and that you'll feel a tingling sensation when the controls are turned on. The controls will be adjusted to specified settings or to those most comfortable and effective. You'll be asked to use the device for at least a week before deciding if it helps reduce your pain.

What happens during the treatment?

The physical therapist or specially prepared nurse performs electrical nerve stimulation treatments. The skin at the electrode sites is cleaned with an alcohol sponge and dried well. The area may be shaved, if necessary. A small amount of electrode gel is applied to the bottom of each electrode (unless the electrodes are pregelled) to improve conductivity. The electrodes are placed on the skin at least 2 inches (5 centimeters) apart and are usually secured with tape (some

Positioning electrodes for electrical nerve stimulation

In electrical nerve stimulation, electrodes placed around peripheral nerves (or an incision site) transmit electrical impulses to the brain. The electric current is thought to block pain impulses. The person can influence the level and frequency of pain relief by adjusting the controls on the device.

Typically, electrode placement varies even among people who may have similar pain. Electrodes can be applied by covering the painful area or surrounding it, as for muscle tenderness or painful joints, or by "capturing" the painful area between the electrodes, as for incisional pain.

In nerve injury, electrodes should be placed between the brain and the injury site to avoid increasing pain. Placing electrodes in a hypersensitive area also increases pain.

The illustrations show combinations of electrode placement (black squares) and areas of nerve stimulation (shaded) for low back and leg pain.

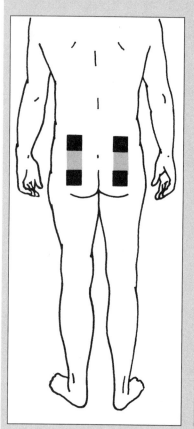 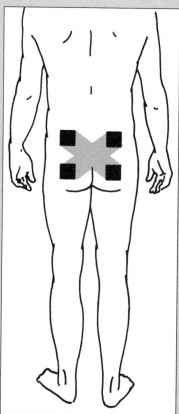 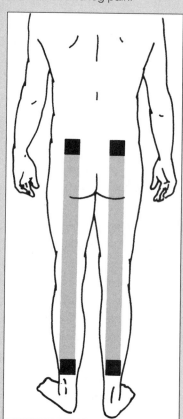

SELF-HELP

Using an electrical nerve stimulator at home

After you've been discharged from the hospital, follow these important guidelines.

Use the device properly
- Follow the instructions provided by the nurse or physical therapist regarding electrode placement, setting the device's controls, electrode removal, and proper care of the equipment.
- Remove the device before coming in contact with water to avoid possible electrocution (unless you're using a battery-powered unit).
- Don't increase the voltage, because this may increase your pain.

- Don't use the device for pain that you haven't discussed with your doctor. Notify the doctor if pain worsens or develops at another site.

Minimize skin irritation
- To help prevent skin irritation, rotate sites of electrode placement. Also, be aware that nonallergenic electrodes are available.
- If skin irritation occurs, keep the area clean and apply soothing lotion. If the problem worsens, notify the doctor.
- To decrease skin irritation, leave the electrodes in place during the day between treatments.

are self-adhering). (See *Positioning electrodes for electrical nerve stimulation* and *Using an electrical nerve stimulator at home.*)

What are the possible complications?

The few side effects of electrical nerve stimulation relate to skin irritation and itching caused by the electrodes, the conductive gel, or the adhesive used to secure the electrodes. Electrical burns can result from improper placement of electrodes.

What happens after the treatment?

The nurse or physical therapist will evaluate your response to each treatment and compare the results.

ACUPUNCTURE

Although primarily used to relieve pain, the ancient Chinese technique of acupuncture is also used to treat symptoms such as diarrhea, hiccups, insomnia, and stress reactions. For this procedure, fine needles are inserted at selected points on the body. Acupuncture provides symptomatic relief that varies from permanent and complete to temporary or inadequate. Typically, several treatments are required.

Many Western pain experts who favor acupuncture explain its effectiveness in terms of the gate theory of pain control. They suggest that the needles used in acupuncture stimulate large sensory nerve fibers that carry pain-inhibiting impulses, thereby blocking impulses from the smaller pain-conducting fibers at the spinal level. Other researchers suggest that acupuncture produces pain relief by triggering the release of naturally occurring substances that relieve pain, called *endorphins*.

Why is this treatment done?

Acupuncture is performed to relieve pain, to regulate certain activities of the nervous system, and to activate the immune system.

Recommended uses of acupuncture

The World Health Organization has published a list of uses for acupuncture therapy. The list includes acute and chronic gastritis, colitis, and pharyngitis; acute sinusitis; acute bacterial dysentery; acute tonsillitis, conjunctivitis, rhinitis (runny nose), and acute bronchitis; AIDS; bronchial asthma (in children and in adults without other coexisting diseases); cataracts (without complications); central retinitis; chronic duodenal ulcer; common cold; constipation or diarrhea; facial paralysis; excess production of acid in the stomach; headache; hiccups; neuralgia between the ribs; lumbar back pain; Ménière's syndrome; migraine; nearsightedness (in children); neurologic problems affecting the bladder; bedwetting; pain after tooth extraction; paralysis caused by poliomyelitis or after a stroke; bowel obstruction; pain caused by inflammation of tissue between the elbow and shoulder; peripheral neuropathy; rheumatoid arthritis; sciatica; spasms of the esophagus and upper stomach; tennis elbow; toothache; and trigeminal neuralgia.

When shouldn't this treatment be done?

Acupuncture should be avoided in people with bleeding disorders or in those with certain psychiatric disorders (such as paranoia) that may preclude the elective use of any invasive procedure. Acupuncture should also be avoided in pregnant women because of the risk of precipitating uterine contractions. Electrical acupuncture should be used with caution in people with pacemakers.

What happens before the treatment?

- The acupuncturist will explain the procedure, the risks, and the expected outcome.
- The amount of pain you have is evaluated as a baseline for comparison after the treatment.

What happens during the treatment?

The treatment should be performed only by a doctor trained in acupuncture or by an acupuncturist who, depending on state law, may practice independently or with a doctor.

You lie down, and the clinician inserts 4 to 20 fine disposable needles under your skin either directly into the painful area or into remote areas. Insertion of the needles may cause sensations of pinpricks, warmth, and stinging or a dull aching throb. When all the needles are in place, the acupuncturist stimulates them, either electrically or manually. Typically, needles remain in the sites for 15 to 30 minutes before they are removed.

The first treatment may provide only transient relief or none at all, but the pain relief should persist longer with successive treatments.

What are the possible complications?

Acupuncture causes few complications if performed correctly. Possible complications include increased blood flow or bruising at a needle insertion site; fainting, particularly in nervous, tense, or tired people; internal organ injury from deep needle insertion over vital organs, such as the lungs; local infection from improper needle insertion or use of nondisposable needles; and soreness at needle insertion sites.

What happens after the treatment?

- The acupuncturist will observe the needle insertion sites for a bruise. If one occurs, he or she will apply pressure.
- You'll be instructed to sit or stand up slowly to avoid fainting and light-headedness.
- If needles were inserted into your chest, the acupuncturist will watch for signs of a collapsed lung, such as shortness of breath or rapid breathing. (See *Caring for yourself after acupuncture.*)
- Your level of pain will be compared with the pretreatment baseline.

 SELF-HELP

Caring for yourself after acupuncture

After you go home, follow these important guidelines.

Watch for problems
- Check for symptoms of local infection, such as redness, swelling, and discharge. Infection is unlikely but, if it occurs, notify the acupuncturist immediately.
- If you had needles placed in your chest, immediately report any shortness of breath or painful breathing to the acupuncturist.

Monitor pain relief
Note the duration and effectiveness of pain relief, and report these observations at your next appointment. Complete relief of pain may require 8 to 16 treatments. However, if your pain isn't relieved after a reasonable number of sessions, the acupuncturist may stop the treatment.

OTHER TREATMENTS

COGNITIVE PAIN-CONTROL TECHNIQUES

Cognitive pain control refers to "mind over pain" methods, including relaxation, biofeedback, distraction, guided imagery, hypnosis, meditation, and behavior modification, that help the person reduce the suffering associated with pain. The person participates in treatment by using his or her cognitive abilities to achieve a degree of control over pain.

These techniques are virtually risk-free and can be used for almost anyone. However, if the person has a significant psychiatric problem, relaxation techniques should be taught by a psychotherapist.

Why is this treatment done?
Cognitive pain-control techniques are used to reduce pain by promoting relaxation or a behavioral change. Pain-control techniques are helpful for acute and chronic pain and may be used with medications that relieve pain for control of intense pain.

What happens before the treatment?
▪ A health care professional will assess your pain as well as environmental factors, family relationships, and any psychosocial considerations that may intensify the pain.
▪ You'll learn about the technique and the importance of your role in the process.
▪ You'll be told to begin using the techniques when pain is absent or mild because they require concentration. However, if the pain is persistent, you may begin with short, simple exercises and build on your abilities.
▪ You'll remove or loosen restrictive clothing, dim the lights, and keep noise to a minimum.

What happens during the treatment?
You'll learn cognitive pain-control techniques. Teaching should begin when your pain is absent or mild so you can concentrate better.

Relaxation

Relaxation involves using rhythmic, slow abdominal breathing to achieve skeletal muscle relaxation and to ward off fatigue, which lowers pain tolerance and increases intensity of pain. The rate of breathing is about 6 to 9 breaths per minute and the rhythm is slow (in, 2-3, out, 2-3). The nurse may count for you or breathe with you when teaching this technique.

Biofeedback

In biofeedback, you use a relaxation technique (the one you find most helpful) while you are connected to a biofeedback machine. You recognize and control the relaxation process, taking your cues from the device's audible tones, flashing lights, or digital readouts of changes in blood pressure, pulse, or skin temperature. These indicate whether you are becoming more relaxed.

Distraction

Distraction involves having you shift your attention away from the pain. You focus your attention on a sensory stimulus such as music, television, humming, singing, or reading and concentrate on the images these things evoke. You may also visually focus on a specific object, keep time to music, or use rhythmic breathing at this time. You may use a headset when listening to music, increasing the volume when the pain worsens. The more absorbed you become in the activity, the less pain you're likely to feel. This method is most effective when multiple senses are involved.

Guided imagery

In guided imagery, you use your imagination to achieve the specific result of pain relief and relaxation. You concentrate on a peaceful, soothing, vivid image while the nurse describes the sensations associated with it, such as the smell of grass or the warmth of the sun. The more vivid the image, the better the results. This technique requires practice, about three times a day for 5 minutes; several days may pass before some pain relief is obtained. You must have a vivid imagination and excellent concentration.

Hypnosis

Hypnosis must be done by a therapist, who may employ such techniques as symptom suppression to block awareness of pain or symptom substitution, which allows a positive interpretation of pain. You may continue to see the therapist or may learn self-hypnosis techniques.

Behavior modification can improve your self-esteem, activity, and productivity and reduce your preoccupation with pain, suffering, and disability.

Using cognitive pain-control techniques at home

After you've been discharged from the hospital, keep in mind the following:

- If you have serious psychosocial problems, you should seek help in psychotherapy. Any gains in pain management may be quickly lost unless you deal with these issues.
- You may want to continue to use pain-control techniques after your pain has resolved because they may help relieve everyday stress.

Meditation

Meditation involves having you repeat a word or phrase or stare at an object until relaxed. This method also focuses attention away from pain and may be especially useful while waiting for the onset of relief from pain medication. You may feel warmth, heaviness, lightness, or tingling while relaxed.

Behavior modification

In behavior modification, you identify behaviors that reinforce pain, suffering, and disability, such as being too dependent on others or using a cane when it's not medically necessary. Behavior modification also helps you to define your goals, such as decreasing your dependence on others, and to use appropriate reinforcements to achieve desired behavior patterns. Behavior modification can improve your self-esteem, activity, and productivity and reduce your preoccupation with pain, suffering, and disability.

What are the possible complications?

Virtually no complications are associated with these therapies.

What happens after the treatment?

- You'll be encouraged to practice the technique, and your ability to perform it properly will be evaluated. (See *Using cognitive pain-control techniques at home*.)
- If you're using biofeedback, you'll be encouraged to practice your relaxation technique without the machine to avoid becoming dependent on it.
- Your pain level will be evaluated to determine if the treatment has been effective.

SITZ BATH

A sitz bath, also known as a *hip bath*, is the immersion of the pelvic area in tepid or hot water.

The tub or device used is usually shaped to allow the legs to remain out of the water. Most health care facilities have sitz bath basins that fit into toilet seats. Disposable sitz bath kits are also available for single-person use. When special sitz bath devices are not available, a regular bathtub may be used.

Why is this treatment done?

Sitz baths are used to relieve perianal pain, swelling, or discomfort; to enhance healing by cleaning the perineum and anus; to increase circulation and reduce inflammation; and to promote relaxation of the perianal muscles. Sitz baths are commonly used after perianal surgery or childbirth.

What happens before the treatment?

- The tub will be cleaned and disinfected before each use. The water temperature should be checked with a bath thermometer before you get in the tub.
- The nurse will explain the procedure to you.
- You'll be asked to urinate; then any soiled bandages are removed.
- The nurse will ask you to use the safety rail for balance when getting into the tub.

What happens during the treatment?

You'll be assisted to sit in a tub of warm (94° to 98° F [34.4° to 36.6° C]) or hot (110° to 115° F [43.3° to 46.1° C]) water.

Usually you soak for 15 to 20 minutes. The water temperature will be checked periodically to ensure that it has not cooled.

A disposable sitz bath kit includes a basin that is filled to the specified line with water and is placed under the toilet seat. An irrigation bag and tubing allow a stream of water to flow continuously over the wound while you are in the bath.

What are the possible complications?

Complications are rare, but occasionally people develop an irregular or rapid heart rate or experience dizziness when standing up from the bath. These effects are due to blood vessel dilation caused by immersion in hot water.

What happens after the treatment?

- You'll be asked to rise slowly from the bath, using the safety rails for balance. (See *How to give yourself a sitz bath*, page 578.)
- The nurse will apply clean dressings to the perianal area if necessary.
- The tub is cleaned and disinfected after each use.

How to give yourself a sitz bath

Use the following directions when giving yourself a sitz bath. You will need a sitz bath kit (plastic pan and a plastic bag with a tube attached) or a clean bathtub, medication (if prescribed), access to warm water, and towels.

After assembling all the necessary equipment, raise the toilet seat and fit the plastic pan onto the toilet bowl. The pan should be positioned so that the drainage holes are along the back of the bowl. If the pan is placed correctly, a single hole will be visible in the front.

Then close the clamp on the bag's tubing and fill the bag with warm water and medication (if prescribed).

Snap the free end of the tubing into the slot at the front of the pan, and then hang the bag on the door knob or towel bar. Make sure that the bag is higher than the toilet.

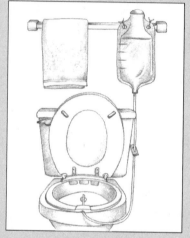

Carefully lower yourself onto the pan and open the clamp on the tubing, allowing the warm water to flow from the bag into the pan to fill it. Don't worry if it overflows because excess water will flow out through the drainage holes

into the toilet. Remain seated in the pan until the water begins to cool.

After the sitz bath, rise slowly and carefully to a standing position because you may experience fatigue and light-headedness. Then dry off completely and apply an ointment or dressing, if ordered.

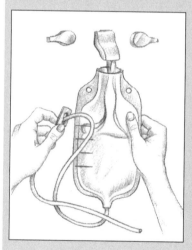

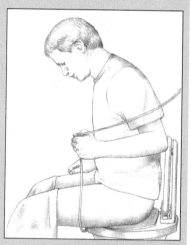

ULTRASOUND THERAPY

For the past 60 years, ultrasound therapy has been used to produce heat in soft tissue. Ultrasonic waves are high-frequency sound waves that penetrate deeply and significantly elevate tissue temperature to depths of 2 inches (5 centimeters). The greatest increase in temperature occurs in tissues with a high protein content, such as muscle, bone, and joint capsules. Thus, ultrasound therapy is an effective way to selectively deliver heat to injured soft tissue.

Why is this treatment done?

Ultrasound therapy is used to increase blood flow to injured soft tissue, to reduce pain and muscle spasm, and to aid in the stretching of joint contractures (conditions in which soft tissue or joints are bent and will not move) and scar tissue. Ultrasound therapy is useful for the management of tendonitis, bursitis, muscle spasm, contractures, scar tissue, and soft-tissue or joint pain. Ultrasound therapy is usually used by the physical therapist as an adjunct to strengthening, mobilization, or range-of-motion exercises in the treatment of these conditions.

Ultrasound therapy is used to increase blood flow to injured soft tissue, to reduce pain and muscle spasm, and to aid in the stretching of joint contractures (conditions in which soft tissue or joints are bent and will not move) and scar tissue.

When shouldn't this treatment be done?

Ultrasound therapy should not be used over areas with poor circulation or acute inflammation or where there is swelling of a vein with clot formation. It should be used cautiously over areas of decreased pain or temperature sensation. An ultrasound transducer should not be applied over the heart because it can cause abnormalities in the electrocardiogram. It should not be applied directly over the eye because this can cause retinal damage; over malignant tissue, because it increases the possibility of cancer spread and can accelerate tumor growth; over the pregnant uterus, because it could injure the fetus; or over the testes, because it can cause temporary sterility. Furthermore, the ends of long bones in children should receive only minimal exposure to ultrasonic waves.

What happens before the treatment?

- The therapist will assess the sensitivity of your skin and the status of your circulation before the treatment.
- The therapist will make sure that your skin is clean, dry, and free from oils and creams.
- You'll be asked to inform the therapist of pain or any changes in tissue temperature.
- The therapist will apply the conduction gel between the transducer and your skin.

What happens during the treatment?

Ultrasound therapy is usually administered by physical therapists, physical therapy assistants, or athletic trainers. Ultrasound treatments are performed in hospital physical therapy departments, outpatient physical therapy clinics, and athletic training facilities. Ultrasonic waves are delivered through a transducer. Piezoelectric crystals within the transducer generate the ultrasonic waves. Air between the transducer and the surface to be treated is eliminated by means of a conduction gel so that sound waves can be transmitted to the surface. The conduction gel usually consists of mineral oil and water-soluble gels. Treatments involve slow, sweeping motions of the transducer over the area to be treated and typically take 5 to 10 minutes.

What are the possible complications?

Correctly used, ultrasound therapy is safe and has few complications. It is important that soft tissue not be overheated because ultrasonic waves can cause thermal injury. The therapist depends on your feedback about any changes in pain and temperature during treatment. For this reason, ultrasound therapy must be used cautiously over areas with reduced sensation.

19

TREATING MENTAL & EMOTIONAL PROBLEMS

DRUG THERAPIES

ANTIPSYCHOTICS

Sometimes called major tranquilizers or *neuroleptics,* antipsychotic drugs help control the symptoms of psychoses and may help persons with these disorders become more receptive to psychotherapy. The major classes of antipsychotic drugs include the butyrophenones, phenothiazines, the butyrophenones, the thioxanthenes, and some miscellaneous drugs.

Most of these drugs appear to act by altering the activity of certain neurotransmitters within the central nervous system. Antipsychotics treat a wide variety of disorders, including schizophrenia, psychoses, and the manic phase of bipolar disorders. They're also used for acute psychotic symptoms, such as paranoia, hostility, combativeness, hallucinations, and persistent delusions. Some also may be used as antinausea medications.

What are antipsychotics used for?
- To relieve psychotic symptoms
- To provide sedation

What are some commonly used antipsychotics?
Butyrophenones
- haloperidol, known by the brand names Haldol and (in Canada) Peridol

Phenothiazines
- acetophenazine, known by the brand name Tindal
- chlorpromazine, known by the brand names Thorazine and Thor-Prom
- fluphenazine, known by the brand names Permitil and Prolixin
- mesoridazine, known by the brand name Serentil
- perphenazine, known by the brand name Trilafon
- prochlorperazine, known by the brand name Compazine
- thioridazine, known by the brand name Mellaril
- trifluoperazine, known by the brand names Stelazine and Suprazine

Thioxanthenes
- chlorprothixene, known by the brand name Taractan
- thiothixene, known by the brand name Navane

Miscellaneous drugs
- clozapine, known by the brand name Clozaril
- molindone, known by the brand name Moban

What are the possible side effects?
- Excessive sedation, movement disorders (including some symptoms resembling Parkinson's disease)
- Fainting, dizziness
- Altered heart rhythms
- Nausea, dry mouth, vomiting, abdominal pain, gastric irritation
- Visual changes
- Skin eruptions
- Sensitivity to light
- Blood disorders

What are the guidelines for taking antipsychotics?
- Call your doctor if side effects develop. Movement disorders are most common with haloperidol, thiothixene, and molindone. Sedation is most common with chlorpromazine. Dizziness occurs with chlorpromazine and thioridazine; dry mouth occurs most often with chlorpromazine and thioridazine.
- Parkinsonian symptoms are reversible. An antiparkinsonian drug, such as diphenhydramine or benztropine, may be used to decrease the symptoms, which usually subside within 3 months. If they persist, the doctor may discontinue the antipsychotic or reduce its dosage.
- During prolonged therapy, you may experience rhythmic, involuntary movements of the tongue, face, mouth, jaw, and extremities. If so, notify your doctor immediately.
- Avoid activities that require alertness, especially early in therapy, because sedation may be a problem.
- Dizziness may be minimized by rising slowly from a lying or sitting position and avoiding hot showers.
- If you suffer from dry mouth, try sugarless hard candy or sugarless gum. If it becomes a serious problem, consult your dentist. Chronic dry mouth can increase the risk of cavities.
- To relieve constipation, increase fluid intake and use a stool softener. Eat low-calorie foods to combat weight gain and to maintain adequate nutrition.

- Expect the doctor to periodically monitor your blood count throughout therapy in order to detect the early signs of drug toxicity. Because these drugs can cause liver damage, watch for jaundice.
- Take a missed dose if you remember within 2 hours of the scheduled administration time. If more than 2 hours elapse, omit the dose and take the next scheduled dose. Don't double the next dose.
- Report a sore throat, fever, or weakness immediately. These symptoms may indicate blood problems.
- Tell the doctor about all medications you are currently taking, including nonprescription medicines.
- Avoid excessive exposure to the sun to reduce the risk of a skin reaction from sensitivity to light.
- If you take antacids and a phenothiazine, separate doses of these drugs by at least 2 hours.
- If you are taking a liquid phenothiazine, guard against skin contact with the drug because it may cause skin reactions.
- Avoid alcohol because it can cause additive sedation.

What else you should know
Check with the doctor before discontinuing any antipsychotic. People using these drugs are usually weaned gradually; abrupt withdrawal may cause nausea, vomiting, trembling, and dizziness.

MONOAMINE OXIDASE INHIBITORS

Monoamine oxidase inhibitors are used to relieve depression by increasing levels of neurotransmitters in the central nervous system.

Monoamine oxidase inhibitors, also known as *MAO inhibitors,* are used to treat depression. These drugs act by preventing the breakdown of certain neurotransmitters in the central nervous system. As these neurotransmitter levels rise, symptoms of depression subside. Although some doctors prescribe these drugs only when other therapies fail or can't be used, many use them as first-line agents.

What are monoamine oxidase inhibitors used for?
Monoamine oxidase inhibitors are used to relieve depression by increasing levels of neurotransmitters (dopamine, norepinephrine, and epinephrine) in the central nervous system.

What are some commonly used monoamine oxidase inhibitors?

- isocarboxazid, known by the brand name Marplan
- phenelzine, known by the brand name Nardil
- tranylcypromine, known by the brand name Parnate

What are the possible side effects?

- Restlessness, drowsiness, dizziness, headache, insomnia
- Constipation, nausea, vomiting, dry mouth
- Loss of appetite, weakness, joint pain
- Blurred vision
- Swelling of the hands or feet
- Urine retention, transient impotence
- Rash

What are the guidelines for taking monoamine oxidase inhibitors?

- Tell your doctor if you have a history of heart or blood vessel disease or impaired kidney or liver function.
- Certain foods may interact with monoamine oxidase inhibitors and cause a condition known as *hypertensive crisis,* an emergency marked by high blood pressure. It is important that you review with your doctor the foods to avoid. These foods include coffee, chocolate, cheese, alcohol, or any nonprescription drugs.
- Always check with your doctor before taking monoamine oxidase inhibitors with any other drugs, including nonprescription drugs.
- Be alert for symptoms of a hypertensive crisis, which is characterized by severe headache, palpitations, nausea, vomiting, neck stiffness or soreness, fever, clammy skin, or other visual disturbances. (In extreme cases, bleeding within the brain may occur.) Go to a hospital emergency department immediately if such signs occur.
- Return for regular monitoring of your blood pressure and liver function; long-term use of monoamine oxidase inhibitors can cause low blood pressure and hepatitis.
- Report to the doctor any unusual sweating; fever; cold, clammy skin; enlarged pupils; increased sensitivity to light; and an unusually rapid or slow heart rate. Also report severe dizziness or chest pain, nausea, vomiting, a stiff or sore neck, persistent constipation, urine retention, light-headedness, drowsiness, or dry mouth.
- Avoid constipation by drinking more fluids and taking a stool softener. Use throat lozenges to help relieve dry mouth.

- Don't change the dosage or discontinue taking the drug. Therapeutic effects may take several weeks to develop.
- Take a missed dose if you remember it within 2 hours of the scheduled administration time; otherwise, skip the missed dose.
- Don't take the drug close to bedtime because it may cause insomnia.
- Know what foods to avoid, even when dining out. You must maintain the restricted diet for at least 2 weeks after monoamine oxidase inhibitor therapy ends to allow for regeneration of the enzyme monoamine oxidase. You mustn't, under any circumstances, drink Chianti or similar red wines. Doing so could cause a deadly reaction.
- Avoid dizziness by not getting up suddenly from a kneeling, sitting, or lying position.

What else you should know

Check with your doctor before elective surgery or dental work. Some doctors prefer you wait until 2 weeks after discontinuing the drug before surgery. Carry a medical identification card in case of an emergency.

ANTIDEPRESSANTS

Antidepressants are used to treat major depression and mood disorder. Major depression, sometimes called *endogenous depression,* differs from the reactive depression that often accompanies life's trials, such as the death of a loved one, changes in the environment, or other stressful events.

Endogenous depression often has no easily identifiable cause. Instead, scientists believe that this form of depression stems from a biochemical imbalance in the brain. Most of the drugs that are used to treat endogenous depression enhance the availability of certain neurotransmitters — most notably serotonin, norepinephrine, and dopamine.

What are antidepressants used for?

- To relieve depression
- To treat obsessive-compulsive disorder (clomipramine and fluoxetine)
- To treat bedwetting in children age 6 and older (imipramine)
- To manage severe chronic pain (amitriptyline, desipramine, doxepin, imipramine, and nortriptyline)

What are some commonly used antidepressants?

Tricyclic antidepressants

- amitriptyline, known by the brand names Elavil and Endep
- amoxapine, known by the brand name Asendin
- clomipramine, known by the brand name Anafranil
- desipramine, known by the brand name Norpramin
- doxepin, known by the brand name Sinequan
- imipramine, known by the brand names Tipramine and Tofranil
- nortriptyline, known by the brand name Aventyl
- protriptyline, known by the brand name Vivactil
- trimipramine, known by the brand name Surmontil

Miscellaneous antidepressants

- bupropion, known by the brand name Wellbutrin
- fluoxetine, known by the brand name Prozac
- sertraline, known by the brand name Zoloft
- trazodone, known by the brand names Desyrel, Trazon, and Trialodine

What are the possible side effects?

- Dizziness, drowsiness
- Dry mouth, constipation
- Elevated blood pressure, rapid heartbeat
- Urine retention
- Sweating

What are the guidelines for taking antidepressants?

- Be sure to tell your doctor if you have a history of seizure disorders. Although most antidepressants may lower the seizure threshold, bupropion appears to pose a greater risk to seizure-prone persons than other antidepressants.
- Also tell the doctor if you have diabetes, urine retention, or a history of heart or blood vessel disease.
- Suicide is an inherent risk in the depressed person. Because an overdose can occur with as little as 10 times the regular daily dose, many doctors limit the number of antidepressants dispensed at one time.
- Expect some improvement in 10 to 14 days after the start of therapy; full effect usually takes 30 days. However, keep in mind that side effects, such as dry mouth, dizziness, and drowsiness, can begin immediately.

Suicide is an inherent risk in the depressed person. Because an overdose can occur with as little as 10 times the regular daily dose, many doctors limit the number of antidepressants dispensed at one time.

- Avoid driving or other hazardous activities requiring alertness and fine-motor coordination until the side effects of the drug on your central nervous system are known.
- If you are taking a tricyclic antidepressant, the entire daily dose may be taken at bedtime. If you are taking Prozac or Zoloft, take the drug in the morning. These drugs may interfere with sleep if you take them later in the day.
- If the drug causes constipation, increase your fluid intake and take a stool softener, as prescribed.
- Rise slowly from a sitting or lying position and sit momentarily before rising in order to minimize dizziness. This effect will subside after a week or so.
- Don't take any other drug, including nonprescription drugs, without first checking with your doctor.
- Most side effects subside within 2 to 3 weeks after therapy begins. Continue taking the drug as long as these effects don't worsen. Don't stop the drug abruptly.
- Take a missed dose as soon as you remember, unless it is almost time for the next dose. Never double the dose.
- Avoid alcohol while taking an antidepressant because the combination can cause central nervous system depression.
- Weight changes can occur during therapy. Some drugs such as tricyclic antidepressants are associated with weight gain; others such as Prozac are associated with weight loss. Weigh yourself weekly; tell the doctor about changes in weight of 5 pounds (2.3 kilograms) or more.
- Use sugarless hard candy or sugarless gum to relieve dry mouth. If dry mouth persists, check with your doctor or dentist. Persistent dry mouth increases the risk of tooth decay.

ANTIMANICS

Antimanics are used to treat manic depression, a disorder characterized by swings of mood from excitment (the manic phase) to depression. Because the moods tend to be opposite, the disease is sometimes referred to as *bipolar disorder*.

Lithium carbonate acts as a mood stabilizer, reducing the severity or frequency of manic episodes. Under proper supervision, lithium may prevent up to 80% of manic and depressive episodes. Episodes that occur during lithium therapy are usually less severe and shorter than those that might occur without it.

Lithium's mechanism of action is not fully understood; however, it may replace sodium ions and alter the way that nerves conduct their impulses.

What are antimanics used for?
Antimanics are used to prevent or control mania.

What are some commonly used antimanics?
- lithium carbonate, known by the brand name Eskalith

What are the possible side effects?
- Fatigue, muscle weakness, headache, confusion, restlessness, stupor, blackouts, coma, seizures, worsened psychotic symptoms, hyperexcitability
- Hand tremor
- Nausea, vomiting, bloating, loss of appetite, diarrhea, abdominal pain, dry mouth
- Weight gain
- Increased urine output

What are the guidelines for taking antimanics?
- Take the drug as ordered. If you miss a dose, take it as soon as you remember, unless it's almost time for the next dose. Never double the dose.
- Tell your doctor if you think you are pregnant. Lithium should not be used during pregnancy because of the risk of birth defects.
- Tell your doctor if you have a history of heart, liver, or kidney disease or high blood pressure, or if you have been told to follow a salt-restricted diet.
- Expect the doctor to take blood samples frequently during the first few weeks of therapy. Close monitoring of blood levels of the drug are needed to ensure therapeutic effects and avoid toxicity.
- Tell your doctor about all of the other medications that you are taking, including nonprescription drugs. Don't take any other medications without first checking with the doctor.
- If you are a diabetic, check your blood sugar levels regularly. Lithium may cause transient increases in blood sugar, requiring increased dosage of an antidiabetic drug. Report nausea, increased urination, increased thirst, mild weakness, and hand tremors.

Under proper supervision, lithium may prevent up to 80% of manic and depressive episodes. Episodes that occur during lithium therapy are usually less severe and shorter than those that might occur without it.

- If you experience persistent hand tremors, ask the doctor about taking most of the daily dose at bedtime. Also, reduce caffeine intake.
- Drink about ten to twelve 8-ounce glasses (2,500 to 3,000 milliliters) of fluid daily and avoid excessive salt intake, which enhances lithium excretion and reduces the drug's effectiveness. Don't take sodium-containing antacids.
- If you experience an upset stomach, take the drug with a glass of water after meals or snacks.
- Contact the doctor if vomiting, diarrhea, or excessive perspiration occurs. Excessive loss of body fluids can require lithium dosage adjustment. For this reason, guard against strenuous exercise, particularly in hot weather.

What else you should know
- Lithium produces its full effects 1 to 3 weeks after the start of therapy.
- Because lithium causes weight gain, you should weigh yourself daily. If you gain weight, reduce your caloric intake while maintaining adequate nutrition.

STIMULANTS

Stimulants increase the activity of nerve cells in the brain by promoting the activity of norepinephrine, a neurotransmitter. Although these drugs enhance alertness, they have a high potential for abuse.

Stimulants are often used to treat attention deficit disorder with hyperactivity, a behavioral disorder that primarily affects children. Beginning 2 to 3 weeks after therapy starts, stimulants produce a calming effect in the child. This calming effect increases the child's attention span, curbs impulsiveness, and assists socialization. Relieving the distressing symptoms of attention deficit disorder also helps the child respond better to psychotherapy and educational modifications. Before such treatment, the child should have a complete physical exam and a detailed psychological history taken. During treatment, close supervision is required because of the potential for drug dependence.

At one time, stimulants were used mainly as appetite suppressants, but the Food and Drug Administration has recommended that such use should be limited to short-term weight control and only as an adjunct to calorie restriction and behavior modification. Many experts feel that these drugs have no place in weight-control programs.

Stimulants are also used to treat narcolepsy, a rare disorder characterized by inappropriate sleepiness. They may also be used to combat the drowsiness produced by high doses of narcotic pain relievers in patients with cancer.

What are stimulants used for?

- To produce a calming effect in children with attention deficit disorder with hyperactivity
- To provide a stimulating effect in narcolepsy
- To assist in the short-term treatment of obesity

What are some commonly used stimulants?

- amphetamine (generic)
- methylphenidate, known by the brand name Ritalin
- dextroamphetamine, known by the brand names Dexedrine and Robese
- pemoline, known by the brand name Cylert

What are the possible side effects?

- Restlessness, hyperactivity, talkativeness, insomnia
- Palpitations, high blood pressure
- Nausea, vomiting, cramps, diarrhea, loss of appetite, weight loss
- Decreased growth (with prolonged use in children)
- Physical or psychological dependence (with prolonged use)

What are the guidelines for children taking stimulants?

- Tell your doctor if your child has heart or blood vessel disease, overactive thyroid, kidney problems, angina, high blood pressure, agitated states, a history of substance abuse, or diabetes. Long-term therapy should be avoided when possible because of the risk of psychological dependence or habituation.
- Have your child take the drug at least 6 hours before bedtime to prevent insomnia and, if appropriate, after meals to reduce appetite suppression.
- Give your child a missed dose only if you remember more than 2 hours before the next scheduled dose. Never double the dose.
- Restrict hazardous activities that require alertness or good motor coordination until your child's response to the drug has been determined.

At one time, cerebral stimulants were used mainly as appetite suppressants. But the Food and Drug Administration recommends that such use be limited to short-term weight control and only as an adjunct to caloric restriction and behavior modification.

- Avoid coffee, chocolate, colas, and other caffeine-containing products. These substances enhance the effects of most stimulants.
- Don't suddenly discontinue the medication after long-term use. Acute rebound depression will occur unless the dose is decreased gradually.
- Cerebral stimulants are addictive and should be stored in a secure location.

What else you should know
- If a child is receiving long-term therapy, check height and weight regularly to detect growth retardation.
- Occasionally, these drugs may be in short supply. If your child will be taking these agents on a prolonged basis, tell your pharmacist so he or she may ensure adequate supplies are on hand.

COUNSELING

PSYCHOTHERAPY

Psychotherapy, a form of counseling, refers to the psychological treatment of mental and emotional disorders. It attempts to uncover the reasons for problem behaviors and promotes effective coping and adaptation skills.

Psychotherapy aims to change a person's attitudes, feelings, or behavior. To promote such changes, the therapist may use methods such as reinforcement, persuasion, suggestion, reassurance, and confrontation. Success of therapy depends largely on the compatibility of person and therapist, the treatment goals selected, and the person's commitment. Therapy may be brief or may span several years.

Why is this treatment done?
Psychotherapy is used to bring about positive changes in a person's attitudes, emotions, or behavior. Psychotherapy is useful for a wide range of mental and emotional problems. Individual therapy may be used when the person develops personal distress or dissatisfaction with self or in relationships with significant others, coworkers, friends, or family.

What happens before the treatment?

- The therapist will review the person's psychiatric history, treatment history, and current psychiatric status to help understand his or her needs.
- The therapist explains the therapeutic technique to the person and helps the person establish a treatment goal.
- The person is informed that the therapist will maintain the confidentiality of information shared, unless the person plans to harm himself or herself or someone else. Typically, the therapist will share only that information that the person wants shared.

What happens during the treatment?

Depending on the therapist's beliefs and training, he or she selects an approach to meet your needs. For instance, the therapist may choose reinforcement, which strengthens the appropriate behavior by fear of punishment or the anticipation of a reward. Or, if a strong rapport exists between you and the therapist, he or she may use suggestion (or persuasion) to implant an idea or belief in your mind as a means of bringing about change. The therapist may also direct discussion of your feelings by helping you to mentally relive or bring into consciousness a long-suppressed, painful experience. Therapists often combine these and other techniques to achieve treatment goals.

The four types of psychotherapy are individual, crisis, group, and family therapy. In individual therapy, the therapist seeks to change the person's behavior through individual counseling sessions. This involves mutually agreed-upon goals, with the therapist mediating the person's disturbed patterns of behavior to promote personal health and development. It can be short- or long-term.

In crisis therapy, the person works on developing adequate coping skills to resolve an immediate, pressing problem. Crisis therapy usually involves just the person and therapist but may also include the person's family. Crisis therapy can range from one session to 6 months of treatment.

In group therapy, a group of people (ideally 4 to 10) with similar emotional problems meet to discuss their concerns as a means of making positive behavioral changes and promoting personal growth. Duration of therapy can range from a few weeks to several years.

Family therapy seeks to alter unhealthy relationships within a family to change the problematic behavior of one or more members. Like individual therapy, family therapy can be short- or long-term.

SELF-HELP

Caring for yourself after psychotherapy

After you've completed therapy, follow these important guidelines:
- Ask your therapist to refer you to an appropriate self-help group.
- Contact your therapist immediately if you experience any recurring symptoms, such as distress, depression, anxiety, or restlessness.

What are the possible complications?

During therapy, the person may experience increased distress, depression, anxiety, and restlessness. If the person feels uncomfortable with the therapy, he or she may experience loss of appetite, irritability, or insomnia. Aggressive or self-destructive impulses may be triggered by the recollection of some memories.

What happens after the treatment?

- The therapist will observe you for mood changes, such as increased distress, depression, anxiety, and restlessness. (See *Caring for yourself after psychotherapy*.)
- The therapist will reassure you that talking about feelings will help relieve distress.

BEHAVIOR THERAPY

Behavior therapy assumes that problem behaviors are learned and that they can be unlearned and replaced by acceptable ones through special training. Unlike psychotherapy, behavior therapy doesn't attempt to uncover the reasons for problem behaviors. In fact, it de-emphasizes the person's thoughts and feelings about them. The goal is to unlearn destructive or unproductive behaviors that result from faulty learning and to enhance effective social and adaptive behaviors. This type of therapy requires a motivated person willing to work at positive change and a cooperative therapist who must understand and respond consistently to specified behaviors.

Behavior therapy can change a negative behavioral pattern through various techniques, such as positive or negative reinforcement, shaping, modeling, punishment, or extinction.

Why is this treatment done?

Behavior therapy is performed to eliminate problem behaviors or replace them with more appropriate and acceptable behaviors; to remove or reduce behavioral excesses, such as compulsive behaviors and rituals; and to reduce behavioral deficits, such as memory impairment or limited social skills. Behavior therapy is used for many types of maladaptive behaviors, including phobias, smoking, alcoholism, and temper tantrums, and for certain disorders, such as migraine headaches and hyperactive bowel syndrome. It is suitable for adults or children and can be used for individuals or groups of persons with a similar behavior problem.

What happens before the treatment?

The therapist will counsel you about what behaviors need changing, the goals of therapy, and the techniques that will be used to accomplish them. The therapist will make clear what is expected of you and what you can expect from the therapist.

What happens during the treatment?

The behavioral therapist, who may be a psychologist, specially skilled nurse, or other specially educated individual, works with you to identify the specific behavior creating the problem. The analysis is based on your strengths, deficits, culture, and environmental influences. Therapy goals are mutually determined by you and the therapist. Once goals have been identified, the therapist — after considering additional factors, such as your age and family status — decides which behavioral therapy or therapies to use. (For more information, see *Comparing types of behavior therapy,* page 596.)

Positive reinforcement increases the likelihood of a desirable behavior being repeated by promptly praising or rewarding the behavior. By contrast, negative reinforcement removes a negative stimulus only after a desirable response is provided. Punishment discourages problem behavior by inflicting a penalty, such as temporary removal of a privilege. Although difficult to sustain, extinction is a technique that simply ignores undesirable behavior — provided, of course, that the behavior isn't dangerous or illegal. Another technique — shaping — initially rewards any behavior that resembles the desirable one. Then, step by step, the behavior required to gain a reward becomes progressively closer to the desired behavior. Modeling provides a reward when you imitate the required behavior. Relaxation techniques include muscle relaxation, biofeedback, and self-hypnosis.

What are the possible complications?

Occasionally, a technique or a therapy prompts an undesired behavioral change.

What happens after the treatment?

▪ The therapist will review the initial goals and your progress during treatment.

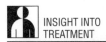
INSIGHT INTO
TREATMENT

Comparing types of behavior therapy

Behavior therapy is a broad term that includes assertiveness training, desensitization, flooding and implosion, positive conditioning, social skills training, and token economy.

Assertiveness training

Using the techniques of positive reinforcement, shaping, and modeling, assertiveness training aims to reduce anxiety through improved communication. It teaches the person acceptable ways to express feelings, ideas, and wishes without feeling guilty or demeaning others. The person learns how to make requests in a frank way and how to refuse unacceptable or unreasonable requests. Assertiveness training is often helpful to people who feel inhibited and unable to express their feelings.

Desensitization

The treatment of choice for phobias, desensitization slowly exposes the person to something he or she fears. It's most successful when used with other psychological treatments because phobias typically reflect unresolved conflicts. Desensitization is also used to treat other problems that produce fear of failure or embarrassment, such as frigidity or impotence. In practice, desensitization teaches the person to use deep-breathing or another relaxation technique when confronting a staged series of anxiety-producing situations. During desensitization, the person requires reassurance and practices relaxation techniques. The person's response to each anxious situation is monitored and he or she doesn't proceed to the next stage until ready.

Flooding and implosion

Flooding and implosion therapy can provide rapid relief of phobias such as travel phobias. It is also used to treat obsessive-compulsive disorder and behavior problems such as compulsive hoarding. Like desen-

sitization, it involves direct exposure to an anxiety-producing situation. Unlike desensitization, it doesn't employ relaxation techniques. Instead, it assumes that anxiety and panic can't persist and that confrontation helps the person to overcome fear.

Positive conditioning

Building on the principle of desensitization, this therapy attempts to gradually instill a positive or neutral attitude toward a phobia. Used effectively for people with sexual problems, positive conditioning first introduces a pleasurable stimulus by associating other pleasurable experiences with it. Next, the therapist introduces the phobia stimulus along with the pleasurable one. Gradually, the person develops a positive response to the phobia.

Social skills training

Using shaping and modeling techniques, this therapy helps people develop or regain skills for forming relationships. Commonly used for institutionalized, acutely ill, and mentally retarded persons, its success depends on consistent reinforcement.

Token economy

Also called operant conditioning, this treatment reinforces acceptable behavior with rewards (tokens), which the person can use as currency for some privilege or object. The therapist can also withhold or rescind tokens as punishment or to avert undesirable behavior. This therapy is often effective treatment for those with behavioral problems who do not respond well to verbal therapy techniques.

- You'll need to make follow-up appointments with your therapist to ensure continual effectiveness of the therapy. (See *Caring for yourself after behavior therapy*.)

MILIEU THERAPY

Milieu therapy refers to the use of the person's environment as a tool for overcoming mental and emotional disorders. It can be used in the hospital or in a community setting. Specifically, the person's surroundings become a therapeutic community, with the person involved in goal setting, which includes planning, implementing, and evaluating the treatment, as well as in sharing with staff and other people the responsibility for establishing group rules and policies. The person may then progress to a transitional or halfway house. Then, if the person continues to improve in this less structured environment, he or she may return to the outside community ready to apply the positive behaviors and skills that have been learned. Or the person may be discharged directly to home with psychiatric follow-up care.

The candidate for milieu therapy must be able to participate in group activities and must show a willingness to accept responsibility for daily activities.

Why is this treatment done?
Milieu therapy is performed to promote behavioral change and personal growth in a controlled therapeutic community. Milieu therapy is used when a person needs to learn or relearn how to function in a socially and emotionally appropriate way.

What happens before the treatment?
- The therapist will explain the purpose of milieu therapy to you, including what is expected from you and how you can participate in the therapeutic community.
- You'll be familiarized with the community's routines, such as the schedule for various activities, and will be introduced to the other people.

 SELF-HELP

Caring for yourself after behavior therapy

After you've completed therapy, follow these important guidelines:
- Keep in mind that by learning the basic techniques of behavior therapy, family members may be able to help you correct problem behaviors.
- Consider asking your therapist to refer you to an appropriate support group so you can build a strong, supportive network with your peers.
- Seek additional therapy if problem behaviors recur.

What happens during the treatment?

You'll follow a schedule of therapeutic programming that includes individual and group therapy sessions as well as group meetings. You'll learn to interact appropriately with staff and other people and participate in other forms of therapy such as art, music, and occupational therapy.

In many cases, milieu therapy allows exploration of the aspects of your environment that seem to contribute to your behavior either by their presence or absence. New strategies may help you develop healthy coping behaviors.

What are the possible complications?

As the type of milieu or environment can vary, so can the complications. In a restricted environment, you may lose some autonomy and decision-making abilities. If the hospitalization is prolonged, you may become dependent on the setting for your care.

OTHER TREATMENTS

DETOXIFICATION

Detoxification refers to withdrawal from the effects of prolonged dependence on alcohol or other drugs. Detoxification programs are designed to help the person maintain abstinence and to provide a relatively safe alternative to self-withdrawal, which is difficult and often dangerous. Provided in outpatient centers or in special hospital units, detoxification programs offer treatment of symptoms as well as counseling or psychotherapy for an individual, group, or family.

Why is this treatment done?

Detoxification programs are used for the treatment of alcohol and drug dependence. They help the person achieve abstinence from alcohol or drugs while providing supportive and symptomatic care.

What happens before the treatment?

- The nurse or doctor will reassure the distressed person, along with the family, that the person will receive immediate treatment.

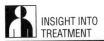
INSIGHT INTO
TREATMENT

Treating drug intoxication

Sometimes drug abusers enter detoxification programs requiring emergency treatment, typically for an overdose of narcotics, barbiturates, cocaine, amphetamines, or tranquilizers.

Narcotic overdose
The immediate goal is to prevent shock and maintain breathing. The doctor inserts a breathing tube and gives the person oxygen and intravenous fluids. A narcotic antagonist medication is also given to combat depression of respirations.

Barbiturate overdose
Like treatment of narcotic overdose, treatment of barbiturate overdose aims to prevent shock and maintain breathing. It may also include stomach flushing or induced vomiting if the person ingested the drug within the previous 4 hours. Or it may include administration of activated charcoal, followed by a laxative, to eliminate the toxic drug. Extreme intoxication requires dialysis.

Cocaine intoxication
Because cocaine can cause an abnormal heart rhythm, the person's electrocardiogram is monitored. Cardiopulmonary resuscitation may be necessary during treatment of cocaine intoxication. Other sup-

portive measures include administration of aspirin or acetaminophen to reduce fever, an anticonvulsant to prevent seizures, and medication to treat a fast heart rate.

Amphetamine overdose
If the drug was taken by mouth, vomiting is induced or the stomach is flushed. A laxative and diuretic are given to hasten elimination, sedatives are given to treat agitation and to prevent or control seizures, and medication is given to lower blood pressure.

Tranquilizer overdose
If the drug was taken orally, vomiting is induced when ingestion is recent and the person is fully conscious. If the person is sleepy or comatose, the stomach may be flushed after the airway is protected with a breathing tube. After induction of vomiting, activated charcoal and a laxative are given to remove residual drug from the gastrointestinal tract. A specific benzodiazepine antagonist is given to awaken the person.

- The doctor or nurse will ask about the person's medical history, noting especially any history of psychiatric disorder, seizures, and specific substance dependence.
- The nurse will take blood samples and urine specimens for alcohol and drug screening.

What happens during the treatment?
Alcohol withdrawal requires total abstinence and usually proves more severe and hazardous than drug withdrawal. The procedure for alcohol detoxification involves providing a safe, softly lit environment to avoid overstimulation and agitation, which can cause tremors, and removing any potentially harmful objects from the person's room. The person is usually treated symptomatically with antianxiety and anti-

SELF-HELP

Caring for yourself after detoxification

After you've been discharged from the hospital, follow these guidelines.

Know what to expect
- If you must return to an environment where substance abuse is common, be aware that you're likely to have a relapse. For this reason, you and your family will need continuing professional support after the detoxification program ends.
- For successful rehabilitation, you must ultimately accept responsibility for avoiding abused substances.

Join a support group
For continued support and encouragement, join an appropriate self-help group, such as Alcoholics Anonymous or Narcotics Anonymous. Your spouse or mature children may accompany you to group meetings.

nausea agents, anticonvulsants, and antidiarrheals. The person who hallucinates may need to be reminded who and where he or she is, and may require short-term use of restraints for combative behavior. Seizure and suicide precautions are usually taken.

Detoxification from narcotics, tranquilizers, depressants, or other drugs is achieved by gradually lowering the dosage of the abused drug or by substituting a drug with similar action; for example, methadone may be substituted for heroin and cocaine addiction may be treated with bromocriptine or naltrexone. The person may be taught relaxation techniques, encouraged to perform mild exercise, and provided with nutritional support.

Some drug abusers who enter detoxification programs require emergency treatment, typically for an overdose of narcotics, barbiturates, cocaine, or amphetamines. (See *Treating drug intoxication,* page 599.) This treatment is aimed at preventing shock and maintaining breathing. Stomach flushing or induction of vomiting may be used if the drug was ingested within 4 hours of treatment. Dialysis and cardiopulmonary resuscitation may also be required.

What are the possible complications?
During withdrawal from prolonged abuse of alcohol, the person experiences a fast heart rate, high blood pressure, fever, flushing, and sweating. Other symptoms include anxiety, tremors, and irritability, which may progress to seizure activity. Loss of appetite, nausea, vomiting, and diarrhea may also occur. Alcohol withdrawal syndrome, an acute toxic state characterized by agitation, confusion, delusions, hallucinations, and tonic-clonic seizures, is a life-threatening response to withdrawal.

What happens after the treatment?
The doctor will encourage you to participate in a rehabilitation program and self-help group. (See *Caring for yourself after detoxification.*)

ELECTROCONVULSIVE THERAPY

Electroconvulsive therapy, also referred to as electroshock therapy, was first used in 1937 as a treatment for various emotional disorders. During electroconvulsive therapy, an electric current travels through electrodes placed on the temples, causing a generalized seizure. Exactly how electroconvulsive therapy works remains unclear, but it seems to produce biochemical changes in the brain that increase levels of two substances that send nerve signals: norepinephrine and serotonin.

Despite its controversial history, electroconvulsive therapy is now considered a relatively simple procedure. Decisions regarding its use are based on the risks and benefits of all available treatments.

Why is this treatment done?

Electroconvulsive therapy is performed to relieve major depression or other severe mental disorders in people who do not respond to or cannot tolerate drug therapy or its side effects. It is also used for actively suicidal people who could die while waiting for antidepressant medication to become effective.

When standard therapies produce inadequate results, electroconvulsive therapy also may be used to treat other mental disorders, reduced pituitary hormone levels, seizure disorders, and Parkinson's disease. Other candidates for electroconvulsive therapy may include people with manic disorders, schizophrenia, or catatonic syndromes.

When shouldn't this treatment be done?

Electroconvulsive therapy shouldn't be used in people who have increased pressure within the skull, a brain tumor or an unstable blood vessel abnormality such as an aortic or brain aneurysm, or in those who have had a recent stroke, heart attack, or congestive heart failure. Such people are at higher risk for complications from the electroconvulsive therapy-induced seizure and the anesthesia. This treatment should be used cautiously during pregnancy and in elderly people.

What happens before the treatment?

- The doctor or nurse will explain the procedure to you and your family, correcting any misconceptions and answering your questions.
- You or a responsible family member will sign a consent form.
- The doctor will complete a thorough medical evaluation before treatment including a physical exam, standard lab tests, electrocardiogram, electroencephalogram, and X-rays.
- Because depressed people may experience sleeping and eating disturbances, the nurse will assist you in maintaining adequate nutrition, proper elimination, and effective sleeping patterns.
- The nurse restricts food and fluids for at least 4 hours before the treatment and asks you to wear loose-fitting clothes.

SELF-HELP

Recovering from electroconvulsive therapy

After you've been discharged from the hospital, follow these important guidelines.

Know what to expect
Be aware that temporary amnesia and mild confusion may follow electroconvulsive therapy. However, these symptoms usually diminish or disappear.

Other instructions
- Follow your doctor's instructions regarding use of antidepressant medication.
- Avoid driving and other potentially hazardous activities until confusion and drowsiness disappear.
- Don't resume your daily activities until you're physically able to do so.
- Make and keep follow-up appointments with your doctor.

- Medications taken to treat depression or other psychological problems will be discontinued the day before electroconvulsive therapy to prevent any interactions.
- The nurse may administer a sedative 30 minutes before the treatment to assist with anesthesia and help you to relax.

What happens during the treatment?

Accompanied by a nurse, you'll go to a treatment room equipped with specialized electroconvulsive therapy and emergency resuscitation equipment. You lie on a padded bed and may be gently restrained. An intravenous catheter is inserted to deliver medication as needed. An oxygen mask is used for respiratory support. Electrocardiogram electrodes are applied to monitor heart function, and electroencephalogram electrodes are applied to monitor brain electrical activity. Usually, the electroconvulsive therapy electrodes are placed on each temple, although some psychiatrists prefer to place both electrodes on the nondominant side because it produces less memory disturbance. An alternating current of 400 milliamperes and 70 to 120 volts is passed between the electroconvulsive therapy electrodes for 0.1 to 0.5 second.

A psychiatrist administers the electroconvulsive therapy and is supported by a specially trained anesthesia and nursing staff. Typically, a short-acting general anesthetic and a muscle relaxant are administered. Treatments vary depending on the severity of symptoms and your responsiveness to treatment. Usually, electroconvulsive therapy treatments are given on alternate days, 3 to 4 times a week. An average of 6 to 10 treatments are given for depression; 20 to 30 treatments may be given for schizophrenia.

Electroconvulsive therapy is not used indiscriminately or for a long time. Medication and psychotherapy may be used as adjunctive therapy.

What are the possible complications?

The two most common side effects of electroconvulsive therapy are temporary memory loss and confusion. These effects are transient and are related to the number of treatments, the technique of electrode placement, the voltage used, and the person's age and mental status before therapy. Memory and cognitive function routinely return to normal 1 to 6 months after treatment. (See *Recovering from electroconvulsive therapy.*)

Heart complications include a fast or slow heartbeat and blood pressure changes, which are related to the use of muscle relaxants, anesthesia, and the induced seizure.

Historically, fractured bones and strained muscles of the neck, back, and extremities were common with the use of electroconvulsive therapy. The use of muscle relaxants and anesthesia has virtually eliminated these problems. Some clinicians report that people who have received electroconvulsive therapy have suffered social stigmatization because of others' negative perceptions of them.

What happens after the treatment?

- The anesthetist will provide respiratory support until you can breathe unassisted.
- The nurse will monitor your vital signs and neurologic status every 5 minutes until you are awake and then every 15 minutes until you are alert.
- The nurse administers medications for headache or nausea as necessary.

LIGHT THERAPY

Light therapy, also called *phototherapy*, is therapeutic exposure to artificial light containing all the wave frequencies present in sunlight. Although ordinary indoor lighting provides 300 to 500 lux (units of illumination), the recommended full-spectrum artificial light — available from several manufacturers — provides 2,500 lux or more. This is 5 to 10 times brighter than the light in a well-lit office.

The exact mechanism of light therapy is not well understood, but it is thought to reduce the activity of melatonin, a hormone that appears to inhibit numerous endocrine functions. When injected, exogenous melatonin causes drowsiness. Correctly used, light therapy has many beneficial effects.

Why is this treatment done?

Light therapy is used to elevate the person's mood, to cause an antidepressant effect, and to reset and synchronize the human biological clock (circadian rhythm) with the solar clock during seasons of shortened sunlight. Light therapy is primarily used to treat seasonal affec-

Caring for yourself during light therapy

If light therapy has been prescribed for you, follow these important guidelines:
- Be aware that seasonal affective disorder may require adjustment of work and personal schedules.
- Make and keep follow-up appointments with the doctor or mental health professional to evaluate treatment and make recommendations regarding therapy.
- Contact the National Organization for Seasonal Affective Disorder (P.O. Box 40133, Washington, DC 20016) for information on a local support group.

tive disorder, also known as SAD. Seasonal changes and limited exposure to bright light may induce depression in sensitive people. Seasonal affective disorder is characterized by a mild depression during the shortened daylight seasons of fall and winter. People with this disorder experience fewer symptoms or remission of symptoms as the days get longer with increased sunlight and warmth. (See *Caring for yourself during light therapy*.)

Light therapy may also be used for other conditions, including delayed sleep-phase syndrome (marked by difficulty in getting to sleep and waking up at conventional times), premenstrual syndrome, circadian disruption caused by shift work, and jet lag.

What happens before the treatment?
- The caregiver may recommend mental health counseling, which may be beneficial to both you and your family.
- Antidepressants and other psychotropic drugs may be administered along with light therapy.
- You'll be encouraged to use the treatment exactly as prescribed.

What happens during the treatment?
A light box for phototherapy can be assembled by an electrician or purchased commercially. It consists of a box containing a high-lux lighting system. You should sit about 3 feet (1 meter) away from the source and may read, write, or watch TV during treatment. The optimal time and duration of therapy remain controversial, but some clinicians recommend early-morning exposure to the bright light for 2 to 3 hours. You should glance at the light a few times every minute or so. Typically, people who are going to respond to light therapy will experience improvement within 3 to 4 days. If the response is inadequate, evening hours may be substituted or added to the schedule.

What are the possible complications?
No long-term side effects of phototherapy have been identified. However, if you have eye problems, you might be at risk for visual side effects. Appropriate precautions should be taken to avoid eye trauma. The most common reactions are eyestrain, headache, and insomnia, which can be managed by decreasing the duration of exposure or increasing the distance from the light.

TREATING COSMETIC PROBLEMS

SURGERIES

BREAST RECONSTRUCTION

Breast reconstruction is an option available to any woman who's had a breast removed for treatment of breast cancer. Dramatic developments in plastic surgery make breast reconstruction more feasible, more appealing, and less costly than in the past. Health care insurance companies are covering the costs as rehabilitative surgery rather than as cosmetic surgery.

Reconstructive surgery can bolster a woman's self-esteem and self-confidence, which may have been lost because of her breast removal. Most women who choose to have breast reconstruction are satisfied with the cosmetic results. The procedure eliminates the need for a prosthesis (an artificial breast) and restores a sense of well-being and wholeness even though it won't restore the sensation lost through breast removal. Any surgery on the breast can damage the sensitive nerves in that area.

Breast reconstruction must be tailored to meet each woman's individual needs. Five types of reconstructive procedures are available; which one is appropriate depends on the type of breast surgery performed. (See *Breast reconstruction methods.*)

Why is this surgery done?
Breast reconstruction is done to replace breasts removed by radical surgery for breast cancer and to restore an acceptable body image. Reconstructive breast surgery can be performed on any woman who has had a breast removed for breast cancer. However, some types of breast removal or adjunctive treatments may require complicated reconstructive surgeries to achieve optimal results.

Breast reconstruction can help relieve the emotional distress caused by breast removal for treatment of cancer. It can improve the person's self-image and restore her sexual identity.

When shouldn't this surgery be done?
Breast reconstruction shouldn't be performed after breast removal for cancer when metastasis (cancer spread) is possible, when healing is

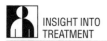

INSIGHT INTO
TREATMENT

Breast reconstruction methods

Simple reconstruction without a flap

This method of breast reconstruction requires insertion of the implant in a pocket created between skin and muscle. An incision of approximately 2 inches (5 centimeters) is made along the lower border of the breast. If the incision for breast removal was low enough, it can be used again, leaving only one scar. The procedure takes 1 to 2 hours and is performed under general anesthesia.

Tissue expansion

The purpose of this procedure is to stretch the skin so that an implant that matches the opposite breast can be inserted. Under local or general anesthesia, an incision is made and the deflated tissue expander is inserted under the skin and muscle. (This can be done at the time of breast removal.) After its placement, the expander is filled with a small amount of sterile fluid. The procedure takes 1 to 1½ hours.

Over the next 8 to 12 weeks, the doctor will inject additional fluid once a week during an office visit. Gradually, the enlarged expander will stretch the tissue over it. When the tissue has stretched enough to hold the desired size implant, the surgeon removes the tissue expander and inserts the permanent implant. The last step can be done as an outpatient procedure under local anesthesia.

Latissimus dorsi flap

The latissimus dorsi flap or myocutaneous flap is a technique in which skin, tissue under the skin, and muscle are transferred to the site of breast removal from another body site. The area most often used is the latissimus dorsi muscle of the back — a broad, flat muscle covering one side of the back below the shoulder blade. This muscle is freed from the spine and pelvic bone and is tunneled forward under the skin to the chest wall, then positioned in place. This surgical procedure is dependable and successful.

It takes 3 to 4 hours and leaves a scar on the back and on the chest.

Rectus abdominis flap

This procedure requires the transfer of one of the rectus abdominis muscles — either the left or right muscle of the abdomen — with the overlying skin and a section of fat. The surgeon moves this flap to the breast area and contours it into the shape of a breast. The artery supplying blood to this muscle is also carried with the flap to the chest to ensure that the muscle will be viable.

Free flap

This new technique uses a wedge of tissue, including skin, fat, and a little muscle and a small artery and vein from the abdomen, buttock, or thigh, which is transplanted into the chest wall; the artery and vein are attached to existing blood vessels that had nourished the real breast tissue. Then the tissue is shaped into a new breast that closely resembles the natural breast.

Reconstruction of the nipple and surrounding pigmented area

Several weeks or months after reconstruction of the breast, women may elect to have surgery to create a nipple and surrounding pigmented area. The surgery takes 1 to 2 hours.

The most common technique for reconstructing the pigmented area surrounding the nipple is to use skin from the upper inner thigh or skin from behind the ear. The nipple is formed from tissue from the newly created breast or by grafting a piece of nipple from the natural breast. Another technique creates the nipple and surrounding area from vaginal skin. If the reconstructed area around the nipple isn't dark enough, ultraviolet light may be used to improve the color match.

Understanding breast implants

The implants used in breast reconstruction are soft, fluid-filled sacs. They're round and shaped like a teardrop. Implants can be punctured by a sharp object but, under normal conditions, are very durable. There are three types of implants.

Silicone gel implant
This implant, the focus of recent controversy about its safety, comes in a variety of sizes.

Inflatable implant
An empty silicone bag is inserted into the incision and filled by injecting saline through a valve in the bag. This implant requires a smaller incision than a pre-filled implant and can be filled to the volume needed for the best fit. Leakage may occur and requires replacement of the implant.

Double-lumen implant
This is a combination of an inner bag containing silicone gel surrounded by an outer bag filled with saline solution. The outer bag's size can be adjusted to achieve the appropriate size.

impaired, or when the person has unrealistic expectations of the effects of surgery.

What happens before the surgery?
- The doctor or nurse will explain the procedure and answer any questions you may have.
- Your food and fluids will be restricted for 8 to 12 hours before the procedure.

What happens during the surgery?
Breast reconstruction involves creation of a pocket between the skin and muscle for placement of a prosthetic implant. (See *Understanding breast implants*.)

Simple breast reconstruction, without a flap, uses the woman's remaining tissue at the surgical site and requires a healthy pectoral muscle and an ample amount of good healthy skin. Skin that has been irradiated, is tight, or is too thin may not be suitable for this procedure.

Tissue expansion is used for women whose skin and muscle is of good quality but insufficient to cover an implant that will match the opposite breast.

Creation of a flap using the latissimus dorsi muscle located on the back of the body is used for women whose skin is tight or thinning and for women whose remaining pectoral muscle is inadequate for other methods of breast reconstruction. Women who need this type of reconstruction commonly have had radiation treatments or skin grafting.

The rectus abdominis flap procedure reduces and tightens the abdominal area much like a "tummy tuck." This is an appealing option for many women. It also can be used for women who've had radiation treatments or skin grafting.

Free flap surgery, the newest technique, can be used for most women who've undergone breast removal. This technique also provides the cosmetic advantage of a "tummy tuck" if the fatty tissue used in the reconstruction is taken from the abdomen.

What are the possible complications?
All surgery entails risks or complications, such as bleeding or infection. Special concerns during breast reconstruction are infection at the breast site, decreased blood circulation to the skin, and capsular contracture. The implant might have to be removed temporarily un-

til any infection at the breast site clears. If circulation to the skin is insufficient, removal of the implant and skin grafting may be necessary. After surgery, scar tissue forms around the implant, causing the breast to look firm and spherical. Sometimes, this scar tissue causes the implant to be displaced. This problem, known as *capsular contracture*, occurs in about 25% of all implants. It can be corrected but usually requires further surgery.

Infection and decreased blood circulation to the area are less likely to occur if the reconstruction isn't done at the same time as the breast removal. Recent studies have shown that silicone implants can leak and possibly burst, causing the release of silicone into the surrounding breast tissue and resulting in pain and hardness in the area.

What happens after the surgery?

- The nurse will monitor the drainage from tubes inserted into the wound during surgery. (See *Caring for yourself after breast reconstruction.*)
- The nurse will administer antibiotic therapy, if prescribed by the doctor.
- You'll be encouraged to walk soon after the surgery to decrease the risk of lung complications.
- Circulation to the skin around the implant and the arm on the affected side will be monitored. Any sign of decreased circulation will be reported to the doctor immediately.

Caring for yourself after breast reconstruction

After you're discharged from the hospital, follow these important guidelines.

Take special precautions
- Observe the nurse's instructions on how to empty and care for drainage tubes in the incision.
- Regularly massage the implant and perform specified exercises as instructed by the doctor or nurse.

Other points to remember
- Avoid swimming, tennis, bowling, or other strenuous activities until your doctor lets you return to unrestricted activity.
- After reconstruction, you should continue to examine your natural breast and the reconstructed breast once a month to note any changes.

BREAST REDUCTION OR ENLARGEMENT

Surgery to change breast size is also known as *mammoplasty*. Breast reduction removes excess breast skin and underlying tissue and reshapes the contour of large breasts. It also includes repositioning the nipple and surrounding pigmented area. Breast enlargement increases breast size. These procedures are usually performed after breasts are fully developed, and they're not recommended for women who want to breast-feed.

Why is this surgery done?

Surgery to change breast size is done to remove excess breast skin and tissue, to reshape the breasts to a smaller size in proportion with the rest of the body, and to enlarge the breasts. Breast reduction is usually done because of physical discomfort, such as backache, shoulder aches, irritation, or fungal infections under the breasts. However, breast reduction or enlargement can also be performed for a woman who's self-conscious about the size of her breasts. The effect of breast surgery is permanent, but breast size can increase because of weight gain, use of birth control pills, or pregnancy.

What happens before the surgery?

- The doctor will ask you to donate several units of your own blood so that it can be kept for you in case you need a blood transfusion during surgery.
- You'll be told to stop taking aspirin or any medication containing aspirin 1 week before surgery.
- The doctor or nurse will explain the procedure to you and inform you that you may have drainage tubes inserted into the incision after surgery.
- You'll be reminded that the surgery will relieve physical discomfort and alter the size of the breast but won't solve your sexual or social problems.

What happens during the surgery?

Surgery is usually performed under general anesthesia and takes 3 to 4 hours, depending on the extent of the procedure. For breast reduction, incisions may be made around the edge of the nipple or in the crease below the breast, following the natural contour of the breast. A vertical incision in the shape of a keyhole may be made in the area surrounding the nipple to allow the nipple to be repositioned. Excess tissue, fat, and skin are removed from the breast. The nipple, surrounding area, and underlying tissue are then repositioned to a normal location on the breast. If the breasts are extremely large, the nipple and surrounding area may be completely detached and then relocated after the tissue is removed. Finally, the skin is brought together to reshape the breast.

For breast enlargement, the surgeon makes a small incision under the breast to insert an implant.

What are the possible complications?

Breast reduction causes scars on the breasts. Sensitivity of the breast and nipple decreases and may not return for as long as 6 months.

Clotted blood may collect under the skin, or blood flow may be reduced in the nipple and surrounding area.

Complications of breast enlargement depend on the type of implant. Recent studies have shown that silicone implants can leak and possibly burst, causing the release of silicone into the surrounding breast tissue. This results in pain and hardness in the tissue.

What happens after the surgery?

- You'll receive pain medications.
- The nurse will encourage you to walk and move your arms the day after the procedure. (See *Recovering from breast surgery*.)
- Your vital signs will be monitored.
- Your bandages will be checked for any bleeding, and drainage tubes will be removed on the 2nd or 3rd day after surgery.

CLEFT LIP AND PALATE REPAIR

Cleft lip and cleft palate are two birth defects that may occur separately or together in various degrees of severity. A cleft lip can range from a slight dimpling in the lip area to large clefts on both sides of the lip. Cleft palate (roof of the mouth) can range from a small defect to clefts on both sides that can extend the entire length of the soft palate (the soft back part of the roof of the mouth) and the hard palate (the upper bony part of the roof of the mouth). It may also involve the nasal cavity. (See *Variations in cleft lip and palate,* page 612.)

Surgical repair of a cleft lip is typically done within the first 3 months of life, although the type and degree of cleft may necessitate several operations to complete cosmetic closure. The best time for cleft palate repair depends on the child, but the procedure is usually done between ages 6 months and 18 months. The goal is to repair the defect before faulty speech habits develop. Methods used to repair the defect vary according to the degree of the defect and the doctor's preference.

Why is this surgery done?

Cleft lip repair is performed to restore the function and cosmetic appearance of the face and mouth and to prepare the gums for teeth eruption.

SELF-HELP

Recovering from breast surgery

After you're discharged from the hospital, follow these important guidelines.

Know what to expect

- Expect swelling and skin discoloration of the breast; both signs will subside in several days.
- Scars will remain visible for up to 1 year and then will gradually fade.
- You'll need to make an appointment with your doctor to have the stitches removed 2 to 3 weeks after surgery.
- After 1 week, the bandages will be removed; a soft bra should be worn at all times for several weeks.

Follow instructions

- Take pain medication as prescribed by your doctor so that you can follow his or her instructions to move your arms regularly.
- Avoid excessive movement and all overhead lifting for 3 to 4 weeks or as advised by your doctor. You may return to work 2 weeks after surgery.
- You should wear a support bra for the first month after surgery.

Variations in cleft lip and palate

Cleft lip and palate can occur alone or together. Cleft lip (shown on the left side) may range from a simple notch to a complete cleft; cleft palate (shown on the right side), from partial to complete.

INCOMPLETE, ONE SIDE

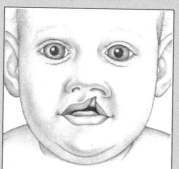

SOFT PALATE ONLY

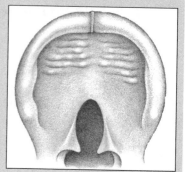

COMPLETE, ONE SIDE

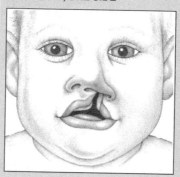

COMPLETE, ONE SIDE

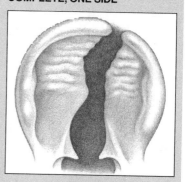

COMPLETE, BOTH SIDES

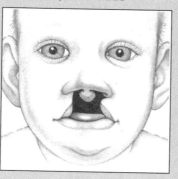

COMPLETE, BOTH SIDES

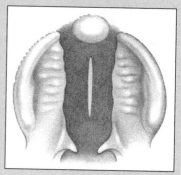

Cleft palate repair is done to restore normal function of the hard and soft palates; to improve speech patterns and eating ability; to avoid hearing loss and fluid buildup within the ear caused by displacement of the eustachian tubes; and to allow for normal development and eruption of the teeth.

What happens before the surgery?

- The doctor explains the procedure to the parents and answers any questions they have.
- The parents sign a consent form.

What happens during the surgery?

For cleft lip repair

Before closure of the cleft, the surgeon removes minimal amounts of lip tissue to preserve soft tissue and mucous membranes. Bilateral cleft lip repair is almost always done in two stages to provide less tension on the incision and to improve the accuracy of measurements for the second repair.

For cleft palate repair

Until palate closure is performed, the infant is fitted with a prosthesis to allow feeding, speech development, and fewer respiratory tract infections. To repair the defect, the surgeon uses tissue adjacent to the defect to close the cleft. The repair may be done in one operation or may require several stages of repair, depending on the severity of the defect.

What are the possible complications?

Hemorrhage, shock, and breathing difficulties may occur immediately after surgery. A simple suture on the tongue may be used to ensure that the tongue doesn't block the airway.

What happens after the surgery?

- The child will lie on one side or on the abdomen to prevent blood or drainage from the incision from going down the windpipe. Gentle suctioning of the back of the throat may be necessary.
- The child will be monitored closely for signs of hemorrhage and difficulty breathing.
- The nurse may apply restraints at the elbows to prevent the child from disturbing the sutures, removing one restraint at a time at fre-

ADVICE FOR CAREGIVERS

Caring for a child after cleft lip or palate repair

When your child is discharged from the hospital, follow these important guidelines.

Watch the child closely

- Watch the child for signs of ear infection, such as fever and pulling on the ear.
- Try to prevent crying until the incision has healed.
- You may need to use wrist restraints to keep the child's hands out of his or her mouth.
- Follow the doctor or nurse's instructions about appropriate diet, feeding techniques, and care of the incision.

Get more help if needed

- The child may need referral to speech and hearing therapists, orthodontists, or reconstructive surgeons — depending on the degree of the defect and the type of repair required.
- Ask the doctor for the names of local support groups where you can obtain additional information and reassurance.
- You may want to seek genetic counseling because you have a greater-than-normal risk of similar defects in future children.

quent intervals for exercise. A jacket restraint may be used for infants who can roll over.

- The nurse will try to prevent crying, which causes tension on the suture line. (See *Caring for a child after cleft lip or palate repair*.)
- After cleft lip repair, the infant will be fed only liquids with a medicine dropper or syringe in the side of the mouth. Breast-feeding or bottle feedings may be resumed 24 hours after surgery.
- After cleft palate repair, only a cup or the side of a spoon will be used for feeding; nothing should be put into the mouth. The child will receive only fluid or semifluid feedings.
- The nurse will apply petroleum jelly or topical antibiotic ointment to the incision, if prescribed by the doctor.
- Mild pain relievers may be given to the child.

LIPOSUCTION

Liposuction is the removal of fat cells from various areas of the body by suction. Body areas that can benefit from liposuction are the face, breasts, abdomen, hips, thighs, posterior upper arms, upper midback, knees, calves, and ankles.

Like other cosmetic procedures, liposuction requires thorough assessment of the person's attitude and expectation about the outcome. It shouldn't be performed on people with unrealistic expectations or on those who are 30% over ideal body weight; it isn't an alternative to weight loss.

Why is this procedure done?

Liposuction is done to remove fat from body areas that are resistant to diet and exercise. It's also performed to reshape a part of the body. The procedure is used to improve or enhance the appearance. It isn't a treatment for obesity and won't remove cellulite. People who are in good physical condition and have a history of rapid healing but who are unable to trim certain areas by dieting are good candidates for this procedure. Liposuction is frequently combined with soft-tissue surgery and can remove fatty cysts, resulting in a much smaller scar.

What happens before the procedure?

- The doctor will ask you to stop taking aspirin and other anti-inflammatory medications 2 weeks before surgery.
- You'll need to be adequately nourished and must avoid following a starvation diet, which will interfere with healing.
- You should stop smoking at least 2 weeks before surgery because smoking can impair the healing process.
- The doctor will recommend that you stay out of the sun before the procedure because sunburn may lead to infection.
- The doctor or nurse will explain the procedure to you.
- You'll be informed that you may need a follow-up procedure and you'll be told about the costs before the first liposuction procedure.
- You'll have blood tests, including screenings for HIV, hepatitis, and blood-clotting disorders.
- You'll sign a consent form.

What happens during the procedure?

Typically, a dermatology surgeon or a cosmetic surgeon performs liposuction. Photographs of the area are taken before and after the surgery to document results. The most frequently used method of liposuction is the wet technique. A newer method, the tumescent technique, requires less anesthetic and offers a faster recovery.

The *wet technique* is performed under general anesthesia or heavy sedation. The area to be suctioned is marked, and a local anesthetic is injected into the designated fatty area. An incision is made in the area, and a catheter is introduced to remove the fat. The size of the catheter largely depends on the size of the area of fat to be removed. Suction is applied through the catheter to remove the fat.

The *tumescent technique* is performed under local anesthesia combined with sedation. A long-acting local anesthetic is injected into the fatty tissue, producing an anesthetic effect that may last as long as 10 hours. One advantage of local anesthesia is that it allows you to stand during the procedure to facilitate comparison of liposuctioned areas with nonsuctioned areas.

Blood transfusions are commonly required, especially with the wet technique. Several units of your own blood are collected before the procedure and reinfused if necessary. After the procedure, an elastic dressing is placed over the site to prevent swelling, bleeding, and fluid shifts.

Recovering from liposuction

After you're discharged from the hospital, keep in mind the following.

Know what to expect
- Remember that bruising, swelling, numbness, tenderness, and redness at the incision site are normal after this procedure. You're also likely to feel tired.
- Be aware that asymmetry of the involved body part may require a follow-up procedure.
- Know that ultrasound treatments to bruised areas may be recommended two to three times weekly to smooth out irregularities and resolve bruises.
- Pink-tinged drainage from the liposuctioned area is common. You can use absorbent bandages to collect the drainage. Sanitary pads are useful to collect abdominal drainage, which can be profuse.

Other instructions
- Take antibiotics if prescribed by your doctor.
- Wear compression garments over the liposuctioned area as recommended by your doctor.
- Follow your doctor's instructions on the type and amount of activity and exercise you're allowed. This will depend on the size of the area suctioned and the technique that was used.
- Inform your doctor if you notice increased pain, fever, or bleeding.
- Make and keep follow-up appointments with your doctor.

What are the possible complications?

Blood loss and fluid loss are possible with both liposuction procedures but are less common with the tumescent technique. Other complications may include a collection of clotted blood or serum in the tissues, shock due to blood loss, nerve damage, dents or waviness over the surgical area, wound separation, and wound infection. Rarely, a fat or blood clot may travel to the lungs.

What happens after the procedure?

- The nurse will monitor your vital signs and watch for signs of reduced blood volume.
- You'll be given pain medication.
- You'll stay in bed for 24 to 48 hours after the surgery.
- You'll be encouraged to drink lots of fluids. (See *Recovering from liposuction*.)

INDEX

i refers to an illustration; t, to a table

i refers to an illustration; t, to a table

i refers to an illustration; t, to a table

i refers to an illustration; t, to a table

i refers to an illustration; t, to a table